KETO
METABOLIC
BREAKTHROUGH

David Jockers, DNM, DC, MS

Victory Belt Publishing Inc.

Las Vegas

First published in 2020 by Victory Belt Publishing Inc.

ISBN-13: 978-1-628603-67-5

Author photos by Robert Halliday

Recipe photos by Megan Kelly, Chene Sonnekus, and Tatiana Briceag

Cover design by Justin-Aaron Velasco

Interior design by Elita San Juan and Justin-Aaron Velasco

Printed in Canada

TC 0120

This book is dedicated to all those who are passionate about their full God-given potential in life and health.

TABLE OF CONTENTS

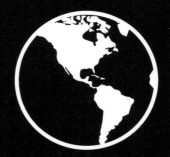

INTRODUCTION

A COUNTRY IN CRISIS

We are living in the Information Age. With a few clicks on our phones, we can find more information on diets, disease, supplements, and exercise than we could ever hope to digest in a lifetime. According to recent reports, 80 percent of Internet users in this country, which is about 93 million Americans, have searched online for a health-related topic.[1] So many people are actively searching for answers because they're overweight and besieged by chronic disease, and they're hoping a source on the Internet can provide a solution to those problems.

It's no secret that our society is facing an epidemic in the form of metabolic disorders. It's one of the reasons I've devoted my career to helping people alleviate the metabolic disorder–related discomfort and chronic illnesses that plague our nation and, increasingly, the world. The obesity rates in westernized countries are steadily climbing, but the United States still tops the list with a whopping 40 percent of the population falling into the obese category. That means more than 130 million Americans are walking around with a body mass index (BMI) of 30 or higher.

BMI is calculated by dividing a person's weight by his height.

Translation? America is fat—really fat.

I wish that having excess adipose tissue and the not fitting into our clothes from high school were the most significant issues we face. Our greater concern is that Americans' weight problem correlates with an alarming rise in autoimmune diseases, neurodegenerative disorders, heart disease, diabetes, cancer, and other life-threatening conditions.

Right now, you may be suffering from one or more of these ailments. You may also be overweight or obese. Even if you're not overweight, you may feel poorly, and you're ready to feel better. You'd like to go an entire workday without feeling the need to lie down next to your desk and take a nap. You no longer want to carry the burden of sleepless nights, mood swings, and lagging energy.

The good news is this: No matter what situation brought you here today, it's not too late. I want to help you achieve your goals. I also want you to know that your current situation is not your fault. For years, we've all gone to our doctors for help and left with more problems than we started with. The medical "solutions" seem to be making us sicker and fatter.

The reality is finally sinking in that the professionals to whom we're supposed to entrust our lives can no longer be trusted. Yes, I'm generalizing. Some physicians *are* trustworthy, but a growing number of people are doubtful that most traditional medical professionals have their patients' best interests at heart.

When you hire a lawyer, you expect to win your case. When you hire a mechanic, you assume that person will fix your car. When you hire a plumber, you expect your toilet to leak no more. But the expectation often isn't the same with doctors. When you visit a doctor, you often expect to leave the visit with a prescription to address some of the symptoms you're experiencing, but you don't necessarily think you'll be cured forever. Can you imagine your mechanic telling you the answer to fixing your car's broken suspension and failing transmission is to put some expensive chemical additives into the fuel tank? You'd laugh, leave his shop, and never look back.

The human body is way more complicated than a car engine, and to address problems, we need to look at how the body works as a whole rather than how each system functions. That's precisely why we can no longer look to traditional medical doctors. They don't treat the human body with the holistic, comprehensive approach needed to address health problems at the root.

Doctors are trained to treat what they see. Symptoms equal diagnoses. Diagnoses equal Band-Aid treatments. Band-Aid treatments lead to more symptoms. And the cycle repeats.

However, it *can* be different. The cycle can end now. In this book, I show you how you can reclaim your body and your life. The information I provide will help you reach your best weight, overcome chronic illness, and stop the cycle of prescription medication that keeps you trapped in a flawed and failing system.

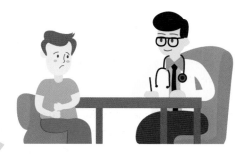

Symptoms equal diagnoses.

Doctors are trained to treat what they see.

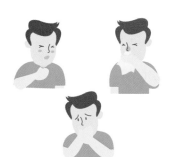

Band-Aid treatments lead to more symptoms.

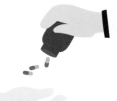

Diagnoses equal Band-Aid treatments.

A Lifestyle or a Fad?

You may be suspicious of the word *keto*, which is short for *ketogenic*, because it's a buzzword. It's plastered all over our social media feeds. For the past several years, it's been the fastest-growing search term in the health and wellness space. The odds are that you have a friend or family member who has "gone keto."

Is keto a fad? The modern-day Atkins Diet? A quick fix for rapid weight loss? You can call keto a *diet*, but weight loss isn't the real point of keto, although you may lose weight as you revamp what you do to fit within the ketogenic way of living. Keto isn't a fad, either. Keto is a lifestyle that gives your body the fuel on which it was designed to thrive. The principles of keto are based on science, and in this book, I share the facts that will empower you with life-changing information.

One of the most significant driving factors for the rise in the incidence of chronic disease and insulin resistance is the overconsumption of the wrong types of foods. The diet you've followed for most of your life is known as the *standard American diet* (aptly nicknamed the SAD). The SAD is heavy on sugar, carbs, and unhealthy fats while being light on *real* nutrition. The result is systemic inflammation and oxidative stress that adversely affect your body at a cellular level.

The ketogenic diet holds incredible promise as a foundational nutritional approach to reducing inflammation, improving fat-burning, and enhancing mental function. An abundance of research and case studies demonstrate the effectiveness of a well-formulated, high-fat diet. The keto diet creates a metabolic shift that helps you become better equipped to burn your stored body fat, transforming you from being a "sugar burner" to being a "fat burner."

Despite what you learned in school, carbs are not the only game in town when it comes to energy. By burning stored body fat instead of burning sugar, you become more energy-efficient, and inflammation and oxidative stress is significantly reduced. Do you like the idea of using your own fat as fuel? Then you need to eat fat to lose fat!

If that advice seems counterintuitive right now, keep an open mind—and also know you're not alone in your doubts. On the surface, eating fat to lose fat may not seem like it makes sense because it's the opposite of everything you've learned about nutrition. By the time you get to the end of this book, though, you'll understand. You need a nutrition revolution, and this book contains the keys to a lifestyle that can free you from your health struggles and lead you to the land of healing and abundant life.

Myths and Misconceptions About Keto

Unfortunately, those of us who are proponents of the keto diet are fighting an uphill battle. Old habits die hard, and food addictions are real. Sugars and carbs reign supreme on America's dinner plate, partly because the media has done such an excellent job of convincing us that fat is bad. In fact, a low-fat, "healthy grains" diet is the one prescribed to most Americans who are dealing with chronic disease, but this is backward! People need *more* fat and *fewer* grains if we ever hope to end the chronic disease and obesity epidemics.

People have some preconceived notions and believe several myths about the ketogenic diet that make them think that keto isn't for them. Here are some of the things I hear from people who've been misled by the media's portrayal of a ketogenic approach to eating.

"But I don't eat meat."

My good friend Eric is a popular health blogger. He's unwilling to consider a keto plan because his diet is mostly plant-based, with less than 10 percent of his calories coming from animal products. He thinks keto is all about eating meat (a modern-day Atkins diet). He tells his readers that keto is a fad diet, and it'll go the way of all the others before it. What Eric doesn't know is that there are many ways to follow a ketogenic diet, including one that is entirely plant-based!

"But keto is dangerous for thyroid patients."

My patient Teresa was diagnosed with hypothyroidism eight years ago, and she had mixed results with a prescription drug called Synthroid. She was 50 pounds overweight and became interested in the ketogenic diet after hearing numerous weight-loss success stories. In her research, she stumbled onto a blog post about how a ketogenic diet is dangerous for those with thyroid issues, so she decided it wouldn't be the right approach for her. Little did she realize that a ketogenic lifestyle has helped thousands of individuals with thyroid conditions improve their health.

"But I'm already thin."

Sheryl had a diagnosis of early-stage dementia, and her family brought her into my clinic to meet with me. In our initial consultation, one of the foundational strategies we discussed was starting Sheryl on a ketogenic diet. Sheryl and her family shook their heads and told me they thought it would be dangerous for Sheryl because she was very lean and didn't have any extra weight to lose. They assumed that keto is a weight-loss-focused nutritional approach. Because of this misinformation, Sheryl is missing out on the incredible neuroprotective benefits that come with keto-adaptation.

"But my doctor said fat is bad."

Jim was 100 pounds overweight and on blood pressure and cholesterol medications. His parents both died of heart disease. Jim's doctor told him he was also at risk and advised him to avoid dietary fat as much as possible. Jim ate the way his doctor recommended for another year with no improvements. He grew increasingly frustrated by the lack of progress in his health journey. Jim decided to do some research and came across my website. He contacted my office, and he and I discussed the benefits of keto for patients with high blood pressure. After our discussion, he started a keto plan. In the first month, he lost 20 pounds. Within sixty days, he also stabilized his blood pressure and stopped all medications!

"But now I feel even worse!"

After just three months on a ketogenic diet, Erica's friend Patty lost 25 pounds and cleared her chronic acne. Erica was 30 pounds overweight and struggled with hypothyroidism and high blood pressure. After seeing Patty's success, Erica couldn't wait to get started with a ketogenic diet. Within days, Erica felt dizzy, fatigued, bloated, and irritable. She also experienced severe headaches.

To make matters worse, she gained two pounds the first week. She felt discouraged and decided keto wasn't for her. What Erica didn't realize is that she was experiencing common side effects that occur when someone shifts to a strict low-carb eating style too quickly. Techniques exist for reducing, or eliminating, these symptoms. You can transition to keto gently, increase hydration and electrolyte levels, and use supplements such as digestive enzymes to support the body as it adapts to its new fuel source.

Some people who start a ketogenic diet see great results right away. Others do not. The keto diet doesn't work like other nutritional plans. You don't just track your calories or "points" for a week or two and expect to step on the scale and see a few pounds gone. Keto isn't a weight-loss app. It's a lifestyle change.

Those people who don't see immediate results often assume keto isn't for them or that they don't have the willpower to do it. Both assumptions are destructive and can lead to depression, binge eating, and other poor lifestyle habits that further derail their efforts.

I wrote this book for people like Eric, Teresa, Sheryl, Jim, and Erica who want to live a healthy lifestyle but are either hindered by myths about keto or unfamiliar with the best practices for transitioning into a low-carb, high-fat lifestyle. I wrote this book for people like you who are ready to experience the health, healing, and happiness that can come only from adequately fueling your body.

Don't let myths and misconceptions stop you from living the life you're designed to live.

Who I Am and How I Got Here

I loved sports as a kid. I was always athletic, and in my twenties, I became a personal trainer. On the outside, I appeared fit and healthy. On the inside, however, I was struggling.

I wrestled with chronic constipation and unpredictable bouts of diarrhea. I would have periods of extreme intestinal cramping that sent me to the ground, writhing in pain. I was already living a much healthier lifestyle than anyone I knew, so what more could I do? I thought my lot in life was to struggle with these issues.

I was a lacto-ovo vegetarian (meaning I ate eggs and dairy but no other animal products), and I also ate fish. I never consumed junk foods. No fast food. No candy or desserts. I lifted weights, ran, and trained daily. I thought I was doing everything right.

What I didn't know was about to hurt me. By ignoring my problems and assuming they were normal, I allowed them to worsen and eventually spiral out of control.

By the time I got into graduate school, my digestive system was chronically overworked and overwhelmed. I lost 30 pounds in six months, dropping from 165 pounds to a gaunt 135 pounds. I was so thin that my family and colleagues became concerned. My blood pressure was alarmingly low, and I experienced frequent bouts of dizziness.

I researched my symptoms extensively and eventually understood that I was suffering from both irritable bowel syndrome (IBS) and leaky gut syndrome. Something had to change. I heard about a book written by my friend Jordan Rubin called *The Maker's Diet*. It appealed to me as a Christian, and the information was truly transformational.

The Maker's Diet

The Maker's Diet, written by Jordan Rubin, was published in July 2004 and became a *New York Times* best seller. More than 2 million copies are in print.

The Maker's Diet discusses a nutrition plan based on biblical principles and practices of the Hebraic people of the Bible along with discoveries made through modern science. Rubin advocates consuming real foods from the earth and promotes a higher fat, lower carbohydrate template with fermented foods, bone broth, pasture-raised meats, herbs, and natural sweetening agents.

The Maker's Diet is not a ketogenic diet, but it was one of the first books to promote a higher fat, lower carbohydrate diet before either the Paleo or keto movements became popular.

I removed as many toxins as possible from my life, practiced stress-reduction techniques, ate a low-carb diet, and practiced intermittent fasting. I ate two meals between 2:00 p.m. and 7:00 p.m. and fasted for the rest of the time. I noticed that when I abstained from food in the morning and focused on consuming tons of clean water, I had much more energy throughout the day than I'd had when I ate on a more traditional schedule. I was implementing this plan in 2005 when the terms *ketogenic* and *intermittent fasting* were not well known. I referred to my new lifestyle as my "healing diet."

In less than six months, I gained my muscle weight back and felt significantly better. I was stronger, slept better, had more energy, and was in a better mood. In the process of changing my lifestyle and developing new, healthier habits, my eyes were opened. I realized just how many damaging things I'd been consuming even though I thought I was the fittest guy on the block. Here were some of the issues:

- **Unhealthy water:** I was drinking a lot of water, at least a gallon a day, but the water contained chlorine and fluoride, which are both detrimental to the digestive system.

- **Artificial sweeteners:** I knew better than to eat pounds of sugar, so I had opted for processed protein bars and protein powders that contained Splenda, utterly unaware of how much damage that sweet chemical additive was doing to my gut.

- **Hidden sugars:** I regularly ate foods I thought were healthy, such as commercial smoothies, processed protein bars, dried fruit, yogurts, and other things that contained far more sugar than I realized.

- **Pasteurized dairy:** Every day, I consumed skim milk, yogurt, and cottage cheese. None of the dairy products were organic, which meant they contained added hormones and antibiotics, not to mention that the pasteurization process creates dangerous chemicals that cause inflammation. Conventional dairy also comes from grain-fed cows— and products derived from grain-fed animals are highly inflammatory because of their high omega-6 fat content.

- **Farm-raised fish:** I ate a lot of salmon, but it was always farm-raised. I didn't even know the difference between farmed and wild-caught fish. Farmed fish feed on grains grown from genetically modified organisms (GMOs), which are laced with pesticides and herbicides that damage the gut lining.

- **Gluten and grains:** My daily breakfast was oatmeal or cold cereal. I also consumed tons of whole wheat bread, pasta, and brown rice. These were healthy grains, right? Not really. These pseudo-healthy choices increase blood sugar and promote inflammation.

- **Processed proteins:** I loved my processed protein bars, protein shakes, and commercial smoothies. I even drank packaged nutrition shakes for extra protein and vitamins. These products are synthetically created and have loads of additives, preservatives, and artificial flavorings that are linked to toxicity and digestive issues.

- **Nonsteroidal anti-inflammatory drugs (NSAIDs):** I had suffered from headaches for most of my life and frequently took ibuprofen and other NSAIDs such as acetaminophen. I also took them to help with pain associated with frequent sports injuries. NSAIDs have a detrimental effect on the liver and kidneys and wear down the intestinal lining.

Once I removed these insidious dangers from my life, I felt like a new man.

Fast-forward five years. By the time I was twenty-eight, I had healed my gut and recovered from IBS, and I was in the best shape of my life. I had also finished my education and was respected as a health leader in my community. I had it all figured out.

Until I didn't.

One day, I noticed a red nodule on the side of my nose. I thought it was a pimple and assumed it would fade in a few days. It only got larger. I remembered learning the ABCDs of assessing skin issues:

A: Asymmetry—one half of a mole or birthmark does not match the other.

B: Border is irregular, ragged, notched, or blurred.

C: Color varies (brown, black, red, white, blue).

D: Diameter is larger than ¼ inch (the size of a pencil eraser).

When I examined the nodule on my nose, I could check all the boxes. That's when it dawned on me that I may have had skin cancer.

During my teen years, I lived in Florida, where I would spend countless hours at the beach and outside playing sports. Skin cancer also ran in the family; my grandfather had numerous "suspicious" moles removed throughout his life, and he eventually died from metastatic melanoma.

My relentless pursuit of higher education and furthering my career also had done me no favors. I had spent the last decade pushing myself beyond healthy limits to become educated on nutrition, health, and wellness. (The irony does not escape me.) I spent nine years getting my degrees while working two jobs to pay for school. After I graduated, I financed opening my clinic with credit cards. I had no business experience, and I worked eighty-plus hours per week to make sure all of my sacrifices would not go to waste.

I wore myself ragged, but I kept pushing because I knew the immense calling God had for my life. My adrenals were shot, and my immune system was compromised. But I didn't complain; I just worked.

To make matters worse, I had gradually drifted away from my healing diet. I knew better than to start using artificial sweeteners, drinking commercial smoothies, or consuming processed protein bars again, but I still didn't understand what my body was trying to tell me.

I thought I was eating healthy. I had a protein shake made with coconut milk, berries, and grass-fed whey protein in the mornings after my workouts. Instead of ordering pizza or eating a bag of chips when I was working late, I'd "binge" on sprouted grain bread topped with coconut oil and blueberries. They were healthy indulgences, or at least that's what I told myself. Eating at night gave me a stress hormone buzz and enabled me to keep pushing, sometimes until midnight.

Unfortunately, the constant influx of carbohydrates from the bread and berries increased my blood sugar and insulin production. Higher insulin levels activate inflammatory gene pathways and increase cell reproduction. Both of these things can increase the risk of cancer development.

I didn't know what I didn't know.

It was time for a life inventory. I took some immediate steps to change my path. First, I focused on improving my mental, emotional, and spiritual walk to overcome the fear of failure that had been my constant companion for more than a decade.

Next, I made the adult decision to buy a house and stop living out of my office. For two years, I had been trying to save money by sleeping on a mattress in the back office and showering every morning at a fitness center across the street. I never slept well, and I was showering in unfiltered water every day. I bought a shower filter for my new home to remove the chlorine from the water and focused on getting seven to eight hours of sleep a night.

I also knew I had been overtraining. I needed less exercise and more rest, so I limited myself to four days a week at the gym and prioritized things like sleep, prayer, and meditation.

I researched the best nutrition for combating cancer and came across the term *ketogenic*. Fascinated, I studied it and began applying the same fasting strategy I had used in graduate school, along with a nutrient-dense, low-carb, high-fat diet. Within a few days of following my new eating plan, I had significantly more energy and mental clarity.

In just four months, my cancer nodule had all but disappeared; only a vague scar remained. Better yet, I felt terrific—my mood and outlook were positive, and I was excited to share what I had learned with the world.

I began teaching ketogenic nutrition principles at my clinic, local churches, and businesses—and word spread. I also took continuing education classes on functional medicine to learn how to use various lab tests to find the root cause of metabolic and chronic inflammatory health conditions.

In 2012, I started my website, DrJockers.com, and began writing articles and producing videos. I wrote three to five well-researched articles each month. Writing these articles gave me a new level of mastery on a variety of health topics. I now have more than 1,000 researched articles on my site, and more than 1 million monthly visitors from around the world come looking for evidence-based information to help them improve their health.

Your Unique Metabolic Makeover

Working with thousands of patients over the years has given me a unique perspective. I know there is no cookie-cutter approach to health that will work for everyone. We're all different, and we should be treated accordingly.

Nutrition and functional medicine must be personalized to the individual. Some people experience the benefits of a ketogenic lifestyle more quickly than others. The important thing to remember is that if the results don't happen rapidly for you, it doesn't mean a keto lifestyle is wrong for you. I believe *everyone* can benefit from a personalized keto metabolic makeover that can lead to a keto metabolic breakthrough.

The goal of this book is to dispel the most common myths about keto and give you the real science behind the diet and lifestyle. I discuss how to overcome the challenges you may experience as you go through keto-adaptation. I also cover how to transition from the SAD into the keto diet safely and gently. Finally, I explain how you can stock your fridge and pantry with nutrient-dense foods, plan your meals, and cook delicious recipes.

God did not design our bodies to be appeased by medication. He created them to run optimally through the right fuel.

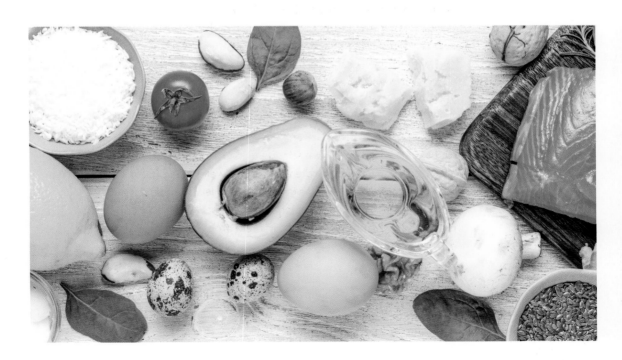

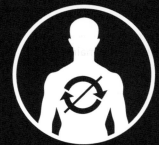

CHAPTER 1

THE WIDESPREAD IMPACT OF METABOLIC DYSFUNCTION

Once upon a time, an *epidemic* represented a crisis such as a plague or terrible famine. These catastrophic events still happen throughout the world today, but in the United States, there is a new kind of terror. Our country is sick and in the grips of a massive health epidemic—one that is entirely preventable.

People like to joke that they are "feeding their cravings" when they indulge in sweet treats or make an impulsive fast-food stop. But the situation created by these indulgences is no laughing matter. Those cravings are very real; we've become a nation of people who are afflicted with an addiction to sugar and processed carbs. A body that's addicted to any substance demands more and more of that thing, regardless of how you feel about it and even though you know better.

That's how we've become trapped in a chronic sugar-burning, sugar-craving cycle and become dependent on a near-constant inflow of high-carb meals and snacks to maintain enough energy and stamina not to fall asleep at work.

You eat sugar
- You like it; you crave it.
- It has addictive properties.

Blood sugar levels spike
- Dopamine is released in the brain = addiction
- Mass insulin is secreted to drop blood sugar levels.

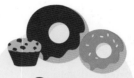

Sugar addiction
The perpetual cycle

Blood sugar levels fall rapidly
- High insulin levels cause immediate fat storage.
- Your body craves the lost sugar "high."

Hunger & cravings
- Low blood sugar levels cause increased appetite and cravings; the cycle repeats.

How did it come to this? Why is it that we have more information available to us than ever before, but we're still sicker and fatter as a nation than we've ever been? The short answer is that we've chosen the wrong fuel.

The body has to be fueled by something. When you choose an inferior fuel source, metabolic dysfunction is the result. *Metabolic dysfunction*, also referred to as *metabolic syndrome* and *metabolic disorder*, is the inability of the body to burn fat efficiently as energy.

If you've never heard of metabolic dysfunction, that doesn't mean it hasn't already affected you. In fact, most of the people in your life are in some stage of it right now. The condition is reasonably easy to spot because it causes a closely correlated group of symptoms, such as excess fat (especially around the waist), high blood pressure, insulin resistance, and abnormal cholesterol and triglyceride levels. However, metabolic dysfunction can be sneaky, such as when it's the cause of the lack of energy you can't explain or the mood swings that you shrug off and always blame on stress or lack of sleep.

The consequences of chronic metabolic dysfunction are far-reaching and deadly. A host of diseases, illnesses, and autoimmune disorders are all potential outcomes of this significant enemy of health. Chronic disease is robbing us of our health and vitality, and it's also robbing our bank accounts via skyrocketing healthcare costs.

Metabolic disorders and their side effects affect us on the cellular level by causing mitochondrial malfunction. In case you don't remember the details of high school biology, *mitochondria* are found within our cells and are home to the biochemical process known as *respiration*, which is the process through which cells convert fuel into energy. In other words, our mitochondria are pretty darn important. The following issues are signs of metabolic dysfunction and mitochondrial disorders:

- Parkinson's
- Autism
- Huntington's
- Chronic fatigue
- Mitochondrial disease
- Muscular dystrophy
- Lou Gehrig's
- Alzheimer's
- Epilepsy
- Cerebral palsy
- Developmental delay
- Diabetes
- Cardiomyopathy
- Atypical learning disability
- Fibromyalgia

Because of metabolic dysfunction, our bodies are out of balance. When a body is out of balance for long enough, disease develops. We need to learn how to identify metabolic dysfunction and then learn what we can do to rebalance our bodies and reverse the damage while we still can.

Sick and Fat:
The New Normal

Obesity is the result of eating a diet rich in carbs, the wrong kinds of fats, and denatured protein, which is problematic because those are the three staple ingredients of the American diet in the forms of processed carbs, inflammatory vegetable oils, and factory-farmed meats.

The United States is leading the world in the metabolic dysfunction caused by being overweight or obese. The most recent National Health and Nutrition Examination Survey from the CDC confirms the spiraling rate of obesity in America. In 2016, the prevalence of obesity was near 40 percent in adults and 19 percent in youth. One out of two American adults will be obese within the next few years—and the kids aren't far behind.[1]

As processed convenience foods have become more prevalent, other parts of the world are now experiencing trends in health similar to what we see in the United States. The World Health Organization (WHO) reports a tenfold increase in childhood and adolescent obesity over the last four decades. By 2022, the number of obese children and adults across the world is expected to outnumber those people whose weights are within a healthy weight range.[2]

AMERICA IS FATTER THAN EVER:

Obesity prevalence among adults and youths in the U.S.

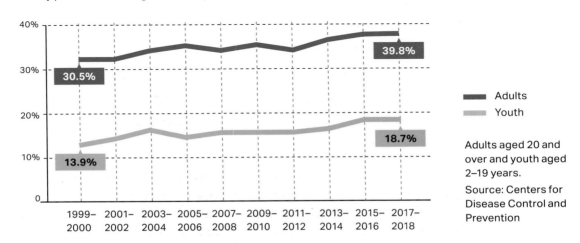

Adults aged 20 and over and youth aged 2–19 years.
Source: Centers for Disease Control and Prevention

Obesity is dangerous, costly, and avoidable. Being significantly overweight is associated with the world's most threatening conditions such as heart disease, diabetes, and cancers, including endometrial, breast, ovarian, prostate, liver, gallbladder, kidney, and colon cancers. Neurodegenerative diseases such as Alzheimer's, Huntington's, and Parkinson's disease are also on the rise. The National Institutes of Health reports a connection between metabolic dysfunction and these neurodegenerative diseases.[3]

The chronic diseases I've mentioned are the leading cause of death and disability in the United States. Around 45 percent of the population, or 133 million Americans, are currently dealing with at least one chronic illness. These diseases are responsible for seven out of every ten deaths, killing more than 1.7 million Americans every year.[4]

No doubt there is a genetic component to many conditions, but many people fail to realize that genetic pathways can either be *supported* or *inhibited* by the environment, which includes what we consume, what environmental toxins we're exposed to, how much sunlight exposure we get, and how we manage our sleep habits, stress levels, and exercise.

When you consume the kind of real food I discuss throughout this book (and in detail in Chapter 9) and engage in healthy lifestyle activities, you can lower your chances of being afflicted by metabolic dysfunction or succumbing to a degenerative disease.

The Perilous Pyramid

People have been vilifying fat for years. They've been blaming it for a host of diseases and health problems. *Fat* is the "four-letter word" of professional dieters.

We can trace the origins of the war against fat back to the findings of Ancel Keys, an American physiologist who studied the influence dietary choices have on health. He theorized that dietary saturated fat causes heart disease, and people should avoid it. His conclusions began the mass exodus away from natural, healthy fats.

In the wake of Dr. Keys's report, Americans started consuming large amounts of refined carbohydrates and added sugars (as long as the food was fat-free, of course) and avoiding healthy fats. Fast forward to today, and we now have widespread metabolic dysfunction syndrome characterized by a rise in triglycerides and LDL (the bad cholesterol), a decrease in HDL (the good cholesterol), and sugar-induced weight gain and diabetes.

For many decades, Americans have been schooled about the best food choices for optimum health. What we learned became the basis for the standard American diet (SAD). This misinformation—dare I call it medical propaganda?—also gave rise to the creation of the USDA-sponsored Food Pyramid, which is in the next illustration.

FOOD PYRAMID

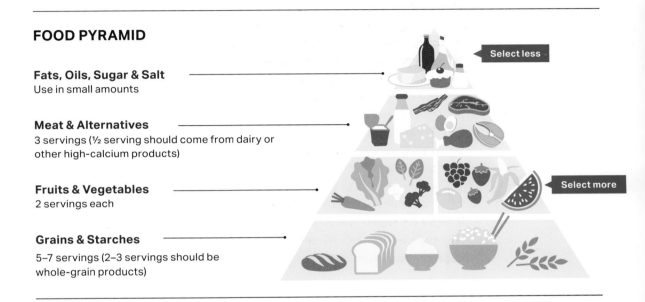

Fats, Oils, Sugar & Salt
Use in small amounts

Select less

Meat & Alternatives
3 servings (½ serving should come from dairy or other high-calcium products)

Fruits & Vegetables
2 servings each

Select more

Grains & Starches
5–7 servings (2–3 servings should be whole-grain products)

It's Upside Down

According to official government recommendations, our bodies need an abundance of carbs and very little fat. If you've ever stopped and examined the Food Pyramid (which our children learn in school), there can be no doubt as to why we as a nation are so overweight and sick. The foundation of the Food Pyramid is bread, cereal, pasta, rice, and whole grains, which are carbs. Unfortunately, those carbs break down quickly into glucose, causing a spike in blood sugar followed by a rapid crash, which leads to cravings for more carbs that provide inferior fuel for energy. It's a vicious cycle that results in exhaustion, weight gain, and sickness.

Carbs are easy to find, and they taste good, but we pay a high price when we eat them; the cost is our good health. The SAD has now been unquestionably linked to weight gain, metabolic dysfunction, and chronic disease. Try eating bread, pasta, cereals, and flour-based products seven times a day (the number of servings recommended by the Food Pyramid) and see how you look and feel in a year. You won't like the results.

The next largest level on the pyramid includes fresh fruits and vegetables, which are far superior choices to grains. However, there is a caveat—not all fruits and vegetables are equally healthy from the standpoint of blood sugar balance and weight management. Some fruits and vegetables are higher in sugar and starch and lower in nutrients—bananas, pineapples, and potatoes are examples of less-desirable fruits and vegetables. I discuss this more in Chapter 9.

Long story short, the Food Pyramid could not be more misguided!

Flip the Narrative

Not everyone jumped on the fat-is-bad bandwagon, even though the fat-free/low-fat dogma became an official part of the USDA dietary guidelines in the early 1970s. There are many thought leaders, scientists, and health experts who have kept digging and spreading the truth. For example, American science writer Gary Taubes wrote an article in *The New York Times* in 2002 about how Dr. Robert Atkins, the legendary founder of The Atkins Diet, had been right all along in promoting a high-fat diet with minimal carbohydrates. [5]

Despite health crusaders who have tried to dispel the myth that fat is terrible, the flawed low-fat advice that swept the country following Keys's research was and continues to be one of the worst trends in the health of our nation.

To be closer to unlocking the secrets to a healthy weight and life, you need to flip that pyramid on its head and remove the sugar. The ketogenic lifestyle provides the template for you to make that flip by favoring healthy fats as the primary fuel for your body.

Steps to Reverse Metabolic Dysfunction

There are only three categories of macronutrients that your body can use: protein, fat, and carbohydrates. There is an endless array of food choices, but at the most basic level, every food you eat is made from some combination of those three macronutrients, or *macros* for short.

As a doctor who has worked with thousands of individuals with chronic health conditions, I've noticed a common link—a poor diet consisting of processed convenience foods that are predominantly carbs, denatured protein, and unhealthy fats such as canola oil.

This type of diet is devoid of the key ingredient for health! The ketogenic diet, which is a far superior alternative to the SAD, is designed like so:

A ketogenic diet consists of 60 to 80 percent healthy fats, 20 to 30 percent clean protein, and 5 to 10 percent (or less) carbohydrates.

Eating according to this formula teaches the body to burn fat as a primary energy source. Fats provide a more efficient and sustainable energy source than carbohydrates.

A ketogenic lifestyle initially places minor stress on the body as it discards dysfunctional mitochondria. But this stress is a good thing! The weak mitochondria will be replaced with stronger and more resilient ones as your body transitions from being a sugar-burner to being a fat-burner.

The positive changes of a keto diet are also observable from a clinical standpoint. Comparing the functional lab analyses of a person before starting a keto lifestyle with the lab analyses after the person has made the transition show improvements in the areas of cholesterol balance, inflammation, and insulin levels. Furthermore, people in pain and suffering from preventable diseases report that a ketogenic lifestyle produces almost universally positive and drastic shifts in how they look, feel, and experience their daily lives.

Your food choices will either weaken or strengthen your immune system; they will either rob you of your health or help your body repair itself at a cellular level.

The principles of a healing diet aren't tricky or particularly profound. And if you're like most of my patients, you're excited to jump right in. I love the enthusiasm—but before you can get started, I want to set you up for success.

I want you to begin to do the following:

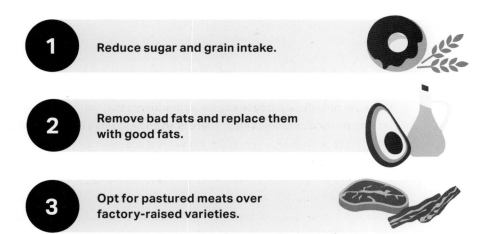

1 Reduce sugar and grain intake.

2 Remove bad fats and replace them with good fats.

3 Opt for pastured meats over factory-raised varieties.

Notice I said that you should "begin" to do these three things. You don't have to do all or nothing from day one. One smart choice prompts another intelligent decision, which then prompts another one. If you have the choice between a hamburger on a bun versus a fresh ground beef patty wrapped in lettuce, choose the bunless burger. As you prepare dinner for your family, start using coconut oil instead of canola oil.

Your taste buds are used to unhealthy stuff. You can retrain them, but it takes time and patience. Believe me, though—it's worth it. Small changes lead to significant results, and by significant, I mean genuinely life-changing. Here are just five benefits of a healing, ketogenic diet:

- **Reduces inflammation:** Inflammation is present in every major chronic disease process.

- **Stabilizes blood sugar:** Elevated blood sugar is a precursor to diabetes and heart disease.

- **Decreases the toxic load on the body:** Toxins in the body overload your systems and prevent them from working correctly.

- **Provides full-spectrum nutrition:** Your body needs all three macros and many micronutrients to thrive, and the SAD doesn't provide the body with an ideal balance of nutrients.

- **Supports the optimization of fat-burning hormones:** Hormonal imbalance is one of the greatest enemies of our health and our waistlines.

I cover each of these benefits in more detail throughout this book to help you understand the *why* behind making the right food choices. In the next chapter, I talk about the dangerous metabolism mistakes you may be making right now and discuss the primary hormones that govern fat-burning in the body. I also give you key action steps to balance your hormones and become a fat-burning machine!

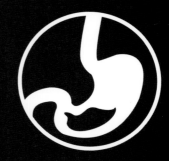

CHAPTER 2

THE BIGGEST METABOLISM
MISTAKES

Metabolism may be a buzzword, but don't gloss over the term just because you've seen it a lot over the years. Metabolism is *everything*. It dictates your ability to create energy. It also plays a primary role in your ability to burn fat and achieve your ideal weight.

In most cases, people are unknowingly engaging in metabolism-destroying behaviors. When you make fat your fuel, your body transforms into a metabolic powerhouse. That is why my goal in working with my patients is to ignite the metabolic process.

In this chapter, I reveal the top five mistakes that are keeping your body from efficiently burning fat as fuel.

Focusing on Calories

One of the oldest and most pervasive myths about diet is that your weight is tied solely to the number of calories you consume. This viewpoint is an outdated way to look at food choices and metabolism. The truth is that the type of food you eat is what affects your metabolism and hormones.

The primary macronutrient you consume, regardless of total caloric intake, determines the effect on your body and your results. For example, eating 500 calories of broccoli doesn't have the same effect on your metabolism as eating 500 calories of donuts. Most people clearly understand that eating junk food like donuts slows down metabolism and turns on fat storage in the body, whereas eating the broccoli helps people burn fat and lose weight.

Earlier I said, "metabolism is everything," but there's something else that plays a big role. When it comes to weight gain and metabolic dysfunction, hormones also are exceptionally important. Weight gain is the most noticeable symptom of hormonal imbalance, but it's certainly not the most severe symptom. Other indicators include fatigue, depression, anxiety, and decreased libido. Some women may also experience severe PMS, infertility, irregular menstrual cycles, and early onset of menopause. More serious conditions that can result from hormone imbalances include autoimmune diseases, cancer, leaky gut syndrome, thyroid issues, and degenerative brain disorders.[1, 2]

Five essential hormones control fat-burning in the body: adiponectin, ghrelin, insulin, leptin, and cortisol. A variety of factors influence these hormones, including stress levels, sleep quality, exercise routine, diet, and hydration. Let me explain each hormone and its crucial roles in maintaining your health.

Hormone	Produced By	Major Functions
Adiponectin	Fat cells	Lowers blood sugar and burns fat
Grehlin	Stomach cells	Stimulates hunger and fat storage
Insulin	Pancreas	Lowers blood sugar and stimulates fat storage
Leptin	Fat cells	Stimulates satiety and fat-burning
Cortisol	Adrenal glands	Increases blood sugar and cravings

Adiponectin: Burning Fat as Fuel

If you're struggling to burn fat and lose weight, your body may not be producing enough adiponectin. Studies show the higher the levels of circulating adiponectin an individual has, the bigger the potential for weight loss.[3] Adiponectin can directly lower blood glucose levels, break down triglycerides, and increase the oxidation of fat in the liver and muscle tissue.

Fat tissue is responsible for the production of adiponectin, which is released through insulin signaling pathways. When a person consumes a high-calorie diet that is rich in carbs and unhealthy fats, this lowers the body's ability to synthesize and secrete adiponectin due to insulin resistance.

KETO PRO TIP

One of the best ways to increase adiponectin and enhance metabolism is to drink green tea. Drinking one to two cups of organic matcha tea every day boosts your metabolism, immunity, brain health, and circulation. (See the Matcha Tea recipe on page 348 for one option.)

Ghrelin: Nurturing the Gut-Brain Connection

The stomach is the primary producer of ghrelin. This hormone triggers the emptying of stomach contents, signals hunger in the brain, and increases fat accumulation by slowing down processes that break down stored fat. Ghrelin overproduction activates a series of events that make it harder to eat right and make sensible food choices. In fact, research shows that ghrelin concentration directly correlates to stomach size.[4]

This powerful hormone is also involved in regulating metabolism because it plays a role in triggering human growth hormone (hGH) secretion. Obese individuals have significantly reduced hGH secretion compared to individuals of average weight.[5] Excess ghrelin production can severely diminish weight loss in overweight and obese individuals who are actively trying to lose weight.[6]

THE HUNGER TRAP

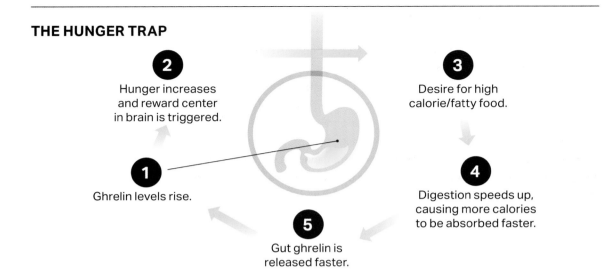

2 Hunger increases and reward center in brain is triggered.

3 Desire for high calorie/fatty food.

1 Ghrelin levels rise.

4 Digestion speeds up, causing more calories to be absorbed faster.

5 Gut ghrelin is released faster.

Insulin: Managing Fat Storage and Inflammation

We all know insulin as the "diabetes hormone." But do you really know what insulin is and the roles it plays in your body? Insulin is secreted by the pancreas to help normalize blood glucose, and it officiates the metabolism of macronutrients.

When you take in a healthy amount of carbohydrates, insulin works to regulate energy for cells and promote muscular activity.[7] However, high insulin levels contribute to chronic inflammation and fat storage. Insulin resistance prevents glucose from being transported into cells, resulting in elevated blood sugar levels and diminished impact of the fat-burning hormones.

Also, higher levels of insulin activate immune system receptors called *inflammasomes*. When inflammasomes are activated, they cause widespread inflammation that accelerates the degenerative processes of every tissue of the body, which is why virtually all degenerative disease is associated with chronically elevated insulin levels. Repetitive spikes or extended periods of unrelenting insulin production can lead to food cravings, metabolic dysfunction, and insulin resistance, as seen in conditions such as type 2 diabetes and Alzheimer's disease.[8]

I share strategies in this book for optimizing your insulin levels and shutting down inflammasome secretion to slow the aging process and prevent or potentially heal chronic inflammatory conditions.

Leptin: Feeling Satiated and Energetic

Leptin is often referred to as the "satiety hormone" because it influences metabolism and controls appetite. It's a critical hormone to consider when addressing obesity because it suppresses the desire for food intake and drives energy output. Leptin normalizes glucose and insulin levels, controls appetite and body weight, and stabilizes endocrine hormones that could otherwise incite physiological imbalances that lead to weight gain.[9]

Having the right amount of leptin is the key to managing your appetite and energy levels. Low leptin levels can stimulate both a decrease in adiponectin and an increase in fatty tissue. However, high leptin levels are linked to a significant reduction in hGH, which suggests that individuals with high levels have chronic inflammation that is affecting the leptin receptor and causing leptin resistance.[10]

Following an anti-inflammatory diet (one that is low in grains, sugars, and refined fats and high in healthy fats and micronutrients, such as the keto diet) and sleeping well are vitally crucial steps toward optimizing leptin sensitivity and stimulating the fat-burning hormones.[11]

GHRELIN AND LEPTIN

When ghrelin levels are elevated, you naturally feel hungry. When leptin levels are elevated, you should feel satiated.

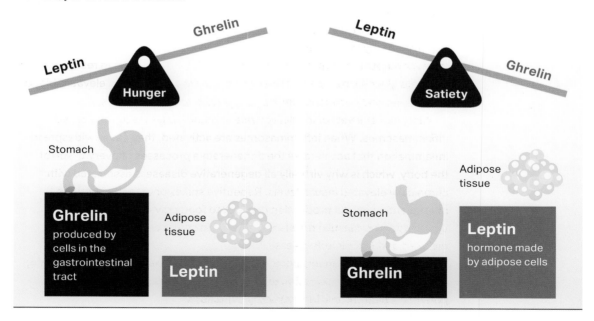

Cortisol: Feeling Stressed, Wired, and Tired

When cortisol is out of balance, life can get rough. People often refer to cortisol as the "stress hormone." Its overproduction is linked to physiological processes in the body that increase a person's propensity to gain weight. Left unchecked, it causes symptoms of fatigue and blood sugar imbalances that create central nervous system dysfunction, which can lead to addictive behaviors, an uncontrolled appetite, and unhealthy food cravings.[12, 13]

The adrenal glands secrete cortisol, which subsequently slows down the production of testosterone. The long-term results of cortisol overproduction creates a *catabolic* state in which the body breaks down bone and muscle and stores fat. Reduced lean body tissue slows down the body's metabolism and causes increased fat storage, which then leads to elevated insulin and insulin resistance.

Here's how things are *supposed* to work: We should have our highest cortisol production in the morning. As the day progresses, cortisol levels are designed to drop until the evening when they're at their lowest. This trend allows us to have steady energy during the day and then be relaxed enough to fall asleep quickly at night.

Unfortunately, most people exist in a state of cortisol dysregulation where they have too little or too much cortisol at the wrong times of the day. Consequently, we feel tired throughout the day but wired at night, which harms our chances of getting restful sleep—and so the savage progression continues. In this case, "vicious cycle" seems like an understatement.

 Symptoms of high cortisol levels

- Wired or fatigue
- High blood pressure
- Hypoglycemia
- Worsening memory and concentration
- Difficulty sleeping (insomnia)
- Decreased sex drive
- Erectile dysfunction
- Weight gain and obesity
- Weakened immune response

 Symptoms of adrenal fatigue (low cortisol levels)

- Fatigue
- Worsening memory and concentration
- Difficulty sleeping (insomnia)
- Sugar and salt cravings
- Decreased sex drive
- Depressed mood
- Weight gain
- Bone and muscle loss
- Anxiety
- Irritability

Not Consuming Enough Micronutrients

A lot of people spend their time focusing only on the three macronutrients: carbs, protein, and fat. Although the percentage of each in your diet is an essential factor in a healthy nutrition plan, what may be even more critical for your metabolism is the proper intake of micronutrients. *Micronutrients* include vitamins, minerals, antioxidants, enzymes, fatty acids, and other vital compounds you receive through your diet.

Vitamins are organic compounds that our bodies need to function correctly. They serve many purposes in the body that include providing protection from free radical damage, supporting the immune system, and contributing to brain development and bone health.

Vitamins can be either water-soluble or fat-soluble. Fat-soluble vitamins accumulate in the body's tissue and need a source of fat to be absorbed. They include vitamins A, D, E, and K. Water-soluble vitamins—such as B vitamins and vitamin C—do not readily accumulate in the body's tissue; your body loses them through urine and body fluids, and therefore you need to take them in more frequently.

Minerals are inorganic, naturally occurring substances that enable the cells to carry out essential functions. Minerals can be further divided into major minerals (macrominerals) and trace minerals (microminerals).

Macrominerals include calcium, magnesium, phosphorus, sodium, potassium, chloride, and sulfur. They perform many functions in the body, including maintaining proper fluid balance and keeping bones and teeth healthy. They also are crucial for muscle contraction, nerve transmission, and immune system health.

Trace minerals are necessary for health, but we need them only in small (trace) amounts. These minerals include iron, copper, iodine, chromium, manganese, molybdenum, selenium, and zinc. Even marginal trace mineral imbalances are considered risk factors for several diseases.[16]

Effects of Micronutrient Deficiency

There are several ways micronutrient deficiencies can negatively influence your metabolism. For example, nutrients such as iodine, selenium, and zinc play critical roles in thyroid hormone conversion. Inadequate intake of these micronutrients can result in decreased production of thyroid hormones and a slowed metabolism.

Your body uses iron and vitamin B12 to form red blood cells that carry oxygen to all the tissues of the body. If you don't take in enough iron and B12 or don't absorb the iron and B12 you consume, then you won't be able to produce enough red blood cells, and you'll end up with anemia.

Magnesium is used for more than 300 physiological functions and is a common deficiency throughout the world. When you don't get enough magnesium, you end up with lower energy production, metabolism issues, fatigue, headaches, constipation, trouble sleeping, tight muscles, and more.

The Roles of Micronutrients

The body uses dozens of different beneficial micronutrient chemicals every hour of every day to keep us energized, produce enzymes and hormones, and prevent deficiencies.

Low levels of specific micronutrients can result in various problems such as

- Mental impairment
- Poor digestion
- Thyroid problems
- Bone loss

The Jobs of Micronutrients

- Producing digestive enzymes
- Helping keep a strong metabolism
- Breaking down carbs, fats, and proteins into usable energy
- Helping with hormone production
- Slowing oxidation damage or signs of aging caused by free radicals
- Protecting the brain
- Aiding in bone mineralization
- Synthesizing DNA
- Allowing cells to rejuvenate
- Allowing muscles to move and helping with tissue repair
- Facilitating growth

Micronutrients vs Macronutrients

THE CHEMICALS found in trace amounts in foods	The way we classify **CALORIES IN FOODS**
More than one present in most foods	More than one present in most foods
There are three main groups: **VITAMINS MINERALS ANTIOXIDANTS**	There are three main groups: **FATS CARBS PROTEINS**
LESS FAMILIAR because we can't always easily pinpoint which ones are in which foods	**MORE FAMILIAR** because they're how we classify foods
Comprise **"small picture"** food elements because we need them in smaller quantities	Comprise **"big picture"** food elements because we need them in larger quantities

The Best Micronutrient Sources

No single food or macronutrient contains all the vital compounds needed for optimal health. The best sources of micronutrients are whole foods such as fruits, vegetables, herbs, nuts, seeds, and organic animal products. Eating a variety of fresh, colorful foods is essential.

Nutrient density is a key determinant of food quality. *Nutrient density* is a ratio that compares the number of calories the food provides to the number of nutrients it contains. Fruits, vegetables, and pasture-raised animal products are more nutrient-dense than processed foods.

It's essential that you consume the highest-quality whole foods to ensure you're getting the optimal sources of micronutrients. Choose organic fruits and vegetables and grass-fed, pasture-raised, and organic animal products.

Highly processed packaged foods are high in calories and low in nutrition. Companies promote many foods as healthy choices—such as whole grain cereals and "all-natural" products—but those foods aren't healthy. Not only do they not contain adequate nutrients but they also increase your need for nutrients by placing additional strain on your body systems by increasing your blood sugar and exposing your liver to more chemicals. They also feed bad microbes that promote inflammation in your gut. If you regularly consume processed foods, sugars, and nonorganic foods, your body will be exposed to toxins that deplete the nutrients in your body.

Supplementation is one way to meet your micronutrient needs when you aren't receiving adequate nutrients through your diet. If you decide to take a supplement, choose only the highest quality professional grade products.

Consuming Too Many Antinutrients

An *antinutrient* is a substance that either prevents absorption of or depletes beneficial nutrients in the body. A *toxin* is one broad category of antinutrient that includes pesticides, herbicides, antibiotics, heavy metals, artificial sweeteners, and other chemical agents in what you eat and drink.

Consuming certain foods causes stress on your body, and sometimes the nutritional value you get from those foods doesn't offset that stress. Eating foods that are high in antinutrients leads to a net loss in your overall nutrients and cellular energy levels. In other words, those foods are taking more from you than they're providing.

Sugar is a toxin that depletes vitamin D, calcium, magnesium, chromium, B vitamins, and vitamin C when you consume it in excess. Sugar also can contribute to a breakdown in cellular energy production, and it increases oxidative stress at the cellular level.[17] This accelerates the aging process of your cells and tissues and contributes to the development of chronic disease.

From a hormonal perspective, consuming sugar promotes higher levels of insulin, which leads to fat storage and more inflammation and can increase pain, cause mood disorders, and promote fatigue and poor sleep.

THE IMPACT OF SUGAR ON THE BODY

Leads to weight gain

Affects brain health

Gives you sleepless nights

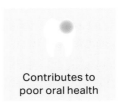
Contributes to poor oral health

Harms the heart

Causes liver problems

Causes anxiety and depression

Raises your risk for type 2 diabetes

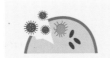
Aggravates pain in the body

Weakens immune system

Increases risk of cancer

Causes chronic inflammation

Nonorganic foods tend to be higher in pesticides, which deplete nutrients from the body and damage the gut. If you can't purchase only organic foods, look for other indicators that the food is free from harmful toxins, such as "non-GMO certified" on the label.

Processed vegetable oils, such as those derived from corn, soy, cottonseed, canola (rapeseed), safflower, and peanuts, are highly inflammatory and serve as inferior fuel sources. They create a significant amount of oxidative stress and trigger inflammatory gene pathways that shut down metabolism and contribute to the development of diseases.

Some plants also produce microtoxins that can be problematic over time. Whereas animals are designed to protect themselves from predators through fight or flight, plants can't sprout legs to run away and thus are stationary. They're also unable to use physical force to fend off predators. Instead, they produce compounds that are toxic to their predators.

Some toxic compounds within plants—such as those found in the roots of water hemlock—cause seizures and vomiting and are potentially fatal to animals that consume them. Microtoxins are subtler; they don't cause death or even an acute inflammatory reaction. Over time, though, the toxin accumulates in the body; the more a person consumes the microtoxin, the more problems it causes.

Some microtoxins are in foods that we consider healthy. Three well-studied and regularly consumed microtoxins found in plants are

- **Phytic acids**, which are high in foods such as grains, beans, and nuts. They're linked to inferior absorption of minerals such as calcium, zinc, and magnesium.[18]

- **Oxalates**, which are highest in spinach, beets, nuts, seeds, chocolate, and raspberries. High oxalate levels can cause kidney stones and joint pain.

- **Lectins**, which are highest in grains, legumes, nuts, seeds, and nightshade vegetables. Overconsuming lectins can cause chronic gut inflammation.

You don't need to avoid these foods altogether, but it may be wise to reduce the quantity if you eat a lot of them, especially if you have gut health issues, kidney problems, or chronic pain.

KETO PRO TIP

Soaking your nuts and seeds overnight in filtered water can significantly reduce their antinutrient content. Soaking the nuts and seeds also makes them more bioavailable and easier to digest. Some nuts and seeds sprout when you soak them, which unlocks an even higher nutritional profile. You can buy presoaked and presprouted nuts and seeds if you have a busy schedule.

Raw cruciferous vegetables also contain antinutrients that are hard on the digestive tract. Steam your vegetables before eating them to gently break down cellulose fibers and make them easier to digest.

Confusing Thirst for Hunger

It's easier than you think to misinterpret thirst as hunger. In fact, dehydration can send a signal that your brain interprets as low blood sugar. This mixed signal makes your body believe that it's time to eat when it's really time to hydrate.

Your hunger and thirst centers are located next to each other in the hypothalamus. Eating stimulates the release of dopamine, endorphins, and other neurochemicals that make you feel good. That's why it's so easy to become neurologically hooked on grazing and snacking; you love that neurochemical reward! The good news is you can retrain your brain to reset its hunger and thirst center.

If you follow a low-carb nutrition plan and frequently get hungry between meals, you're likely not eating enough fat or not drinking enough water. Instead of reaching for a snack, first drink 8 to 16 ounces of water to see what effect it has on how you feel. You'll be surprised how staying well-hydrated keeps you from feeling hungry. If you're still hungry a few minutes after you've consumed a large glass of water, then consider a snack that contains healthy fat.

Eating Too Often

Somewhere in the mid-1990s, eating small, frequent meals throughout the day became all the rage. That was supposed to be the recipe for a fired-up metabolism. Unfortunately, that advice is the opposite of what we now understand is best for human physiology.

The goal is not to stoke your metabolism. Instead, you want to improve your metabolic flexibility. *Metabolic flexibility* is the ease with which your body switches between using fat and sugar as its primary energy source.

When you're metabolically flexible, your body is efficient. It burns body fat for fuel and can go long periods without food, with no decrease in your energy, strength, or mental clarity. You won't need to snack constantly to avoid a crash! You'll also find yourself consuming far fewer carbs and other quick-energy, insulin-spiking foods to get your energy fix. And lower insulin levels mean more fat-burning and less inflammation. The best way to reduce insulin is to follow a keto-style nutrition plan with fewer meals in the day than fad diets and other outdated eating plans recommend.

How Much Water?

I've observed that most people do not drink nearly enough throughout the day. I recommend consuming a minimum of half your body weight in ounces of water. In other words, if you weigh 180 pounds, you should be drinking 90 ounces of water every day.

One of the best hydration strategies is to start drinking early in the day. We go many hours during sleep without drinking; upon waking, we're in a state of dehydration. Starting your day by drinking 16 to 32 ounces of water in the morning before you consume anything else is a great way to flush the body and push yourself out of the dehydrated state. It also helps reset your hunger hormone, ghrelin, to help reduce cravings and stimulate fat-burning.

KETO PRO TIP

Intermittent fasting, also referred to as time-restricted eating, is a practice that's great for building metabolic flexibility. Fasting is often associated with long periods of not eating, but fasting periods don't always have to be extreme. You technically fast every night while you're sleeping. You fast every day between meals. By merely lengthening the window of time between meals, you can train your body to tap into its fat stores and improve your metabolism.

To practice intermittent fasting, start with a twelve-hour break between dinner and breakfast, and eat three meals during the day with no snacking between meals. Try this for two weeks, and then increase the fasting window from twelve to fourteen hours. After your body gets used to fourteen hours, increase the window to sixteen to eighteen hours.

During your fasting time, consume lots of water and herbal teas. You may find you feel best when you eat just two meals per day. Once you incorporate intermittent fasting into your daily routine and "flex" your metabolic muscles, you will be surprised at how much less you think about and depend upon food.

Combining intermittent fasting with a ketogenic lifestyle is one of the best ways to build metabolic flexibility that will enable you to lose weight, have more energy, and stop obsessing about food around the clock. Once you become fat-adapted, you'll have the metabolic flexibility to efficiently use ketones (by-products of fat metabolism) as your body's primary energy source.

In the next chapter, I go into more detail about the three-letter word that we have been led to fear for what seems like forever—F-A-T—as we continue down the road to discovering how to find your ideal weight and the absolute healthiest version of you.

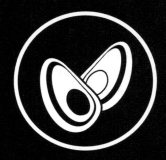

CHAPTER 3

THE UNCENSORED TRUTH ABOUT FAT

It's hard to know what to believe anymore. We live in a fake news era—and we have been living in this era for quite some time. The official and commonly accepted narratives we hear from our doctors and the media often are based on hidden agendas that may not have our best interests at their core, which is why it's vital to trace the facts back to their sources.

Here's an example: the established recommendation for what people commonly refer to as a "heart-healthy" diet.

Back in the 1960s, the sugar industry quietly paid Harvard-based researchers to publish a review on heart disease and its relationship to sugar and fat. The sugar industry funded the research to mask findings that emerged in the 1950s about sugar's undeniable link to heart disease.[1]

The cover-up was successful, and the cause of heart disease was soon shifted squarely onto the shoulders of saturated fat. In the decades following the study, experts, the media, and the food industry universally promoted a low-fat, high-carb diet. This misleading advice was touted as the healthiest way to stave off heart disease.

Food manufacturers took the cue, saw their opportunity for massive profit, and flooded the market with cheap-to-produce, processed foods containing hydrogenated fats and refined sugar. The results were less than ideal. Widespread consumption of trans fat and sugar resulted in epidemic rates of obesity and its related health complications.[2] Diabetes, heart disease, and cancer rates have risen in the past five decades and continue to climb.

The Truth Is Out There

Despite the evidence before us—such as collective America being fatter than ever—the idea that saturated fat is unhealthy and that low-fat, whole grains are a wholesome alternative is still widely accepted. For example, the American Heart Association made a statement in June 2017, claiming that dietary saturated fats and cholesterol are unhealthy. The AHA recommended that people should largely avoid them.

What are people eating instead of healthy fats? Processed vegetable oils, inflammatory carbs, and added sugars.

I'm no conspiracy theorist, but it cannot be a coincidence that much of the funding for the American Heart Association comes from corporations that profit from the sale of processed foods.

Fortunately, the truth about fat will not be contained. Facts continue to come to light as science confirms the many benefits of eating healthy fats. Those benefits include weight loss, reduced inflammation, increased energy, enhanced brain function, and longer, healthier life.

Two recent studies thoroughly debunked the myth that a low-fat, high-carb diet is healthy. In an August 2017 study from *The Lancet*, scientists concluded that excessive carb intake is directly proportional to increased mortality risk, whereas fats (both saturated and unsaturated) are associated with a lower risk of total mortality. Also, the researchers reported the absence of any detrimental cardiovascular effect from fat intake.[3] A September 5, 2017 study published in *Cell Metabolism* echoed the conclusion from *The Lancet* when it stated that a high-fat, low-carb, ketogenic diet extends longevity and promotes health.[4]

Other studies have confirmed the health benefits of following a low-carb diet rather than a low-fat diet. In one study, women lost more weight on a low-carb diet compared to an eating plan that was low in fat.[5] Studies also report that low-carb, high-fat diets help reduce inflammation, lower blood sugar levels, reduce triglycerides, and increase healthy cholesterol levels.[6, 7]

All About Healing Fats

There seems to be an ongoing discussion about "good" fat and "bad" fat in which the leaders of the American Heart Association and other groups proclaim that only unsaturated fats are good, whereas both saturated fats and trans fats are considered bad.

This proclamation is accurate in that there are such things as *bad fats*. However, saturated fat from sources such as virgin coconut oil and organic, grass-fed beef should not be on that list. When incorporating fats into your diet, you must distinguish between healing fats and toxic, processed fats.

Healing fats are nutritious fats needed for vital functions in our body. They are anti-inflammatory, promote muscle growth, and serve as an efficient source of energy. On the other hand, toxic fats are highly inflammatory and contribute to a series of health problems. Learning which fats to consume and which to avoid may be one of the most important things you discover for your health.

You can find many sources of fats that heal rather than harm. Restorative, plant-based fats come from natural sources such as avocados, nuts, coconuts, and olives. Healing animal fats come from foods like organic dairy, grass-fed meats, wild-caught fish, and pasture-raised chicken and eggs.

Incorporating healing fats into your diet has many benefits. First, they provide building blocks for cell membranes and promote an ideal hormone balance. They also function as carriers for essential fat-soluble vitamins such as vitamins A, D, E, and K and aid in the absorption of minerals. In this section, I cover the best types of fats and where you can find them. I also introduce critical terms you need to know as you transition into a keto lifestyle.

KETO PRO TIP

You will see the words *saturated* and *unsaturated* (including monounsaturated and polyunsaturated) quite a bit in the next few pages. In a nutshell, a fatty acid's saturation level is based on the number of hydrogen atoms present. The amount of hydrogen present matters because the more hydrogen, the more saturated the fat is. The more saturated the fat, the higher the melting temperature is. Here's an easy way to tell the difference: If the oil is liquid at room temperature, it's unsaturated.

Omega-3 Fatty Acids

Omega-3 fatty acids are polyunsaturated fats that are liquid at room temperature. They are in fish such as salmon and sardines, nuts, and some seeds, such as chia seeds. Omega-3 fatty acids are well-studied and known to promote health in several ways. They help reduce inflammation and lower the risk of chronic diseases, including heart disease, cancer, and several autoimmune conditions. Omega-3 fatty acids can help lower triglycerides and inflammatory proteins such as C-reactive protein (CRP), and they raise healthy cholesterol levels.[8] They're also essential for brain and eye health.[9]

Omega-6 Fatty Acids

Omega-6 fats also can be healthy as long as you eat them in the correct ratio with omega-3 fats. The proper omega-6 to omega-3 ratio is between 1:1 and 4:1. Like omega-3 fatty acids, omega-6 fatty acids are polyunsaturated fats. Healthy sources of omega-6 fats include nuts, seeds, and various animal products.

   Unfortunately, most people don't eat the correct ratio of omega-6 to omega-3 fats. Corn and soybean oil, two staples of the standard American diet (SAD), contain much higher amounts of oxidized omega-6 fatty acids than omega-3 fatty acids. In fact, refined corn oil has an 83:1 ratio of omega-6 to omega-3! The proportions in safflower, sesame, and grapeseed oils are even worse. Oils with unbalanced ratios are harmful because an excessive intake of omega-6 fats can lead to chronic inflammation.[10]

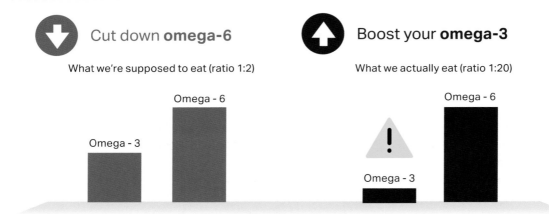

Cut down omega-6

What we're supposed to eat (ratio 1:2)

Omega - 3
Omega - 6

Boost your omega-3

What we actually eat (ratio 1:20)

Omega - 6
Omega - 3

Eat more of these omega-3-rich foods to balance your omega-6 to omega-3 levels and reduce inflammation in your body.

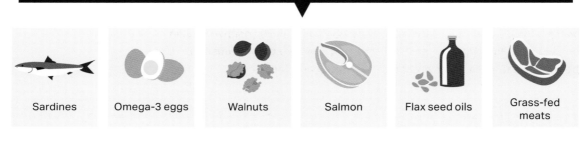

| Sardines | Omega-3 eggs | Walnuts | Salmon | Flax seed oils | Grass-fed meats |

Monounsaturated Fats

Monounsaturated fats are liquid at room temperature but solid when chilled. Foods rich in monounsaturated fatty acids include olives/olive oil, nuts/nut butters, and avocados/avocado oil. Monounsaturated fats may protect from heart disease by optimizing cholesterol and triglyceride levels and improving body composition, the function of blood vessels, insulin sensitivity, and blood sugar control.[11, 12] Oils rich in monounsaturated fats contain vitamin E, which has many health benefits for your brain, immune system, and heart health. Monounsaturated fats have even been linked to a lowered risk of developing certain cancers.[13]

Saturated Fats

Saturated fats are solid at room temperature. They're in animal products such as grass-fed beef and dairy and plant-based sources such as coconut, palm, and MCT oil. (MCT stands for medium-chain triglycerides. Read more about MCT in Chapter 15.) Saturated fatty acids comprise at least 50 percent of your cell walls and offer protection against unwanted materials that attempt to invade the structural integrity of the cells. Saturated fats promote bone health by helping you use calcium. They also help protect the liver from toxicity, fight off microbial infections, and support the immune system.

Grass-fed beef and dairy (including organic cheese, butter, and ghee) and organic, pasture-raised chicken (meat and eggs) are excellent sources of saturated animal fats. Grass-fed beef and dairy are rich in nutrients including protein, omega-3s, conjugated linoleic acid (CLA), creatine, iron, zinc, and vitamins B1, B2, B6, B12, and E.

Coconut oil is a remarkable fat. It has numerous benefits that include aiding digestion, strengthening the immune system, preventing and fighting the overgrowth of candida (yeast), balancing blood sugar levels, nourishing skin and hair, and improving bone health. If it is not already a part of your diet, it will be soon because it's an excellent part of a ketogenic lifestyle.

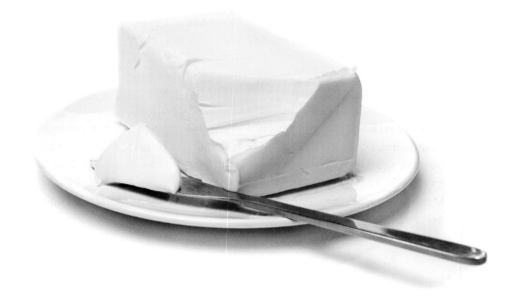

GRASS-FED BUTTER BENEFITS

1 **Contains CLA**

Conjugated linoleic acid (CLA) helps to reduce belly fat and protects against cancer. It also supports muscle growth.

4 **Great Source of Vitamins D and K2**

Vitamin D supports your immune system. Vitamin K2 may reverse arterial calcification and helps to improve bone density.

2 **Great Source of Butyrate**

Butyrate, a short-chain fatty acid, reduces inflammation.

5 **Contains Essential Fat**

Butter is rich in omega-3 fatty acids.

3 **Contains Vitamin A (Retinol)**

Vitamin A is good for the thyroid, adrenals, and cardiovascular health.

6 **Additional Beneficial Nutrients**

Lecithin   Zinc
Selenium   Copper
Magnesium   Iodine and more

All About Toxic Fats

A diet that's rich in the fats we've discussed so far— those healthy fats that come from organic, whole food–based sources and are as close as possible to their natural state—is exceptionally beneficial. The key is to focus on consuming fats that are nondenatured and unrefined because we ruin food when we interfere with and alter it to make it last longer, taste better, or be more cost-effective, as many of the dietary fat sources in the SAD have been altered.

The most common sources of toxic fats are factory-made saturated fats, trans fats, and highly processed unsaturated fats such as canola oil and corn oil. Most respected health authorities now agree that highly processed, factory-made fats are detrimental to the body, and we should avoid them.

Hydrogenated and Partially Hydrogenated Fats

Hydrogenated and partially hydrogenated oils top the list of harmful fats. Although unsaturated vegetable-based fats are inexpensive, they're also liquid at room temperature and less shelf-stable than saturated fats. Manufacturers decided to address the issue of shelf stability by hydrogenating unsaturated vegetable oils by heating the oil using hydrogen as a catalyst. The result is that liquid oil turns into a solid shortening. The manufacturers generally don't add enough hydrogen to thoroughly saturate the fat—hence the term *partially hydrogenated.*

Prevalent hydrogenated fats include hydrogenated or partially hydrogenated cottonseed, palm, soybean, and corn oils. Margarine and shortening are two hydrogenated fats made from cheap oils such as soy, corn, and canola (a genetically modified version of rapeseed).

Hydrogenated and partially hydrogenated fats are associated with cancer, atherosclerosis, diabetes, obesity, immune system dysfunction, low-birth-weight babies, birth defects, decreased visual acuity, sterility, difficulty with breastfeeding, and bone, joint, and tendon issues.[14] Regularly consuming these fats also has been shown to increase the risk of depression.[15]

Ironically, hydrogenated oils are often ingredients in foods that are marketed as health foods because they contain "healthy" alternatives to natural, saturated fats. The reality is that these processed fats are highly inflammatory and offer zero benefits to the human body. To add insult to injury, these unhealthy oils come from large factory farms, which use production methods that are incredibly damaging to the environment.

Trans Fats

During the hydrogenation process, some unsaturated fats become something called *trans fats.* These fats have been linked to particularly destructive effects on the human body. Even "trans-fat-free" soft margarine and tub spreads are still produced from rancid vegetable oils and contain many additives. Although the label may say the processed product is free from trans fats, you should be aware that any oils created in a factory are not good for your health, and you should avoid those products.

Avoiding trans fats can be tricky because food labels are often misleading. Even though the FDA officially banned trans fats, foods with less than 0.5 gram of trans fat per serving don't have to report any trans fat on the label.

To better determine if a food contains toxic trans fats, check the ingredients list for hydrogenated or partially hydrogenated oil. Although 0.5 gram may seem insignificant, eating several portions of foods containing even small amounts of trans fat could be enough to affect your health adversely.

Trans fats are chiefly found in processed foods such as convenience snack foods, chips, popcorn, cakes, and cookies. Ready-made frosting and refrigerated doughs (canned biscuits, pizza and pie crusts, cinnamon rolls) also often include trans fat.

Processed foods with harmful fats make up a large percentage of American diets because they are convenient—but the convenience is not worth the consequences.

HEALTH PROBLEMS ASSOCIATED WITH TRANS FATS

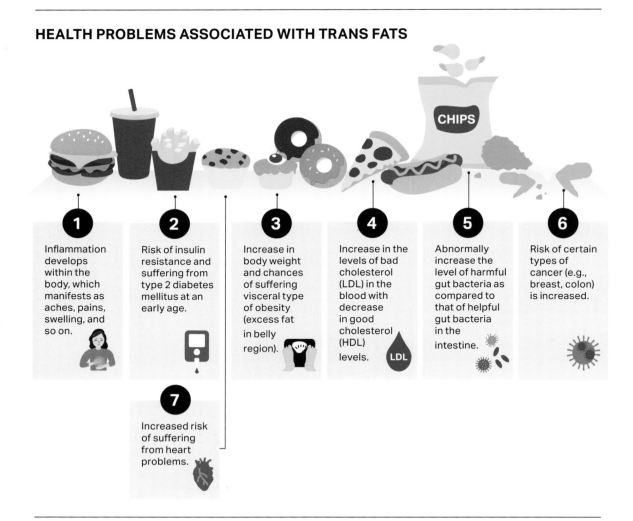

1 Inflammation develops within the body, which manifests as aches, pains, swelling, and so on.

2 Risk of insulin resistance and suffering from type 2 diabetes mellitus at an early age.

3 Increase in body weight and chances of suffering visceral type of obesity (excess fat in belly region).

4 Increase in the levels of bad cholesterol (LDL) in the blood with decrease in good cholesterol (HDL) levels.

5 Abnormally increase the level of harmful gut bacteria as compared to that of helpful gut bacteria in the intestine.

6 Risk of certain types of cancer (e.g., breast, colon) is increased.

7 Increased risk of suffering from heart problems.

Processed Vegetable Oils

Most oils sold and used in the United States are polyunsaturated vegetable oils, which are highly processed and easily oxidized. These oils include canola, corn, vegetable, grapeseed, soybean, sunflower, safflower, rice bran, cottonseed, sesame, and peanut.

Oxidation occurs when oils are exposed to light, air, or heat. Oxidation promotes free radicals, which are chemicals that are highly reactive and have the potential to harm cells, including causing cellular damage that may lead to more serious, life-threatening conditions.

Additionally, more than 90 percent of the soy, corn, cotton (cottonseed), and canola (rapeseed) crops grown in the United States are made from genetically modified organisms (GMOs). GMOs are products that have undergone genetic manipulation to survive environmental or chemical challenges.

Experts suggest there are serious health risks associated with GMO-based foods, including immune system issues, changes in the gut that lead to the development of pathogenic microbes, and faulty insulin regulation. I recommend avoiding GMO-based products. Because food manufacturers aren't required to label which foods are made with genetically modified ingredients, the surest way to avoid GMO-based foods is to buy organic or look for the seal of approval from the Non-GMO Project, a nonprofit organization dedicated to helping consumers make wise, healthy choices.

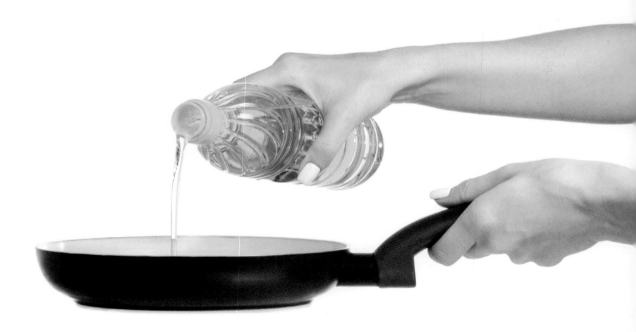

FATS / OILS

Cleaning up your diet by using the right fats and oils is essential to improving your health.

 Which to eat

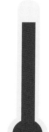

Saturated (for hot uses)

Organic, virgin coconut oil and organic, pasture-raised animal fats.

- **Coconut**
- **MCT oil**
- **Butter**
- **Ghee**
- **Tallow**
- **Schmaltz (chicken fat)**
- **Lamb fat**
- **Duck fat**
- **Grass-fed dairy**
- **Avocado oil**
  (a monounsaturated fat that has a high smoke point and can be used in hot applications)

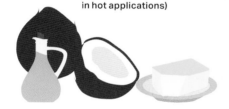

Unsaturated (for cold uses)

Organic, extra-virgin, and cold-pressed forms of these oils are ideal.

- **Olive oil**
- **Avocado oil**
- **Nut oils (walnut, pecan, macadamia)**
- **Flax seed oil**

  Note: Unsaturated fats (typically liquid at room temperature [68°F]) are easily damaged/oxidized when heat is applied to them. You do not want to consume damaged fats.

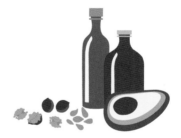

 Which to ditch

Saturated

Man-made fats are never healthy. Trans fats are particularly harmful.

- Margarine
- Hydrogenated or partially hydrogenated oils and manufactured trans fats often found in "buttery spreads."

Unsaturated

These oils are highly processed and oxidize easily via one or more of the following: light, air, or heat. Consuming oxidized oils is never healthy.

- Canola oil (also known as rapeseed oil)
- Corn oil
- Vegetable oil
- Soybean oil
- Grapeseed oil
- Sunflower oil
- Safflower oil
- Rice bran oil
- Cottonseed oil
- Sesame oil
- Peanut oil

Healing Fat in Action

Now I've discussed the good, the bad, and the ugly concerning fat sources. When it comes to oils and fats, it may seem like there are only a few widely available good alternatives, whereas there are plenty of unhealthy choices. If we're talking about processed food, this is true.

Focusing on eating real food helps you naturally make better choices. You have to stay vigilant and educate yourself about reading food labels. In the following sections, I explain ways you can incorporate healing fats into your diet and avoid the bad fats.

Fat and Eating Out

America is obsessed with going out to eat. We love to break bread with family and friends, and our social lives revolve around food. Unfortunately, the food you eat when you're out almost always contains harmful, inflammatory fats. In fact, it's estimated that more than 90 percent of restaurants cook with unsaturated, oxidized oils. Even some restaurants that claim to use only healthy oils have been known to cut healing oils with cheaper alternatives to keep their costs down.

When you go out for dinner, you have the right to ask your server what type of oil the chef uses. If the answer is that the restaurant uses an inflammatory, processed oil, you can ask for steamed vegetables and a side of butter or olive oil to drizzle over them. If you order a salad, ask for olive oil and vinegar and say no to premade dressings and sauces, which almost always contain oxidized oils and added sugars. It's also a good idea to choose grilled protein over deep-fried options; oils with trans fats are typically used in deep fryers because the kitchen staff doesn't have to swap them out as often as they would healthier choices.

The best way to avoid damaging, hidden ingredients is to cook fresh food at home using the healthy fats and oils I discussed earlier. But sometimes, eating out is necessary—and also fun! We connect over food, and with the hectic pace of modern life, most people don't have time to cook every meal from scratch. So, take the time to learn which restaurants use healthy fats, and avoid the restaurants that don't.

Cooking with Fat at Home

Eating home-cooked meals is the best way to promote weight loss, increase energy, and feel great. You need to use healthy fats in your kitchen—on the stove, in recipes, and in your protein sources.

Include grass-fed beef, organic chicken, and wild-caught salmon on the menu. Have a burger with a lettuce wrap for lunch and top it with avocado and grass-fed cheese. For side dishes, try steamed vegetables coated in grass-fed butter or olive oil. These fats taste fantastic and help you better absorb the vitamins and minerals in the veggies.

When it comes to cooking with oil, select the type of fat based on the temperature at which you'll be cooking. For high-heat cooking, avocado oil and ghee are best because they have a higher smoke (flash) point, which is the temperature at which fat begins to break down. It's crucial that you never heat oil to the point that it smokes; when oil is hot enough to smoke, it's emitting toxic fumes and harmful free radicals. For medium-temperature cooking, virgin coconut oil is excellent. Reserve the extra-virgin olive oil only for low-temperature cooking and dressings or sauces. Keep the following list of healthy fats and their smoke points handy when you're preparing meals.

Fat	Cooking Temperature
Avocado oil	520°F
Ghee (clarified butter)	485°F
Extra-virgin olive oil	375°F
Extra-virgin coconut oil	350°F
Butter	302°F

Fat in Dressings and Snacks

Extra-virgin olive oil (EVOO) is the healthiest form of olive oil with the most vibrant flavor. Because of its low smoke point, EVOO is best drizzled over cooked or raw foods or when used as a salad dressing. To give your salad an extra nutrition boost, top it with olives, avocado, grass-fed cheese, and nuts.

Healthy fats are easy to incorporate into snacks and appetizers. Freshly made guacamole served with sliced raw vegetables is one of the best keto snacks around. Other great snack options are a handful of walnuts or other nuts or nut butters with veggies. Grass-fed cheese is a delicious snack if you aren't sensitive to dairy. One of my go-to fat-burning snacks is grass-fed cheese with cucumbers, Dijon mustard, and olives.

Fat in Smoothies and Drinks

Another excellent way to add healing fats to your diet is to include them in smoothies. For example, you can make a smoothie with full-fat coconut milk; high-quality, organic protein powder; and a scoop of almond butter to give it an extra fat (and taste) boost. Other fats that are delicious in smoothies include avocados, flax and chia seeds, coconut, and MCT oil.

KETO PRO TIP

One of my favorite ways to take in more healthful fats is to make Golden Milk (page 351) and Matcha Tea (page 348). I also enjoy adding more butter or olive oil to the veggies I eat for dinner.

Get creative with your cooking! There are lots of delicious ways to incorporate healthy fats into your lifestyle.

KETO PRO TIP

If you see the word "hydrogenated" anywhere on the label, stay away. Also check the ingredients for other oils that are cheap and heavily processed, such as canola, soybean, corn, safflower, peanut, cottonseed, sunflower, and generic "vegetable oil." If the fat source listed on a food label is not from extra-virgin olive oil, virgin coconut oil, butter, ghee, or avocado oil, the chances are high that the oil has been heavily processed.

Embrace the Fat

Your body wants and needs dietary fat, which is essential for health and well-being. The key is to consume wholesome varieties of fat and avoid toxic ones. Your body responds to margarine, shortening, and other factory-made oils in a way that's appropriate for what they are—artificial, enemy invaders. Is it any wonder, then, why they cause an inflammatory response? The body knows what it's doing, so we should listen to it.

Take in real food and ditch the fake stuff. Learn to read nutrition labels, cook with healing fats, consume organic proteins, and add nondenatured fats to your vegetables, smoothies, and snacks.

In the next chapter, I explain the benefits of being in the fat-burning state known as ketosis and tell you how you can transform your physiology to get your body burning fat for fuel!

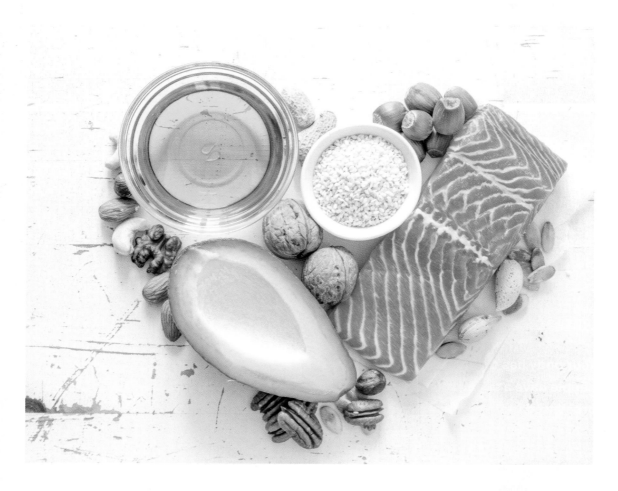

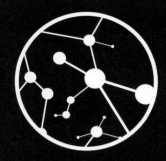

CHAPTER 4

THE KEY TO IT ALL

The idea that eating fat makes you fat is a damaging untruth, and I intend to put an end to that myth in this book.

In this chapter, I talk about the foundation of achieving a metabolic breakthrough. I'm going to give you the keys to losing weight, having more energy, reducing inflammation, and helping avoid (and, in some cases, even reverse) many crippling, preventable diseases. I'm talking about *ketosis*, which is the metabolic state of burning fat as an energy source rather than using sugar as fuel.

Your body has to work with what you give it, which is why most people have a sugar-burning metabolism. When your diet consists of processed grains and sugar, your body adapts to fuel and bases its energy production on it.

When you're in ketosis, however, your body has adapted to a far superior fuel source because you've deprived it of the inferior one. Once you're in ketosis and your body considers fat to be its fuel, stored body fat suddenly becomes a readily available source of energy. In this way, ketosis truly maximizes your fat-burning potential.

To get into ketosis, you must have low blood sugar levels and adequate dietary or body fat to provide a source of ketones. You can enhance your state of ketosis through fasting, following a high-fat, low-carb diet, doing high-intensity exercise, and supplementing with MCT oil, exogenous ketones, and caffeine.

So, it's time to dig in to learn more about each of these things and the science behind this phenomenal process.

What Is Ketosis?

Your cells must make the energy to perform their various functions and to make life itself possible. The body's "energy currency" comes in the form of adenosine triphosphate (ATP), and the mitochondria within every cell in your body metabolize either glucose or ketones to form this critical energy molecule.

For most people, the energy that fuels their bodies is created by the breakdown of glucose, which comes from carbohydrates in the diet. After it digests food, the body burns the glucose for energy, stores it as glycogen, or stores it as fat.

An alternative fuel source is ketones, which are water-soluble metabolites of fatty acids that the liver produces from both dietary fat and body fat. When your body switches to burning ketones for energy, you move into a metabolic state known as *ketosis*. You achieve ketosis after a prolonged period of low insulin and low blood sugar levels.

Based on what we understand about cellular energy metabolism, ketones can create much higher amounts of energy per molecule than glucose can. So when your body begins to convert fat into ketones, those ketones become a much more reliable and sustainable energy source than glucose. Many people report feeling much more stable when they go into ketosis, meaning they no longer experience brain fog, extreme hunger, severe cravings, extreme mood swings, or post-meal energy crashes.

Another appealing aspect of ketosis is that burning fat for fuel doesn't create the same insulin and blood sugar response that burning sugar does. Elevated insulin levels and the insulin resistance that ensues are vital players in the development of many damaging conditions and diseases. When you're in ketosis and aren't experiencing the insulin response prompted by eating carbohydrates, you reap some of the profound benefits of being in ketosis, such as improved hormone balance, lowered inflammation, and enhanced brain health.

HOW DOES KETOSIS WORK?

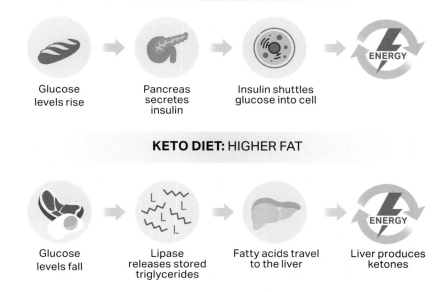

TRADITIONAL DIET: HIGHER CARB

Glucose levels rise → Pancreas secretes insulin → Insulin shuttles glucose into cell → ENERGY

KETO DIET: HIGHER FAT

Glucose levels fall → Lipase releases stored triglycerides → Fatty acids travel to the liver → Liver produces ketones / ENERGY

What Are Ketones?

I've already introduced you to the term *ketosis;* now I can share some specifics. *Ketones* are the by-products of the metabolism of fat. Your liver uses dietary fat or stored body fat and converts it into ketones to be used by the mitochondria in the production of ATP. This fatty acid metabolism results in three different types of ketones:

- Acetoacetate (AcAc)

- Acetate (also called acetone)

- Beta-hydroxybutyrate (BHB)

AcAc is the primary ketone; your body converts it into either energy or BHB. Acetate (or acetone) exhibits the least metabolic effect; your body breaks it down and excretes it through the breath and urine. (The acetone excreted through the breath is responsible for the telltale "keto breath" some people experience during the beginning stages of keto-adaptation.)

Based on its molecular structure, BHB is not an actual ketone. However, its presence is one of the beneficial effects of being in ketosis. BHB modulates brain-derived neurotrophic growth factor (BDNF), which is essential for learning and memory, and it also stimulates the growth of neural tissue.[1]

Nutritional Ketosis and Ketoacidosis: What's the Difference?

If you have friends or family members who've tried following a keto diet, or if you've attempted to go keto in the past, you've probably heard some people say that ketosis is dangerous for your body over a long period—and that it's the state diabetics try to avoid. This is simply *not* true.

The problem is that the state of *nutritional ketosis* is sometimes confused with a state referred to as *ketoacidosis*, which is an extreme condition that occurs only in diabetic populations. When an individual is unable to produce insulin, sugar can't get into the cells. As a response, the body drastically upregulates ketone production.

Type 1 diabetics do not produce any insulin. In contrast, type 2 diabetics produce insulin but have a poor response to it. Ketoacidosis can occur only in people with type 1 diabetes or extreme cases in which a person with type 2 diabetes has lost his or her ability to produce insulin.

When a person is in a state of ketoacidosis, that person's body is experiencing both extremely elevated blood sugar levels *and* elevated blood ketone levels. The result is that the body pH becomes dangerously acidic, which can be fatal. Although this condition is potentially harmful, entering this state is extremely rare. In fact, the condition primarily occurs only in people with type 1 diabetes who unsuccessfully manage their disease.

In ketoacidosis, ketone levels reach 20 mmol/L and beyond. A healthy individual could fast for twenty days and hit a ketone level of 5 to 7 mmol/L, which is still significantly lower than the ketoacidosis range. In other words, unless you have type 1 diabetes, reaching a state of ketoacidosis through dietary changes alone is virtually impossible.

For those people with diabetes, achieving nutritional ketosis can be a safe and healthy goal, as long as they regularly monitor their blood sugar and insulin levels to note any concerning changes.

The real difference between ketosis and ketoacidosis is in blood sugar levels. Low blood sugar is the trademark of nutritional ketosis (along with low insulin levels and a moderate level of ketones). In ketoacidosis, however, high blood sugar is the norm (along with low insulin levels and a high level of ketones). Consequently, people with diabetes who are pursuing a keto diet should test their blood sugar levels regularly.

If you have diabetes, don't let this common misunderstanding keep you from benefiting from one of the best lifestyle changes you could ever make. Just be sure to check your blood sugar and ketone levels regularly and work with your physician to establish the proper medication dosage as your numbers change.

How Do You Achieve Ketosis?

Ketosis will not become the primary metabolic state of your body until you meet three parameters:

- You have low blood sugar.

- You have low insulin levels.

- You provide fat to be used as energy.

To satisfy these criteria, you need to have a plan and use the proven tools required to reach ketosis. In the next sections, I discuss the top six tools for reaching ketosis.

Fasting

Perhaps the quickest way to get into ketosis is through water fasting, which is when you refrain from eating food and consume only water for at least twenty-four hours until your blood sugar becomes low. At that point, your body switches over to burning body fat instead of using glucose for fuel.

There are several benefits to fasting, including easing gut issues, reducing inflammation, boosting fat-burning, improving cognitive function, increasing growth hormone production, and promoting cellular healing. If water fasting is not for you, you might prefer a combination of consuming healthy fats and drinking organic coffee. I recommend drinking Fat-Burning Turmeric Coffee (page 350) to provide enough healthy fats to ease the body into ketosis. Research has also shown that caffeine assists in ketone formation. Another option is to perform a fat fast, where you refrain from consuming proteins and carbs and consume 90 percent or more of your calories from fats.

Read more about how to implement intermittent fasting with your ketogenic lifestyle in Chapter 13.

Ketogenic Diet

Although fasting can help push you into ketosis, you must follow a ketogenic diet if you want to maintain ketosis in perpetuity. A keto diet is made up of 60 to 75 percent healthy fats, 20 to 35 percent proteins, and minimal calories coming from carbs, ideally from 5 to 10 percent. Eating this way ensures the body maintains a fat-burning state.

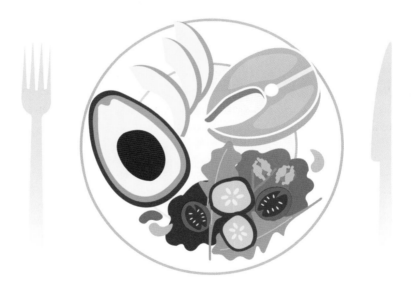

When it comes to carbs, there are four main types: sugar, starch, fiber, and sugar alcohols. Sugar and starch are the ones that most significantly affect blood sugar and insulin levels, whereas fiber and sugar alcohols have little to no effect on blood sugar and insulin levels. The key is to maintain a low net carb amount. The net carbs are the total carbs minus fiber and sugar alcohols. The equation looks like this:

Net Carbs = Total Carbohydrates − (Fiber + Sugar Alcohols)

For example, if you eat 1 cup of broccoli, you'd calculate the net carbs like so:

6 total carbs – 2.5 grams of fiber = 3.5 grams of net carbs

I recommend getting plenty of fiber and limiting your intake of sugar alcohols, even though they don't count as a "carb" in the formula. Sugar alcohols such as xylitol, mannitol, and erythritol cause digestive challenges for some people and elicit a mild insulin response for others. Pay close attention to how your body responds to sugar alcohols and adjust your intake as needed.

High-Intensity Exercise

Fasting and low-carb eating are the best ways to promote ketosis. The next-best trick is performing high-intensity exercise that uses large muscle groups in rapid bursts. This type of exercise is a great way to quickly use sugar stores and switch your body into fat-burning mode.

Some good options for high-intensity exercise include resistance training and HIIT (high-intensity interval training) to burn up your body's stored sugar and activate fat-burning mechanisms. Many health clubs and fitness centers offer this sort of exercise. You also can find info on resistance training and HIIT by searching on YouTube.

KETO PRO TIP

If your goal is weight loss, combine high-intensity exercise with fasting three to four times per week to accelerate your results.

Coffee (Caffeine)

Consuming coffee or another source of caffeine in the morning is one powerful way to spur ketone production. In a recent study, researchers found that caffeine consumption in the morning (especially when combined with intermittent fasting) significantly increased ketones.[2]

If you're sensitive to caffeine, don't worry; it's certainly not the key to maintaining a state of ketosis. However, if you enjoy coffee and tea, start drinking my Fat-Burning Turmeric Coffee (page 350) and Matcha Tea (page 348) to add a caffeine boost and a dose of healthy fats to your day. This combination of caffeine and fat is ideal if you suffer from massive cravings around lunchtime and you're not ready to break your fast.

MCT Oil

MCT stands for *medium-chain triglycerides*, which is a type of fat that occurs naturally in coconuts and palm oil. This kind of fat converts easily into ketones for energy, but coconuts and palm kernel oil contain only small amounts. Fortunately, scientists have been able to extract MCTs into a concentrated form. You can consume this tasteless oil on its own, add it to smoothies, drizzle it over food, or blend it into a fat-burning coffee to provide ketones for energy. Read more about MCT oil in Chapter 15.

KETO PRO TIP

When buying MCT oil, avoid the types that contain lauric acid. Although it's technically an MCT, lauric acid does not easily convert into ketones. I recommend using an MCT oil that is made primarily of caprylic acid (C8) and capric acid (C10). The best option, however, is an MCT oil that's just pure C8 oil.

Exogenous Ketones

One game-changing development in the world of ketosis is supplemental *exogenous ketones*, which are synthetically created BHB that mimic the body's endogenously produced BHB.

MCT oil is excellent for providing a readily available source of ketones, but exogenous ketones take things a step further to help quickly place your body in a state of ketosis. Exogenous ketones also help you maintain a state of ketosis during times when your carb intake is higher than usual.

Combining exogenous ketones with MCT oil helps to raise ketone levels quickly and maintain them for an extended period. This combination is excellent for people who are new to a ketogenic lifestyle, for those who are experiencing keto flu, or for those who are having a hard time getting into ketosis.

In Chapter 11, I provide full details about implementing changes to kick-start your metabolism and regain your fat-burning potential so you can have a keto metabolic breakthrough.

How Do You Know When You're in Ketosis?

I've shared six reliable tools for stimulating ketosis, especially when you use them in combination with each other. Most people enter into light nutritional ketosis (a reading of between 0.5 to 1.0 mmol/L on a ketone meter) within three days to a week after starting a ketogenic eating plan. The following graph illustrates the states of ketosis. Your goal is to reach a state within the optimal ketone zone of 1.0 to 3.0 mmol/L, which usually takes two to three weeks.[3]

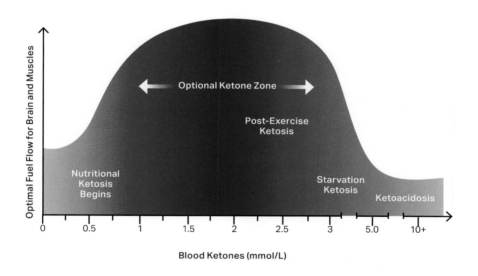

However, everyone is different, and our bodies can respond to lifestyle changes in different ways. Some people can tolerate more carbohydrates, whereas other people must keep net carbs extremely low. Several factors can influence your state of ketosis.

The best way to know whether you're in ketosis is to measure your ketone levels, ideally through the breath or blood. You can also use urine to test for ketones, but urine testing isn't as accurate as the other methods.

Use a Blood Ketone Meter

Blood testing is considered the gold standard for measuring ketone levels. A blood meter measures the BHB level, which is considered to be the most accurate way to determine ketone levels. Unfortunately, this form of testing is pricey and invasive. I don't enjoy having to prick my finger, and I know others feel the same!

If you want to use this method, the Precision Xtra is a blood glucose and ketone meter available online for less than $50. The expensive part is buying the ketone test strips, which can cost as much as $4 each. If you want to test yourself every day, you'll spend $120 a month on test strips.

Keto Mojo is a newer company that offers affordable blood test meters and the least expensive ketone strips ($0.99 per strip). After the initial cost of the meter ($60), the ongoing cost of daily testing is just $30 a month.

Use a Breath Testing Meter

People often prefer breath testing over blood testing because it doesn't require a finger prick, and it's simple to perform. This measurement technique is a great way to test for nutritional ketosis. However, remember that breath ketones are not always a pure reflection of blood ketones because they can be affected by factors such as how much alcohol and water you've consumed. The key is to use the breath testing meter regularly and track your results so you can see what kinds of slight variations occur in reaction to your habits.

Another advantage of breath testing is that there's just a one-time expense for the purchase of a meter. You don't have to purchase any blood strips or lancets because you're analyzing your breath rather than your blood. You can test at home easily.

The two most common options for breath ketone meters are the LevL and the Ketonix. Both offer accurate testing and digital recordings, and they have smartphone apps to help you track your readings over time. See "Resources" at the end of this book for a little more information about these meters.

Use Urine Ketone Strips

The most common way to measure ketones is through the urine (acetoacetate) with simple ketone strips. Urine testing is the most commonly used method because it's inexpensive and convenient. You spend about $9 to get 150 strips, so your total cost per month is $1.80 to $3.60, depending on whether you test once or twice per day.

To do this test, you urinate on the strip and wait up to a minute for the band on the strip to change color. The color indicates what level of ketones you urinated out, ranging from negative (no ketones) to large amounts. The nearby chart shows the color range.

Ketone - Read the test strip at exactly 15 seconds.

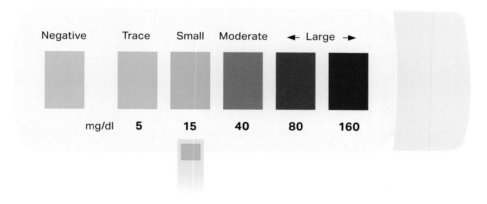

If you've followed a ketogenic diet for more than one day, you should be creating and urinating out ketones that will show up on the test strip. When you first get started on keto, urine ketone strips can be a good tool to see when you begin producing the ketones in large amounts.

Unfortunately, urine testing is not a highly reliable analysis of blood ketone levels. When you start a ketogenic diet, you naturally see high levels of urinary ketones. However, as you become fat-adapted, urinary ketone levels decrease because your body's cells become more responsive to the higher ketone levels, and you use the ketones for fuel. The result is that you throw off fewer ketones in your urine, so you have lower urinary ketone measurements.

So to summarize this point, if you see high ketones on a urine test strip, it doesn't mean you're in ketosis. It only means that you're producing ketones, and your body may not be able to use them as an energy source.

Once you become keto-adapted and you actually begin using the ketones as an energy source, you won't eliminate so many through your urine, and therefore your urine strips will typically show low-moderate levels of ketones.

This information is important. I've had a lot of people tell me they're in ketosis, but they report that they don't feel well. When I ask them how they know they're in ketosis, they tell me that the urine test strips reflect high levels of ketones. They don't realize that means their bodies are not yet adapted to using ketones as a fuel source. They need to allow more time to adapt to using them.

Changes in hydration also can affect ketone concentration in your urine. If you're thoroughly hydrating your system (which I recommend), you have a diluted ketone concentration in your urine. Unusually high ketone readings via urine test strips are often indicative that you're in a dehydrated state. Your other habits—such as fasting states, eating periods, exercising, and your level of hydration when you wake—can affect the reading of a urine test.

Test Blood Glucose Levels

Testing blood glucose levels is a less common testing technique, but for some people, it's an attractive option because it's less expensive than testing blood ketone levels. Glucose strips cost much less per unit than ketone test strips. You can use either of the two blood ketone and glucose meters that I previously mentioned: the Precision Xtra or the Keto Mojo. The least expensive test strips (for both ketones and blood glucose) work with the Keto Mojo meter.

When your body is in sugar-burning mode, it's susceptible to low blood sugar levels (hypoglycemia), and it secretes stress hormones to boost blood sugar if it drops too low. Typically, the critical range when this occurs is 75 to 80 mg/dL, even though hypoglycemia is technically diagnosed by a fasting blood sugar less than 70 mg/dL.[4]

When blood sugar levels drop below 80 mg/dL, your body responds by producing cortisol, which tells the body to break down the glycogen (stored sugar) in the muscle and liver to get more sugar into the bloodstream. This survival response is natural because your body is concerned that sugar (its primary fuel) is scarce, and you're entering a time of famine.

When your body increases cortisol production, you feel a natural high—at first. However, if this cycle becomes repetitive, you eventually get to a state of brain-adrenal fatigue, and your body is unable to maintain high enough cortisol and blood sugar levels for the brain to produce adequate energy.

The result of this pattern is blood sugar imbalance and hypoglycemia. In this state, your brain cells are starving, and they begin to signal you to crave sugar and sweets. You will also experience fatigue and mental lethargy and have sleep and mood disturbances. I think most people have experienced the classic "hangry" mood—the one where you're highly irritable because you've gone too long without food.

When you're in a ketogenic or fat-adapted state, you can maintain a hypoglycemic level (less than 70mg/dL) and feel great! You'll have lots of energy, mental clarity, stamina, good mood, and restful sleep, which are all signs your body has adapted to using ketones and isn't reliant on sugar as its primary fuel source—and so the body is no longer concerned with keeping blood sugar levels up to survive. If your blood sugar is between 50 and 80 mg/dL, and you feel mentally sharp, energetic, and relaxed continually, then you are keto-adapted!

KETO PRO TIP

An HbA1C test looks at the level of *glycation* (indicative of blood sugar levels) in red blood cells over a 90- to 120-day period. The typical HbA1C result on a ketogenic diet is 4.5 to 5.2 percent. A result higher than this range is an indication that you have not been in ketosis enough during the past three to four months.

Monitor How You Feel

The final method for measuring ketones is subjective but *extremely* important. When you're in ketosis, you should feel relaxed and mentally sharp. You'll have energy throughout the day. You shouldn't experience cravings. And—perhaps even better—you'll hardly think about food. Conversely, if you're in sugar-burning mode, you'll feel fatigued, have cravings, and want to snack throughout the day. If you notice these symptoms, you're not in ketosis.

Another thing you may notice when you're in ketosis is the smell of acetone, which has a fruity, sweet odor. You may detect it in your breath, sweat, or urine. This effect is natural while you're in ketosis, but the odor should be faint. If the smell is overpowering, it's a sign you're electrolyte-deficient. Drink more water and increase your sodium, magnesium, and potassium levels.

You also can try eating an avocado, drinking the juice from a fresh lemon each day, and including some pink salt or a seaweed spice mix on your foods to help relieve the acetone smell. These things all provide electrolytes that can help improve your overall breath. Drinking peppermint tea and frequently brushing your teeth can also help reduce the fruity smell.

Side Effects and Other Considerations of Ketosis

Ketosis is a natural metabolic state that our bodies are designed to move in and out of periodically. This fat-burning state has many benefits for the body, including lowered inflammation, improved energy, heightened brain function, and emotional stability. Although being in ketosis is generally safe and well-tolerated by most people, you should consult with your physician if you have a history of pancreatitis, kidney disease, gallbladder disease, or type 1 or 2 diabetes.

Additionally, some people experience symptoms in the early stages of ketosis; we often refer to these symptoms as *keto flu*. During this period, the body is shifting its metabolism from burning sugars to burning fats, and the body reacts with symptoms including hypoglycemia, drowsiness, dizziness, irritability, sugar cravings, and muscle weakness. I cover the keto flu in more detail in Chapter 8 and explain the best ways to mitigate symptoms.

Now that you know what ketosis is, in the next chapter, I explain what benefits living in a state of ketosis has for your body.

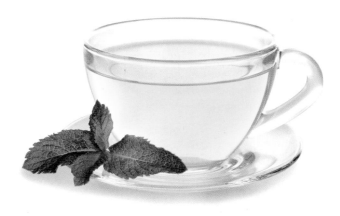

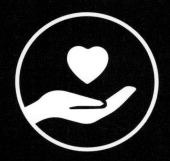

CHAPTER 5

THE BENEFITS OF A KETO LIFESTYLE

If you started this book with limited knowledge of ketosis or what it means to be on a ketogenic diet, now you know some of the fundamentals. But we're far from done. If you're tired of counting calories and gaining all the weight back the moment you stop counting, you're ready for a breakthrough, and you want this to be the last "diet" you ever do, you need to do more digging. A lot of diet evangelists love to give you the *how* of their diets. What you need is the *why* behind the decisions that affect your health! The *why* is what I cover in this chapter as I briefly examine the top twelve most common and well-researched benefits of living a ketogenic lifestyle.

In my experience, most people try keto to lose weight. They've attempted all the popular calorie-restrictive diets, and they've come to the same conclusion:

Calorie restriction just doesn't work.

Here's the thing: Keto is a lifestyle, *not* a fad diet. Keto turns on the proper fat-burning hormones while suppressing the fat-storage hormones. Keto also turns on your mitochondria (which I discuss shortly) and gives you all-day energy without hunger and cravings.

The benefits of a keto lifestyle stretch far beyond weight loss. People who go on a ketogenic plan because they want to lose some weight are often pleasantly surprised to discover that their anxiety levels, skin issues, mental clarity, and more also improve.

So, let's get started with discovering why the ketogenic lifestyle can do so much more than help you lose weight.

Reduced Inflammation

One of the most basic and profound benefits of a ketogenic diet is that it drastically lowers *inflammation*, which is essentially an immune response in the body.[1] I think of inflammation like a fire in your fireplace. It's good in small amounts because it helps you to heal wounds and fend off bacterial and parasitic infections. However, if the fire spreads from the fireplace to the walls, it starts burning down your home. Similarly, when you consume sugar and promote higher insulin levels, you drive up inflammation, and the fire spreads throughout your body.

When you provide ketones to your body's cells and keep both sugar and insulin low, your immune system remains calm and keeps inflammatory pathways suppressed. In this way, it's similar to keeping the fire well controlled in the fireplace.

Reduced inflammation allows for more energy production and a body that functions more efficiently overall. Under these conditions, your body is better able to repair and heal itself. Because of this, a keto lifestyle may be well suited for supporting the fight against certain cancers, autoimmune conditions, neurological disorders, and metabolic disorders.

HOW INFLAMMATION AFFECTS THE BODY

Inflammation is at the root of practically all known chronic health conditions.

Brain

Pro-inflammatory cytokines cause an autoimmune reaction in the brain, which can lead to depression, autism, poor memory, Alzheimer's disease, and MS.

Cardiovascular

Inflammation in the heart, arterial, and venous walls contributes to heart disease, strokes, high blood sugar (diabetes), and anemia.

Muscle

Inflammatory cytokines can cause muscle pain and weakness that can manifest as carpal tunnel syndrome, polymyalgia, or rheumatica, to name a few.

Bones

Inflammation interferes with the body's natural ability to repair bone mass, increasing the number of fractures and leading to conditions like osteoporosis.

Skin

Chronic inflammation compromises the liver and kidneys, resulting in rashes, dermatitis, eczema, acne, psoriasis, wrinkles, and fine lines.

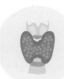

Thyroid

Autoimmunity as a result of inflammation can reduce total thyroid receptor count and disrupts thyroid hormone function.

Lungs

Inflammation induces autoimmune reactions against the linings of airways, which can result in allergies or asthma.

GI Tract

Chronic inflammation damages the intestinal lining and can result in issues like GERD, Crohn's disease, and celiac disease.

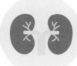

Kidneys

Inflammatory cytokines restrict blood flow to the kidneys. Complications like edema, hypertension, nephritis, and kidney failure can result.

Liver

Buildup of inflammation leads to an enlarged liver or fatty liver disease, and you have increased toxic load in your body.

Accelerated Fat and Weight Loss

By definition, being in a state of ketosis implies the body is using fat for its fuel. Once you're in ketosis, the damaging effects of a high-sugar diet are lessened and eventually reversed as your stored body fat becomes a prime source of energy.

Recent studies have shown that consuming a high-fat, low-carb diet is superior to a low-fat diet for enhancing weight loss and improving risk factors for cardiovascular disease.[2] Most people find that they lose a considerable amount of weight on keto, and many people claim the weight loss was nearly effortless once they got over the initial cravings.

The weight loss is important for physical, mental, and emotional health. People who are overweight are at a much higher risk of heart disease, diabetes, depression, anxiety, and suicide.

When people experience sustained weight loss on a keto diet, they feel very empowered. I've seen many clients on the keto diet lose more than 50 pounds within six months and more than 100 pounds in a year and keep it off years later.

WEIGHT LOSS BENEFITS IN KETOSIS

 Burn more fat
- Fat is utilized for energy instead of carbs.
- The body goes into an extremely high fat-burning state.

 Reduce hunger
- Keto-friendly foods are high in healthy fat, protein, antioxidants, and fiber.
- You feel satiated quicker and longer.

 Stabilize blood sugar
- You eat good sources of fat, protein, and veggies.
- Blood sugar and insulin spikes caused by high-carb and high-protein diets are eliminated.

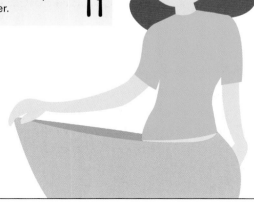

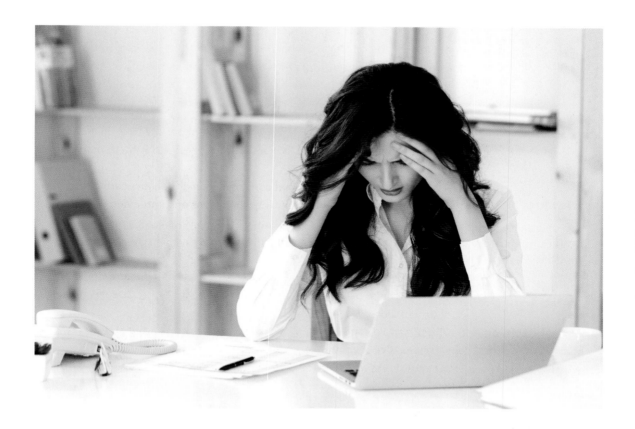

Reduced Oxidative Stress

Oxidative stress is a natural by-product of energy production in the mitochondria, and it's beneficial in small amounts. In excess, however, it can be highly damaging to the mitochondria. Excessive oxidative stress caused by the overproduction of free radicals creates inflammation and mitochondrial damage.

Because oxidative stress causes damage on a microscopic level, it can negatively affect every cell in your body. And because your brain is so reliant on healthy mitochondria, it's the first part of your body to suffer the consequences of excess oxidative stress. When your brain encounters high levels of oxidative stress, you feel anxiety and irritability, and you experience slow cognition and lethargy. Over time, the oxidative stress wears down the brain tissue and increases the risk of neurodegenerative conditions like dementia, Parkinson's disease, and Alzheimer's disease.

Ketone metabolism has been shown to foster much lower levels of oxidative stress in comparison to glucose metabolism, effectively lowering inflammation and reducing oxidative stress, which results in improved energy production.[3] This is why I consider ketone energy production a source of "clean energy," whereas glucose metabolism is a source of "dirty energy." The more you can produce clean energy, the less metabolic stress your body will encounter, and the better you will feel, think, and age.

What Are Free Radicals?

Molecules have electrons, and a double pair of electrons in a molecule helps to create molecular stability. However, free radicals are missing an electron from their outer ring, which makes them unstable molecules that carry a negative charge.

Free radicals are produced as a part of metabolism, and they're "starving" for an extra electron. Consequently, they'll damage other molecules to "steal" one of the outer electrons. An example is the hydroxyl radical (OH-), which is missing an electron on the oxygen atom. Free radicals like this are healthy at normal levels because they help the immune system fend off pathogens and stimulate the body's natural production of antioxidants.

However, an overabundance of free radicals can cause cells and tissues of the body to degenerate faster than normal, which leads to the development of chronic disease. We call this process of cell and tissue damage from free radicals *oxidative stress*, and it's one of the leading theories of aging and the progression of chronic disease.

Antioxidants are produced within the body. We also consume them in foods such as vegetables and herbs, and they offer a free electron to stabilize the free radical and bring harmony to the molecule.

Enhanced Mitochondrial Health

Ketosis mimics a state of starvation. *Starvation* may sound extreme, but for healing and energizing the body, it's actually beneficial. Switching from a sugar-based metabolism to a fat-based metabolism is a mild stressor on the mitochondria. This stress promotes a process called *mitochondrial biogenesis*, which is the process in which new mitochondria form in the cells.[4] The more mitochondria you have, and the more efficiently they function, the healthier you will be.

During the transition phase into ketosis, as cells are stimulated to burn fat, old and weak mitochondria start to die. As a result, this stimulates the growth of new and stronger mitochondria, which can significantly increase energy and mental clarity.

Mitochondrial dysfunction is thought to be at the root of many conditions, including obesity, diabetes, cancer, and many autoimmune disorders. Ketosis is a foundational health strategy for promoting overall health and healing because of its vital role in maintaining the health and growth of mitochondria.

ENERGY: KETONES VS. GLUCOSE

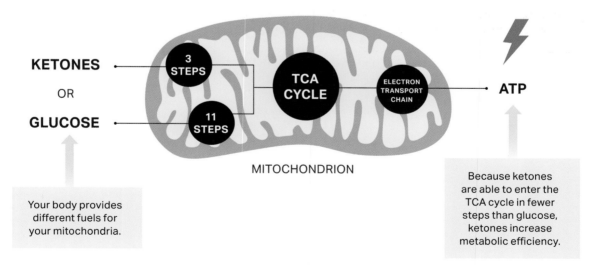

Ketones create more metabolic energy and significantly fewer free radicals and less metabolic waste than glucose metabolism (glycosis). This is equivalent to a vehicle that gets better performance and gas mileage and creates significantly less exhaust and carbon emissions.

Improved Insulin Signaling

Most people burn sugar for fuel, which presents the body with a huge potential problem. For sugar to enter the cell to be made into adenosine triphosphate (ATP), insulin must transport the sugar into the cells. When you're eating a higher carb diet, you can develop unhealthy blood sugar regulation that includes lots of sharp blood sugar spikes and rapid crashes.

These blood sugar swings lead to high levels of insulin and reduced insulin sensitivity. This means that cells are less responsive to insulin, which is something we call *insulin resistance*. Therefore, the body continues to produce higher and higher levels of insulin.

Chronic blood sugar imbalance can damage your brain, promote inflammation, and contribute to weight gain. Signs of poor blood sugar regulation include unstable energy levels, sudden and intense hunger, brain fog, and emotional imbalance. Here are some other symptoms of insulin resistance:

- Tendency to be overweight
- Difficulty losing weight
- Cravings for sweets after meals, but eating sweets doesn't relieve cravings
- Tired feeling after meals
- Frequent thirst and need to urinate
- Hormone problems and issues such as PCOS
- Estrogen or testosterone dominance (for women)
- Skin issues such as acne, skin tags, and changes in pigmentation
- High blood pressure and triglycerides

Ketosis naturally balances blood sugar and stops the vicious cycle of insulin resistance. Using fat as fuel gives your insulin receptors a much-needed rest, allowing them to return to a more responsive and efficient state.[5]

Reduced Risk of Chronic Disease

A ketogenic diet is one of the absolute best defenses against living a life full of pain, discomfort, and pharmaceutical treatments. Most of the lifestyle-induced, chronic diseases are rooted in the chronic inflammation and mitochondrial dysfunction that results from high-sugar, high-carb diets, including

- Cancer
- Depression
- Heart disease
- Anxiety
- Diabetes
- Autoimmune conditions
- Neurodegenerative processes
- Autism
- Fibromyalgia
- Chronic fatigue

The combination of decreased inflammation and improved mitochondrial function promoted by a ketogenic lifestyle allows the body to heal and mitigate disease processes much more effectively than the body does when it's burning sugar for fuel. When the body isn't constantly battling with antinutrients, it can begin to repair and once again find balance.

Increased Mental Clarity

One of the most notable benefits of following a ketogenic diet is how engaged and sharp you feel, thanks in large part to the decrease in inflammation. Inflammation is always present in the body, and some inflammation is necessary and even advantageous. However, too much of it too quickly becomes a problem.

For example, neurological inflammation is insidious and has been linked with depression, anxiety, and reduced cognitive function.[6] Although there are many strategies for addressing inflammation, a ketogenic diet is a powerful tool to combat the onset of various neurological disorders and improve overall mental performance.

In addition, ketones stimulate brain-derived neurotrophic factor (BDNF) and enhance the function of the brain and nervous system cells, which enables you to have sharper and quicker thinking and to perform at a higher level.

NEUROPLASTICITY

The ability of the brain to rewire and rebuild itself to form new neural networks and reinforce familiar neural connections

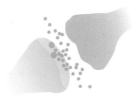

Why should you care about your BDNF?

Brain-Derived Neurotrophic Factor is a key neurochemical responsible for the growth and maintenance of neural connections.

- BDNF helps your brain adapt and learn.
- It improves all forms of plasticity.

YOU control your BDNF levels.

Nutrition

High sugar and trans fat consumption reduce BDNF levels. Intermittent fasting, ketosis, and omega-3 fatty acids all work to improve BDNF levels.

Sleep

Poor sleep reduces BDNF levels.

Exercise

Movement and exercise at any age improves BDNF levels.

Chronic Stress

Imbalance in cortisol and adrenaline lower BDNF levels.

Improved Mood and Emotional Balance

Glutamate and gamma-aminobutyric acid (GABA) are two important neurotransmitters that are responsible for focus and relaxation, respectively. Normal neurological function requires a balanced interplay between the two. An imbalance in these neurotransmitters has been associated with brain disorders such as autism, amyotrophic lateral sclerosis (ALS, sometimes called Lou Gehrig's disease), epilepsy, and mood disorders.

Glutamate is the "gas pedal" of the brain; it helps you think sharply and quickly. You need it to react well in stressful situations, make quick decisions, and maintain a high level of performance, both physical and mental. However, many people suffer from excessive glutamate—a condition called *glutamate dominance*—which results in excess stress and anxiety. Glutamate dominance is a highly inflammatory state in which to exist. Anxiety and depression are characterized by brain inflammation and an imbalance in the glutamate-to-GABA ratio. Those people with excess glutamate and low GABA levels tend to feel anxious, be more irritable and emotionally unstable, have trouble sleeping, and experience frequent brain fog.

Promoting the formation of GABA is an excellent remedy for this imbalance. GABA acts like the "brakes" for the brain; it helps slow down out-of-control trains of thought and allows you to remain cool, calm, and collected under stress. It also helps you to relax and unwind in the evening.

In a healthy person, excess glutamate should be converted into GABA to help balance neural processes—and the good news is that ketones are reported to help improve the process by which the conversion takes place.[7] The immediate effects of a more balanced glutamate-to-GABA ratio are improved focus and decreased levels of stress and anxiety.

Abundant Energy

Fats produce more energy per gram than sugar does, which is the reason so many people talk about the tremendous energy boost they feel from following a ketogenic diet. The increased energy is due to the lower levels of inflammation, improved mitochondrial function, increased efficiency of using fat as fuel, and stabilized blood sugar levels.

However, not every person reacts in the same way to the conversion process. Some people face discouraging challenges in the transition to a ketogenic diet. As your body shifts its metabolism to burn fats, you may not experience endless amounts of energy immediately. Instead, you may suffer from keto flu as you temporarily experience headaches and low energy levels. But be patient and stay the course; those symptoms will fade eventually. In Chapters 7 and 8, I talk about what causes common roadblocks and how to overcome them.

Clearer Skin

Skin conditions such as eczema, acne, and psoriasis are rooted in chronic inflammation and autoimmunity. Often, inflammatory processes arbitrarily attack different structures of the skin, resulting in various dermal conditions. For example, eczema is caused by generalized inflammation of the skin cells, and acne is associated with inflammation of the sebaceous glands in the skin.

Imbalances in gut bacteria, exposure to environmental irritants and allergens, chronic stress, and hormone imbalance can contribute to these skin conditions. If you suffer from skin issues, you should address these factors, but following a ketogenic diet also can help to quickly lower inflammation, accelerate healing, and soothe irritated skin.

Reduced Cravings

Most people don't realize how much their lives revolve around their next meal. Sudden intense hunger pangs and the mood changes that tend to accompany them are typical and expected in our society. There's even a word for it now. When it's been a few hours since your last meal, you become *hangry* (the combo of *hungry* and *angry*).

In reality, these cravings and mood issues are no laughing matter; they're caused by chronic blood sugar instability that tells your brain that you're starving when you're anything but. As a result, you get a sudden urge to eat *now*.

If you find yourself frequently getting hangry, you're likely dealing with blood sugar instability. Ketosis effectively balances blood sugar, provides the brain with a reliable energy source, and eliminates cravings. My keto patients often report that they barely think about food between meals anymore.

Antiaging Effects

There are many theories about what causes aging. Until recently, the commonly held belief was that aging depended solely on the rate at which your telomeres shorten. (*Telomeres* are structures that protect your chromosomes from deterioration.) However, we're beginning to understand that mitochondrial health may be relevant to the question of why we show signs of aging.

Because mitochondria have such a profound impact on energy production, inflammation levels, and gene expression (and the overall function of the body), the *mitochondrial theory of aging* has emerged.[8] Some researchers now think that other known antiaging strategies such as prolonged fasting work by promoting mitochondrial health and biogenesis. As I discussed earlier, the ketogenic lifestyle enhances mitochondrial health, so, once you transition to being keto, you could effectively slow the aging process!

A ketogenic diet can improve your health in virtually every area. Lowering inflammation and improving mitochondrial function can drastically improve your life and reduce your risk of developing many chronic diseases.

Next, in Chapter 6, I dispel some of the myths you may have heard about keto by telling you the truth on those topics.

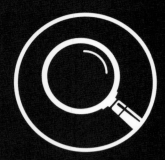

CHAPTER 6

KETO MYTHS
(AND THE TRUTH)

People tend to have a lot of questions about the ketogenic lifestyle. Luckily, we have the Internet to give us all the answers, right?

Well, it's not quite that simple. The information age in which we live can be both a help and a hindrance in people's search for the complete story. So much misinformation is available about keto that it's difficult to discern the facts from the myths.

I've been implementing a ketogenic-style diet for years, long before the keto craze hit. During that time, I've heard every imaginable question, skepticism, and hesitation related to keto. Consequently, I have a great understanding of the general perception of keto and where different concerns arise.

The keto myths in this chapter are some of the most common concerns I regularly encounter in my practice. Most of these ideas are based on misinformation. As I discuss each myth, I'll highlight strategies you can take to mitigate issues so that you can have a truly exceptional experience and enjoy the many benefits of keto.

Keto Is Only for Weight Loss

The most common keto myth is that the diet is beneficial only for people who want to lose weight. Yes, a ketogenic diet has been shown to promote weight loss, but it also provides numerous other benefits, including reducing inflammation, boosting energy, mitigating the risk of chronic disease, reducing cravings, and potentially increasing your life span.[1, 2, 3, 4]

I've been fortunate in that I've always been naturally thin, and I've never needed to follow a weight-loss protocol. In fact, I would love to add another five to ten pounds of muscle. However, over the years, I've found that when I overeat in an attempt to gain weight, I feel sluggish and fatigued. It's not worth it!

If you believe the myth that the ketogenic diet is only for weight loss, you'd think that someone like me—someone who would prefer to gain a little weight—would have no business following this lifestyle. Won't it make me lose even *more* weight? Not at all! My weight is healthy, and I rely on ketosis to optimize my mental focus, memory, and resiliency to stress, which then enables me to perform at an elite level in my roles of husband, father, doctor, business owner, speaker, and author. So although weight loss *can* be a result of going keto, you need not be concerned if you're someone who doesn't need to shed any pounds. You can adopt this lifestyle for its many other benefits without worrying that your weight will drop to an unhealthy level.

Keto Is a Meat-Based Diet

Another faulty keto myth is that you have to consume tons of meat to eat a ketogenic diet.

While some people do great on a primarily meat or carnivore diet, that isn't for everyone, and a ketogenic lifestyle has a wide spectrum. In fact, there are thousands of people all around the world who are practicing a plant-based, vegetarian keto diet and seeing outstanding results.

If you would prefer not to consume meat at all, there are plenty of ketogenic recipes that are purely plant-based. For example, try out the Creamy Lemony Superfood Guacamole (page 285), Key Lime Smoothie (page 343), and Turmeric Coconut Cream Cups (page 330) recipes in this book for a few great-tasting meatless options. It's entirely possible to get into and stay in a state of nutritional ketosis while still maintaining your vegan, vegetarian, or ovo-lacto vegetarian lifestyle.

Keto Is Restrictive and Hard to Sustain

One of the most pervasive myths is that the ketogenic diet is restrictive and therefore difficult to follow as a long-term strategy.

If you genuinely want to transform your health and lose weight, you have to make changes. No magic pill for weight loss exists. (And if it did, it would certainly be dangerous.) If you're accustomed to eating nothing but processed foods such as pasta, bread, and high-carb snacks, I understand that opting for fresh, nutrient-rich foods can seem daunting because it's different than what you're used to.

I have good news, though: The list of ketogenic-friendly foods is massive, and you can find many recipes for keto bread, desserts, and more. I share some with you in the Recipes section of this book. If you're still worried that a keto diet may be too restrictive, check out Chapter 9, where I give you an extensive list of the top keto foods you can eat. In Chapter 12, I guide you through the grocery store to help you discover the wide variety of foods available to you as you embark on your keto metabolic breakthrough.

Here's something else you should know: Living a ketogenic lifestyle doesn't mean that you have to be in ketosis every minute of every day of the rest of your life. I've been living the keto lifestyle for years, and I cycle out of ketosis once every few weeks when I enjoy a high-carb day. After that brief respite, I return to my normal routine. The most important thing is that you keep an open mind and know that you can have both health *and* delicious food!

Keto Is Low in Fiber and Harms the Gut

Many people think that a keto diet is an all-meat-and-cheese diet, and it doesn't contain enough plant food. The truth is, though, that some people find that their guts do better with less fiber, whereas others do better with more fiber. You can personalize your keto diet to get the level of plant-based fiber that you feel best with.

Eating keto means getting the right amounts of healthy fats and moderate amounts of clean protein, and then you round out the remainder of your daily calories with low-carb, fibrous veggies including leafy greens, asparagus, green beans, cucumbers, celery, broccoli, cauliflower, and cabbage.

Most people who follow a nutrient-dense ketogenic plan tend to consume much more fiber than they have on other meal plans because increasing vegetable intake becomes a priority.[5] One of my all-time favorite foods—avocado—is an excellent source of fiber and healthy fats, which makes it a tasty and versatile part of your diet.

On the standard American diet (SAD), carbs are the primary sources of fiber. Unfortunately, those carbs (such as wheat and other grains) establish unwanted microbes, such as candida, in the gut. A keto diet eliminates all the unhealthy sources of fiber and replaces them with plenty of fibrous veggies that are healing and beneficial for the microbiome.

If the word *microbiome* is new to you, or you're not sure of the exact role it plays in your health, let me introduce you to the world living inside your body and, more specifically, in your digestive system or gut.

The gut *microbiome* is the makeup of all the bacteria and microorganisms living within your digestive tract. Our microbiomes are like fingerprints—each of us has a unique system.[6] The balance within our microbiomes is continually changing and easily altered by many things, including stress, over-the-counter medications, and diet.

Research of this intricate ecosystem of microscopic organisms has determined that some strains of bacteria are beneficial, whereas others are harmful. If pathogenic microorganisms are allowed to grow unchecked, they leach nutrients, harm cells, release toxic waste into the blood, and significantly increase inflammation levels.

Chronic inflammatory responses negatively affect digestion, the immune system, and brain function, among other things.[7] Maximizing levels of good bacteria and minimizing the presence of pathogenic bacteria is a crucial strategy for optimizing gut health.

A ketogenic diet positively affects gut health and the microbiome. In the following sections, I share information about three studies that show the desirable changes that occur within the microbiome on a ketogenic diet—and the implications of these changes for specific neurological diseases.

Autism

It's well established that in cases of autism spectrum disorder (ASD), gut microbiome imbalances are common. A recent study published in the *Journal of Molecular Autism* investigated whether a ketogenic diet was able to elicit beneficial changes in the gut microbiome in an animal model of autism.[8] The results were fascinating. After implementing a ketogenic eating plan in the test animals over a ten- to fourteen-day period, researchers observed the subjects' microbiomes and concluded the following:

- The ketogenic diet had a significant antimicrobial effect by decreasing the overall microbial content in fecal waste and the large intestine.

- The ketogenic diet also appeared to increase the ratio of *Firmicutes-to-Bacteroides* species. (A low *Firmicutes-to-Bacteroides* species ratio is standard with ASD.)

- The ketogenic diet helped to lower an overabundant growth of *Akkermansia muciniphila* species, which is a type of bacteria thought to have a link to obesity, diabetes, and inflammation.

In addition to beneficial changes in the microbiome, the researchers concluded that the ketogenic diet also produced a reduction of ASD-associated neurological symptoms. That should be an encouraging conclusion for those who have ASD or have a loved one with the disorder.

Multiple Sclerosis

In a study published in *Frontiers in Microbiology,* researchers observed the connection between the microbiome, a ketogenic diet, and the potential role both of them could play in cases of autoimmune multiple sclerosis (AIMS).[9]

AIMS has been shown to impair the ability of bacteria in the colon to ferment different food materials into beneficial by-products. This fermentation is a vital role for producing essential compounds such as short-chain fatty acids (SCFAs), which protect the gut and help provide energy.[10] In patients with AIMS, their improperly functioning colonic bacteria are more likely to ferment foods into harmful and toxic by-products rather than forming beneficial SCFAs.

The inability of colonic bacteria in AIMS cases to perform the beneficial process of fermentation is likely due to imbalances in microbial species. In the *Frontiers in Microbiology* study, following a keto diet for just six months restored healthy levels of microbes in the colonic microbiome of the test subjects. This news is truly amazing and potentially life-changing for AIMS sufferers.

Refractory Epilepsy

A recent study published in *World Journal of Gastroenterology* investigated refractory epilepsy in young children and its connection to the microbiome. Researchers implemented a keto diet in fourteen epileptic infants and thirty healthy babies and noted the frequency of seizures and gut microbiome balance to identify any notable trends.

They found that infants with refractory epilepsy had substantially different microbiomes when compared to the microbiomes of normally functioning babies. Implementing a ketogenic diet caused a significant reduction in seizures along with a radical reshaping of the gut microbiome in the epileptic infants.[11] The study noted the following specific bacteria species:

- Harmful proteobacteria (including *Salmonella*) accounted for approximately 24 percent of the microbiome of both groups of pediatric patients. This class of bacteria is associated with a surprisingly large number of health problems. These species were reduced significantly after the implementation of a ketogenic diet in both groups.

- A specific class of bacteria called *Bacteroidetes* (typically found in higher percentages in healthy babies) increased in both infant groups once the researchers introduced a ketogenic diet, which is relevant because *Bacteroidetes* may help reduce the severity and frequency of epileptic episodes.[12]

- The presence of *Cronobacter*, which was far more prominent in epileptic infants (found in 23 percent of epileptic infants' microbiomes compared to no presence at all in healthy infants) was reduced significantly after implementing a ketogenic diet. *Cronobacter* is infectious in epileptic infants and has the potential to lead to sepsis or meningitis if left unaddressed.

Now you have more insight into the microscopic world living, working, and interacting inside your gut. As researchers continue to discover more about this unseen ecosphere called the microbiome, we'll more fully understand its prominent and critical role in our overall health and immunity.

Keto Is Harmful to the Thyroid and Adrenals

If you have a normally functioning thyroid and adrenal glands, the ketogenic diet won't cause damage to those glands. However, the idea that a ketogenic diet may not be suitable for those with hypothyroidism or adrenal fatigue has some merit, so it's worth addressing.

First, let's establish that you need insulin to convert *inactive* thyroid hormone (T4) into active thyroid hormone (T3). Second, being in a state of low blood sugar (which happens when you begin a keto diet and aren't accustomed to using ketones as fuel) can be stressful on the body and can overtax the brain-adrenal connection called the *hypothalamic-pituitary-adrenal* (HPA) axis.

These are both scientific facts, and if you have a thyroid or adrenal issue, you might be concerned about how a ketogenic diet will affect your energy, sleep patterns, and brain.

However, there are several reasons why a ketogenic lifestyle can greatly benefit people with thyroid issues, adrenal issues, or both. Here are two primary reasons:

- **Reduce chronic inflammation:** Thyroid and adrenal problems are characterized by chronic inflammation. Inflammation acts as a stressor, affecting adrenal function and inhibiting the conversion of T4 into its active form, T3. A ketogenic diet dramatically reduces inflammation and therefore benefits the adrenals and thyroid. Now, you do need some insulin to convert T4 into T3, but if you produce too much, it triggers inflammation that disrupts healthy thyroid and adrenal hormone function. So, a healthy balance is necessary—and that requires regular monitoring for those dealing with conditions affecting the thyroid.

- **Boost mitochondrial function:** It's common to see those with adrenal or thyroid issues suffer from poor mitochondrial function, which is why boosting mitochondrial performance (as the keto diet does) is critical for improving adrenal and thyroid function.

WAYS KETO IMPROVES THYROID AND ADRENAL FUNCTION

1

Significantly reduces inflammation

By reducing inflammation, a keto diet improves hypothalamus communication with the pituitary and adrenal glands. It also improves communication between the pituitary and thyroid glands.

Reducing inflammation also takes stress off of the thyroid gland, which may have been damaged by chronic inflammation or autoimmunity, as with Hashimoto's thyroiditis or Graves' disease.

Reducing inflammation improves T4-T3 conversion in the liver and gut and at the cell itself.

Reducing inflammation helps to modulate the amount of adrenal hormone released.

2

Improves mitochondrial function

A keto diet improves the number and the functionality of mitochondria, which improves the overall cellular energy.

When the cells produce more efficient energy, the need for both thyroid hormone and adrenal hormone reduces, and it causes less wear and tear on the endocrine system and the intracellular organelles.

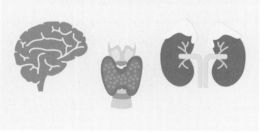

When you compare the benefits of going keto with the potential downsides, the benefits outweigh the risks almost every time. Long-term ketosis could be challenging for some individuals with thyroid and adrenal issues. However, adhering to a keto diet also reduces inflammation, which is critical to the health of the thyroid and adrenals.

If you have a preexisting condition, monitoring your numbers becomes especially important. Those people who naturally have lower insulin levels may need to follow a *cyclical ketogenic diet*, which I cover in Chapter 11. For individuals who have both thyroid issues and insulin resistance, a strict ketogenic diet typically works best.

The first few weeks on a ketogenic diet can be stressful on the body, no matter your current state of health. If you have a thyroid or adrenal issue, I recommend the following guidelines:

- Gradually and safely wean off a carb-heavy diet by using the carb-phasing approach I discuss in Chapter 11.

- When you're not fasting, make sure to consume enough calories. Long-term hypocaloric (low-calorie) diets are problematic for the thyroid and adrenal glands.

- Avoid long fasts in the early stages of a keto transition, and eat every three to four waking hours. Once you feel better and your body switches to fat-burning mode, you can incorporate more intermittent fasting into your daily or weekly schedule.

- Focus on eating plenty of nutrient-dense foods, especially those containing trace minerals. Some of my favorite foods that are rich in trace minerals are broccoli, cauliflower, olives, avocados, grass-fed meats, and fermented veggies like sauerkraut and pickles.

- Consume MCT oils and exogenous ketones to lessen the demand on your body for ketone formation.

- Use carbohydrate cycling (periodically eating a higher carb diet) to support your thyroid and adrenals.

- Take thyroid medication or thyroid glandular extracts and supplement with thyroid-converting compounds such as zinc and selenium.

- Consume adaptogenic herbs such as ashwagandha, Rhodiola, and cordyceps. Adaptogenic herbs are known to stabilize the body and help bring it back into a state of balance. (Read more in Chapter 15.)

As a general guideline, if you have adrenal or thyroid issues, you may need to cycle out of ketosis more often and consume more carbs than people with optimally functioning adrenals and thyroid. When you consume higher amounts of carbs and protein, the body senses that you're in a state of *feasting*, where food is plentiful, which drives up thyroid activity and lowers adrenal hormone output.

However, if you keep feasting, you also drive up insulin and inflammation. Balance is the key. Strive to achieve a mix of keto and a slightly higher carb diet so that you enjoy the benefits of ketosis while also cycling in carbs once in a while to stimulate the thyroid. The optimal frequency of higher carb eating varies from person to person. I offer some general recommendations regarding a cyclical ketogenic diet in Chapter 11.

Keto Is Harmful to the Liver and Gallbladder

Can eating a high-fat diet put stress on your liver and gallbladder? The short answer is yes, but for the longer answer, you have to compare the benefits of keto with its relative risks. To help you better understand, in this section, I give you a brief overview of the vital roles of the liver and gallbladder.

The liver does a tremendous amount of work: It helps deactivate toxins in the bloodstream, stores energy and nutrients, and produces bile for fat digestion (which is critical for the absorption of fat-soluble nutrients and other necessary functions). Because the liver performs these tasks and so much more, some cultures consider it to be the most vital organ in the body.

LIVER FUNCTIONS

✔ Helps your body fight infection by removing bacteria from the blood.

✔ Prevents shortages of nutrients by storing vitamins, minerals, and sugar.

✔ Converts inactive Thyroid Hormone (T4) to active T3 that the cells can use.

✔ Creates cholesterol for hormone production and tissue healing.

✔ Metabolizes, or breaks down, nutrients from food to produce energy when needed.

✔ Produces bile, a compound needed to digest fat and to absorb vitamins A, D, E, and K.

✔ Creates ketone bodies for cellular energy production.

✔ Produces most of the substances that regulate blood clotting.

✔ Removes potentially toxic substances you consume from the environment, such as xenoestrogens, pesticides, herbicides, and medication by-products.

✔ Produces most proteins needed by the body.

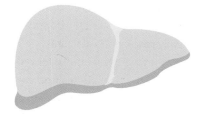

The gallbladder has a much more precise role. The liver produces bile, but the gallbladder stores bile and releases it after you consume a meal. The combined roles of the liver and gallbladder help ensure you properly metabolize fats and excrete unwanted toxins from your body. Pretty important stuff.

Even if you've had your gallbladder removed, your liver still produces bile. However, because you don't have a gallbladder to store bile to assist with efficient fat digestion, the bile slowly seeps into your intestines. The result is that you're unable to digest high-fat meals properly. Reduced bile flow can result in malnutrition and the accumulation of toxins in the body. Because keto is a high-fat diet, it makes sense that people question the effect a keto lifestyle has on liver and gallbladder health.

Let's do some more digging to get to the bottom of this issue.

Bile 101

Bile is a greenish-brown liquid primarily made of cholesterol, bile salts, and bilirubin, and its main job is to emulsify fats for absorption in the small intestine. Bile also helps pass waste products through the digestive tract to be released through bowel movements. Bile serves four primary digestive functions:

- Breaks down fatty acids
- Stabilizes blood sugar
- Inhibits bacterial overgrowth
- Removes toxic waste and cholesterol from the liver for excretion

Given this impressive list of functions, it's easy to understand why a disruption in the bile process is so detrimental to the body.

Fatty Liver and Keto

Non-alcoholic fatty liver disease (NAFLD) is a condition associated with obesity, insulin resistance, diabetes, and metabolic syndrome. The disorder is characterized by large deposits of fat around the liver, elevated liver enzymes, and chronic inflammation that affects the liver, causing scar tissue or fibrosis and eventually resulting in cirrhosis.

We know that ketosis is useful for promoting weight loss and preventing or even helping reverse diabetes and metabolic syndrome. So, it makes sense that being in a state of ketosis can help address NAFLD. A 2007 pilot study examined five obese patients with NAFLD who followed a ketogenic diet for six months. During that time, the patients lost an average of 27 pounds and had marked improvement in fatty liver disease symptoms. In particular, their livers showed decreased signs of fat deposits, inflammation, and fibrosis.[13]

However, the research is still inconclusive; a 2016 meta-analysis and systemic review on low-carb diets and liver function in patients with NAFLD showed mixed results. That study demonstrated that a low-carb diet decreased liver fat significantly, but liver enzyme production did *not* improve. The study also reported that for some individuals, following a keto diet made significant improvements, whereas the results were not as remarkable for others.[14]

It's impossible to know with certainty how other variables (such as food quality, genetics, sleep quality, stress levels, relationship status, microbiome, and activity level) differed among people in the group. Still, the conclusion is an important one: Keto is a smart nutrition strategy, but it isn't a cure-all! Many factors could play a role in affecting the results you may experience.

Steps to Improve Bile Flow for Optimal Results

Since keto is a high-fat diet, it's vital to maintain good bile flow while on a ketogenic nutrition plan. Even if you've had your gallbladder removed, you can improve your bile flow and your ability to emulsify fats and use them as fuel. If you have a compromised digestive tract, the key is to take the following action steps regularly.

1. **Eat bile-stimulating foods.** Food is always our best medicine, and this is particularly true when it comes to promoting healthy digestion. Ginger and radishes are excellent for stimulating the production of stomach acid and bile. Apple cider vinegar assists in thinning bile for a more efficient flow. Artichokes stimulate liver bile production and increase bile flow. Sour foods such as lemons and limes also help stimulate and thin bile, improve your fat tolerance, clean the liver, and improve overall digestion and nutrient absorption. Fibrous veggies and fermented foods and drinks are excellent for promoting a healthy gut and preventing the overgrowth of harmful gut bacteria.[15] Celery and cucumbers are low-carb foods that naturally contain sodium, vitamins B and C, and trace minerals that support liver health. Celery and asparagus help detoxify the liver and improve bile flow.

2. **Drink ginger, peppermint, and dandelion teas.** Ginger, peppermint, and dandelion are "bitter" herbs that increase bile production and bile flow to support healthy liver function. Ginger and peppermint have well-known carminative properties, which means they can help relieve symptoms of

indigestion and prevent nausea and vomiting. These herbs also stimulate the secretion of gastric juices such as hydrochloric (HCl) acid. They have even been shown to inhibit inflammation of liver tissue and aid in the removal of toxins. Dandelion greens are considered a natural source of prebiotics that helps support healthy gut microflora and keep pathogenic bacteria at bay.

3. **Practice good hydration.** One of the most significant differences between those with good bile flow and those with poor bile flow is hydration levels. The better you hydrate your body, the better your bile will flow. When you don't provide your body with sufficient amounts of water, bile production decreases, and the bile becomes thick and sluggish. Take in at least half your body weight in ounces of purified water each day and work to take in at least 48 ounces of that water by noon each day.

THE MIRACLE THAT IS WATER

What does water do for the human body?

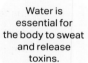

Water is essential for the body to sweat and release toxins.

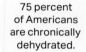

75 percent of Americans are chronically dehydrated.

 Dehydration taxes the heart by causing it to pump faster to get sufficient oxygen to your muscles.

Without the flow of water, there's insufficient water to remove waste and toxins through your stool.

 Lubricates joints and lessens discomfort from arthritis or back pain.

 Slows down the aging process and makes skin smooth.

 Prevents loss of memory as you age. Lessens addictive urges, including to caffeine, alcohol, and certain drugs.

 Cleanses toxic waste from various parts of the body and carries it to the liver and kidney for removal.

 Allows red blood cells to carry oxygen more efficiently, resulting in better muscular function and increased mental acuity.

 Allows efficient cellular repair.

A University of Washington study discovered that one glass of water stopped hunger pangs for almost 100 percent of studied dieters.

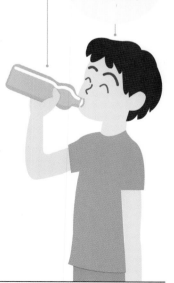

4. **Support stomach acid levels.** The combination of optimal stomach acid and steady bile flow is critical to the detoxification of the liver and gut. It's also a required combo for ensuring you feel healthy and energized while maintaining ketosis without a gallbladder. Stomach acid stimulates liver bile secretion. Adequate stomach acid production supports your body's ability to metabolize fats, absorb essential nutrients, and prevent digestive issues and feelings of discomfort.

You can support ideal stomach acid levels by limiting water intake fifteen to thirty minutes before meals and sixty minutes after meals. I recommend no more than 4 to 6 ounces of water during this time. That quantity is enough for you to take any medications or supplements you may be consuming with your meal. If you drink much more while you eat, you dilute your stomach acid levels and negatively impact your digestion.

High levels of stress also block the secretion of stomach acid, so take steps to relax your mind and body before eating. My family prays before meals and offers gratitude for the food. This mindset moves us into a relaxed state, which activates the part of our nervous systems that enhances the production of stomach acid, bile, and pancreatic enzymes.

10 WAYS TO IMPROVE STOMACH ACID

1 Use liquid nutrition throughout the day.

2 Use ginger.

3 Super hydrate outside of meal times.

4 Drink very little with meals that include meat.

5 Use lemon and apple cider vinegar.

6 Eat protein foods at the beginning of the meal.

7 Use fermented veggies.

8 Use fermented drinks.

9 Hold off on water after a meal.

10 Eat your largest meal when you're most relaxed.

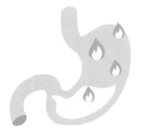

5. **Take digestive enzymes and ox bile.** Supplementing with digestive enzymes and ox bile can significantly support fat metabolism when you're transitioning into a keto lifestyle without a gallbladder. A good-quality digestive enzyme can help you produce sufficient stomach acid. It also inhibits inflammation of the intestines and aids in fat metabolism and the absorption of fat-soluble vitamins. High-quality digestive enzymes typically include natural bile salts, betaine HCl, and herbs that support gut function. Ox bile is particularly helpful for those people who don't produce enough bile on their own. It can help relieve symptoms of indigestion that you may otherwise experience on a high-fat diet without healthy bile concentrations.

6. **Avoid high amounts of long-chain fats.** Long-chain fatty acids are in avocados, nuts and seeds, olives and olive oil, and meats, whereas small- and medium-chain fatty acids are more prevalent in grass-fed butter and coconuts. The longer the fatty acid chain, the more bile, time, and energy required to metabolize the fat.[16] Therefore, it's critical for people without a gallbladder to eat small meals that are light on long-chain fats. I recommend that you consume three to four small-to-medium-sized meals throughout the day. You also can opt for liquid nutrition (homemade shakes and smoothies) that is easy on the digestive tract.

7. **Use MCT oils.** Unlike most fatty acids, medium-chain triglyceride (MCT) oils do not rely on bile to be metabolized; these oils begin breaking down immediately from contact with enzymes in your saliva. MCT oil notably reduces your overall energy dependence on fats, making MCTs easier to absorb for those without a gallbladder or those with impaired liver function. MCTs have also been shown to effectively synthesize ketones and cross the blood-brain barrier to promote healthy brain function.[17]

Although many people believe that coconut oil is the best source of MCTs, you may be surprised to learn that coconut oil is 35 percent long-chain triglycerides and just 15 percent medium-chain triglycerides. The remaining 50 percent is lauric acid, which is utilized as a long-chain fatty acid.[18] Consider finding a high-quality MCT oil that has higher concentrations of the medium-chain triglycerides your body needs.

Keto Will Elevate Your Cholesterol Levels

The majority of us have been raised to believe that eating fat—especially saturated fat—causes high cholesterol and eventually heart disease. This is just not true. The research shows that consuming a lower-carb diet helps to lower LDL (bad cholesterol) levels, raise HDL (good cholesterol) levels, and lower triglycerides.

However, some people see their cholesterol increase on a keto diet. Because this could be a cause of concern for some, I need to address the phenomenon of high cholesterol on keto.

The term *high cholesterol* causes many people to live in fear, despite the reality that most people have a superficial understanding of why cholesterol is "bad" in the first place. The bottom line is that cholesterol is often misunderstood. Knowing how cholesterol works and how to interpret your numbers empowers you to move forward on your ketogenic journey with confidence.

Cholesterol is a vital substance naturally made by your liver or taken in through your diet. Regardless of whether you consume high-cholesterol foods, your liver still produces cholesterol, and for a good reason—it's critical to your overall health and well-being.

Cholesterol acts as a transport molecule to shuttle fat-soluble nutrients into cells. Cholesterol serves as an essential building block for progesterone, estrogen, testosterone, cortisol, and vitamin D. Also, it's a critical structural element in neural tissue; as much as 25 percent of our cholesterol is in the brain!

To further highlight how our beliefs regarding fat and cholesterol have gone awry, it's interesting to note that higher saturated fat intake and higher cholesterol levels are linked with *better* mental function as we age![19]

We've been told for many decades that having high levels of cholesterol, particularly LDL, dramatically increases your risk for heart-related diseases. When we look only at cholesterol numbers, there is undoubtedly some correlation between high cholesterol and the prevalence of cardiovascular-related diseases. However, there are other, more critical measurements to consider.

So, is high cholesterol really the serious problem we've been told to believe it is? Perhaps not.

Cholesterol and Heart Disease Misconceptions

Traditionally, we have thought that elevated blood cholesterol causes *atherosclerosis*, which is the formation of arterial plaque that can ultimately lead to a heart attack or stroke. This conclusion came about because cholesterol is a component of plaques.

However, we now know this is not the full story. Plaque formation is more than just a build-up of cholesterol. It's a result of prolonged inflammation at the site where the plaque forms along with an interaction between calcium, cholesterol, and other biological substances.

Even more surprising has been the evidence that the body uses cholesterol as a kind of internal bandage when chronic inflammation damages the arterial lining over time. Cholesterol buildup in the arteries may be a protective mechanism!

A fascinating and long-running study called the Framingham Heart Study (named after the city in Massachusetts where it started) has been monitoring a group of more than 5,000 participants for heart disease risk factors since 1948. Throughout this study, researchers have made some shocking realizations about cholesterol levels:

- As much as 40 percent of heart attacks occur in individuals with total cholesterol lower than 200 (which is a desirable number according to the American Heart Association).

- Having total cholesterol lower than 180 *triples* your chances of suffering a stroke.[20]

- Overall cholesterol levels below 200 are associated with reduced cognitive function in old age compared with the results for people who are in the borderline-high (200–239) to high (240+) total cholesterol categories.[21]

These findings suggest there is an insignificant difference in heart disease risk relative to total cholesterol being above and below 200. Researchers didn't observe any notable increase in risk until cholesterol reached 240 and higher. Perhaps even more interestingly, having cholesterol more than 180 seems to serve a protective role for both the heart and brain.

Know Your Cholesterol Terminology

It's important to understand the cholesterol terminology so that you understand what's happening with your physiology. This knowledge will help you not to be alarmed by people who think that following a keto diet will cause you to die of a heart attack!

LDL Cholesterol

LDL stands for *low-density lipoprotein*, and it's the form of cholesterol generally deemed to be "bad." In reality, LDL and HDL aren't cholesterol at all. They're the transport vehicles *for* cholesterol.

LDL's primary role is to transport fat-soluble nutrients into cell membranes. LDL particles are categorized based on size. The two LDL particle sizes have significant disparities: pattern A LDL molecules are the largest size and tend to carry more fat-soluble nutrients and antioxidants that protect the body from oxidative stress; that means pattern A molecules are cardioprotective.[22, 23]

On the other hand, pattern B LDL cholesterol molecules are small enough to enter into the endothelial lining of the arteries, where they can become oxidized and are more likely to form plaque. There is a direct correlation between higher quantities of these small, dense particles and cardiovascular disease.

ALP (LDL PATTERN B)

Why is it dangerous?

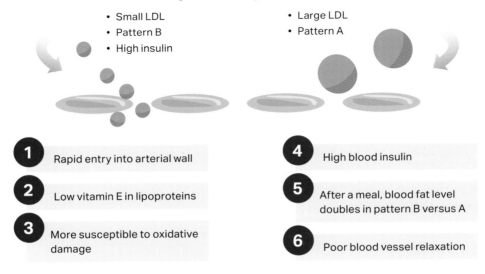

- Small LDL
- Pattern B
- High insulin

- Large LDL
- Pattern A

1 Rapid entry into arterial wall

2 Low vitamin E in lipoproteins

3 More susceptible to oxidative damage

4 High blood insulin

5 After a meal, blood fat level doubles in pattern B versus A

6 Poor blood vessel relaxation

This means that two individuals with identical LDL, HDL, and triglyceride levels could have a vastly different level of heart disease risk depending on the predominant size of their LDL molecules. Fortunately, following a ketogenic diet has been shown to reduce the number of the smaller, pattern B particles present in the blood.[24]

HDL Cholesterol

HDL stands for *high-density lipoprotein*. Its primary role is to sweep up LDL particles and return them to the liver for recycling. LDL is highly susceptible to oxidation and must be cleared from the blood regularly. The longer LDL cholesterol remains in the bloodstream, the more inflammation and the higher the risk of heart disease. Studying inflammation markers and the LDL-to-HDL ratio is the best way to interpret cholesterol panels and what they mean to your health rather than merely considering raw, isolated values. Having balanced proportions suggests that your LDL and HDL are working together correctly.

Triglycerides

Triglycerides are a significant energy source for cells. LDL particles transport triglycerides to cell membranes, where they are metabolized to make ATP (adenosine triphosphate, which is for cellular energy). High levels of triglycerides in the blood are thought to be a sign of insulin resistance, which is often a marker of heart disease, autoimmune diseases, obesity, and cancer. Elevated triglycerides are also a common side effect of insulin resistance. In these cases, a ketogenic diet is an excellent strategy to improve those numbers.

- LDL serves as a transport molecule to deliver nutrients, building materials, and energy (in the form of triglycerides) to your cells.

- LDL is more prone to oxidation than the other forms of cholesterol.

- Size matters—larger LDL molecules provide benefits to the body, whereas smaller LDL molecules are linked to health issues.

- HDL's primary job is to clear LDL from the bloodstream to be recycled, ideally before it becomes oxidized.

- Having balanced ratios of cholesterol types helps facilitate cellular function and minimize oxidation. High LDL isn't necessarily bad as long as you have adequate HDL to help clear those molecules (especially smaller pattern B) from the bloodstream.

- Reducing inflammation may be the most powerful way to mitigate heart disease risk.

The Terrible Triad

A combination of high triglycerides, high LDL, and low HDL is known as the *Terrible Triad*, and it's linked to a drastic increase in heart disease risk. The good news is that following a well-formulated ketogenic diet can help increase HDL and decrease triglyceride levels. On a keto diet, LDL may remain the same or potentially increase to transport triglycerides to cells to metabolize for energy efficiently.

Ketogenic Diet and Cholesterol

Research has shown that following a low-carb, high-fat diet improves cholesterol ratios and reduces your risk of heart disease in four primary ways:

- Increases LDL particle size and makes them less likely to oxidize
- Increases the amount of HDL available to recycle LDL from the blood before it has a chance to become oxidized
- Improves LDL-to-HDL ratio
- Lowers triglycerides and improves the triglyceride-to-HDL ratio[25]

OPTIMAL LIPID PROFILE ON A KETOGENIC DIET

Total Cholesterol	LDL:HDL Ratio	Triglyceride:HDL Ratio
180–200	**3:1 or less**	**2:1 or less**
(The test will flag it as high if it is more than 200, but you don't need to be concerned about it if the ratios are in range.)	(2:1 is great.)	(1:1 is great.)

Triglycerides should be less than 100 and ideally right around the same number as HDL or in the 40–80 range. If these ratios are in order, it's a sign that the LDL particles are the larger fluffy types that are less prone to oxidation.

How the ketogenic diet impacts the lipid profile

1. Increases LDL particle size to the less oxidation-prone state

2. Increases the amount of HDL available to recycle LDL from the blood before it has a chance to become oxidized

3. Improves the LDL to HDL ratio

4. Lowers triglycerides and improves triglyceride to HDL ratio

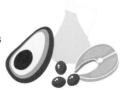

If you do not notice these beneficial changes in your cholesterol once you have been in ketosis for one to three months, you may need to examine whether some underlying cause is preventing the improvements from occurring. Even though a ketogenic diet has been shown to improve cholesterol readings and mitigate the risk of heart disease, in some cases, your cholesterol numbers may surprise you (by drastically dropping or significantly increasing). The following sections outline the key reasons why cholesterol could increase as you transition to a ketogenic lifestyle.

Insulin Resistance

If you have insulin resistance when you start keto, you could experience a temporary increase in total cholesterol. Root causes are related to poor diet, chronic stress, and inflammation. As long as you're working to correct the root causes of insulin resistance, a temporary increase is acceptable because a ketogenic lifestyle helps address all of those issues; eventually, your insulin sensitivity will improve.

Rapid Weight Loss

A notable increase in cholesterol may be typical for people who experience rapid weight loss because fat cells stored in adipose tissue contain high amounts of both triglycerides and cholesterol. Thus, when the stored fat begins to break down so the body can metabolize it for energy, cholesterol in the blood can increase temporarily. The reason is that the triglycerides from fat cells are metabolized, whereas the cholesterol is not. Cholesterol is released into the blood, where it remains until the liver removes it. As a result, it appears that cholesterol has suddenly skyrocketed. People naturally assume this is due to the increase in dietary fat and cholesterol intake. However, this effect should diminish as weight loss reaches a plateau, and cholesterol levels should return to a more normal state.

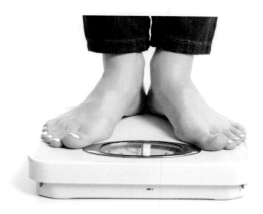

Increase in HDL

High-fat, low-carb diets have been shown to increase HDL cholesterol more effectively than low-fat diets. In fact, in many cases, people notice their LDL cholesterol level remains the same or decreases only slightly, whereas their HDL level increases. Even though an increase in your HDL level doesn't adversely affect your health (and would, in fact, be beneficial), it could cause an increase in total cholesterol. As a general rule, HDL should remain in the range of 50 to 80. You should take action to address anything higher than 90 because that elevated level could be an indication of an infection or leaky gut.[26]

LEAKY GUT SYNDROME

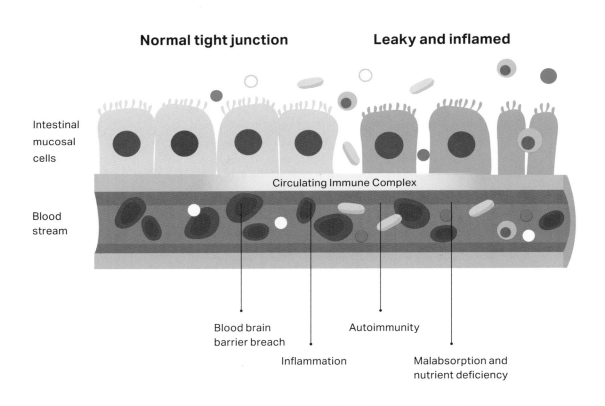

Normal tight junction

Leaky and inflamed

Intestinal mucosal cells

Circulating Immune Complex

Blood stream

Blood brain barrier breach

Autoimmunity

Inflammation

Malabsorption and nutrient deficiency

Poor Thyroid Conversion

The active version of thyroid hormone, T3, plays a vital role in activating the LDL receptors on our cells. However, if something were to inhibit this process, it could lead to an increase in LDL cholesterol. For example, the thyroid predominantly makes thyroid hormone in its inactive form, known as T4. The liver and gut must then convert T4 into active T3. If you have liver or gut issues, then this could inhibit T3 conversion and the ability to activate LDL receptors on cells. This inhibition may cause an increase in LDL cholesterol levels.

Additionally, thyroid hormone plays an important role in removing cholesterol through the bile. Hypothyroidism is a major factor in the development of high cholesterol. (See the nearby graphic.)

THYROID HORMONE EFFECTS ON LIPID METABOLISM

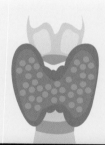

Low thyroid hormone decreases fractional clearance of LDL by liver:	Low thyroid hormone decreases catabolism of cholesterol into bile	Overt hypothyroidism
• Decreases number of LDL receptors • Decreases LDL receptor activity	• T3 negatively regulates liver-specific enzyme cholesterol 7a hydroxylase	• Hypercholestrolemia • Marked increases in LDL and apolipoprotein B • Changes are also evident in subclinical hypothyroidism

- 90 percent of hypothyroid patients had hypercholesterolemia.
- Prevalence of overt hypothyroidism in patients with hypercholesterolemia is 1.3 to 2.8 percent.

Inadequate Sunlight Exposure

Sunlight has an important effect on your cholesterol and vitamin D synthesis. Cholesterol is used to create vitamin D within your body, but it needs to be activated by sunlight exposure on your skin.[27]

Cholesterol and vitamin D are created from a molecule called *squalene*. The sun exposure converts squalene into 7-dehydrocholesterol and vitamin D. Without sunlight, squalene is formed into LDL cholesterol.

Getting outside and in the sunshine for fifteen or more minutes a day may be exactly what your body needs!

Chronic Inflammation

Remember that cholesterol serves as a repair mechanism for cells. Therefore, if your body perceives cell damage (perhaps caused by chronic inflammation), it may increase cholesterol to assist in fixing that damage, which could result in higher cholesterol numbers.

There are multiple ways that chronic inflammation sets the stage for elevated cholesterol and increased risk of heart disease. A diet full of sugars and processed vegetable oils is the primary cause of chronic inflammation. Blood sugar and measurements of insulin resistance are a much more accurate predictor of heart disease risk than are cholesterol readings. Consequently, I prefer to examine values such as fasting glucose, HbA1c, and fasting insulin to most accurately determine the inflammatory state of a patient's body.

The real takeaway here is this: High cholesterol *isn't* the problem.

Chronic inflammation brought on by poor lifestyle choices is the *real* issue—and the solution rests in helping your body find balance through an anti-inflammatory, ketogenic diet.

Food Sensitivities

A food sensitivity is an immune-mediated response to certain foods. When you have a food sensitivity, your immune system reacts to a particular food as if it's a threat to your well-being.

By continually eating food your body is sensitive to, you drive up inflammation in the body. Your lipid metabolism alters as a result, which can cause an increase in LDL and triglycerides and lower your HDL levels.

The most common keto foods to which you may be sensitive include nuts, eggs, dairy products, and coffee. You can try eliminating one or all of these items for a week at a time to observe whether you feel better. You also could try eliminating all of those foods for a month and repeating your lipid panel to see if it changes.

Understanding Your Cholesterol Levels

For too long, we've believed untruths about cholesterol—both what it is and what it isn't. Cholesterol is necessary for good health. When you've been following a ketogenic diet for several months, your cholesterol should fall within the following ranges:

- **Total cholesterol levels:** 180 to 250 (up to 300 is acceptable if LDL-to-HDL and triglyceride-to-HDL ratios are within the ideal range)

- **HDL level:** 50 to 80

- **LDL-to-HDL ratio:** 3-to-1 or less (2-to-1 is ideal)

- **Triglyceride-to-HDL ratio:** 2-to-1 or less (a 1-to-1 ratio or even having higher HDL than triglycerides is optimal)

If you fall outside these ranges, there are likely underlying issues that you need to address. I recommend working with a functional medicine practitioner or naturally minded nutritionist to discover the root of your problems.

There is more than one way to follow a ketogenic diet. Technically, eating cheese wrapped in salami is "ketogenic" because it's high in fat and low in carbs. However, such a meal is far from ideal. To ensure maximum benefits, follow a ketogenic diet that is high in healthy fats, clean-sourced proteins, and tons of antioxidant-rich vegetables and herbs. When you flood your body with nutrient-rich, keto-friendly foods, your lifestyle becomes genuinely healing.

Now that you know more about the myths that swirl around the ketogenic lifestyle, it's time for me to tell you about the most common ketogenic mistakes you can make.

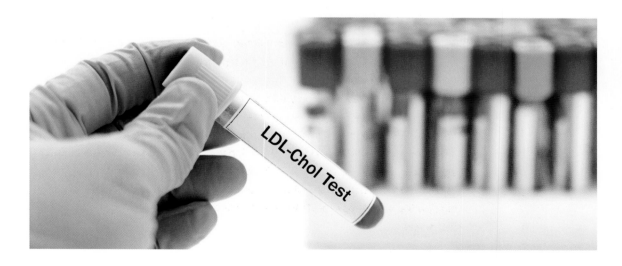

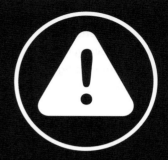

CHAPTER 7

THE BIGGEST KETO MISTAKES

A ketogenic diet is a powerful tool that boosts fat-burning and helps the body heal from chronic disease. I have used the approach both clinically and personally for years with amazing results.

Although the benefits of keto are genuine and attainable, people make a handful of all-too-common ketogenic diet mistakes. If you make the same mistakes, you may not experience the full benefits of living the keto life, but I'm here to help you avoid those pitfalls.

When you're in full-swing ketosis, you should lose weight quickly and have abundant energy. When those two results aren't present, one or more of the following nine mistakes are the likely culprits, and you have to do some investigation to figure out which problem (or problems) might be getting in the way of progress.

The common ketogenic diet mistakes I cover in this chapter can stifle your progress and your motivation to stay the course. That's why you must become a "body detective" if your results are disappointing. We're often our own worst enemies, so be honest with yourself as you examine your daily habits and routines.

If you're not feeling well or feel "stuck" in terms of weight loss or energy level, address the issues I discuss, and you're likely to experience tremendous breakthroughs!

Not Consuming Enough Calories or Fat

This mistake often surprises keto dieters. Many people don't eat enough calories (especially calories from healthy fats) as they attempt to transition to a keto lifestyle. Fasting and calorie restriction have their place, but routinely restricting calories is stressful for your body and can lead to many adverse long-term effects—most notably lethargy and adrenal and thyroid issues.

When keto newcomers first begin their journey, it's easy to get on board with the idea that reducing carbs and sugar is good. However, some people are hesitant to increase their fat intake to 65 to 75 percent of total caloric intake.

As I mention throughout this book, evidence shows that low-carb, high-fat nutrition plans are much more useful than low-fat diets in promoting weight loss and overall health.[1, 2] The message is clear:

Be generous with your fat intake.

Healthy fats (see the nearby graphic) should comprise a significant portion of every meal so that your body can turn fat into ketones for energy. If you find that you're hungry shortly after eating, increase your fat intake per meal.

You should feel satiated and full when you finish eating, and you shouldn't feel hungry for at least four to five hours after consuming a meal. If you do get hungry more quickly, you most likely didn't eat enough. Adding some more fat and protein can help get you to the point of satiation.

If you're worried you'll eat too much, just watch out for the obvious signs of overeating, including bloating, gas, and indigestion after meals. These symptoms may mean you need to cut down your calories just a bit.

GOOD FAT VS BAD FAT

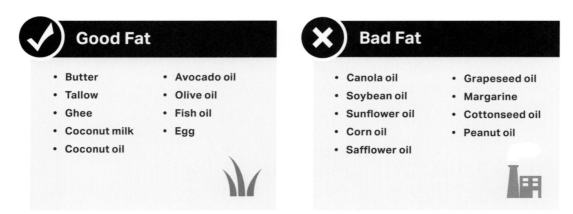

Good Fat
- Butter
- Tallow
- Ghee
- Coconut milk
- Coconut oil
- Avocado oil
- Olive oil
- Fish oil
- Egg

Bad Fat
- Canola oil
- Soybean oil
- Sunflower oil
- Corn oil
- Safflower oil
- Grapeseed oil
- Margarine
- Cottonseed oil
- Peanut oil

Nature doesn't make bad fats, *factories do.*

Not Being Adequately Hydrated

The second mistake is probably just as common as not eating enough fat. You're not drinking enough water! I recommend consuming a minimum of half your body weight in ounces of water daily. One of the most common grievances on a ketogenic diet is constipation. If you're not using the restroom one to three times a day, the reason is likely inadequate water intake.

Do yourself another favor and don't drink your water with your meals. I recommend you stop drinking anywhere from fifteen to thirty minutes before you eat. Then wait at least an hour after your meal before hydrating.

One of the most helpful strategies is to start your day with "super hydration." Upon waking, consume 20 to 32 ounces or more of water. Drinking as soon as you get up will help quell hunger and cravings, stimulate your bowels, and give you more energy. You also will notice that your brain functions better, and you have cleaner, healthier skin.

Here are some other key tips for optimal hydration:

- **Get pure, filtered water:** Drink water that's been processed with reverse osmosis or some other very good filtration system to remove toxins and impurities. You also can drink distilled water.

- **Drink continuously:** Drink at least 4 ounces every thirty minutes throughout the day.

- **Use high-quality salt:** Use a really good sea salt, such as Redmond Real Salt, Celtic Sea Salt, or Himalayan salt.

- **Think "water first":** Before you think about snacking, always drink at least 8 ounces of water to see if your hunger, cravings, or desire for food goes away.

- **Reduce alcohol and caffeine:** You can use alcohol and caffeinated beverages in moderation, but overdoing it (more than two combined servings of alcohol and caffeine per day) can easily dehydrate you.

- **Flavor your water with stevia:** Add stevia drops—which have no calories, have no chemicals, and are natural—to your water to give it great flavor. Most people find it much easier to hydrate with water that includes a few stevia drops.

Not Consuming Adequate Electrolytes

Staying hydrated is about more than drinking enough water. You also need the right minerals. Without them, you will never maximize your fat-burning potential.

Your nervous system uses electrolytes to send messages. When you don't take in enough electrolytes, you experience a decrease in energy, and you may feel dizzy and nauseated.

On a ketogenic diet, your body's insulin sensitivity improves, which results in lower insulin production. Insulin signals the kidneys to hold on to water and minerals, so when insulin levels drop, you excrete excess water and minerals, such as magnesium, potassium, and sodium, which then need to be replaced more frequently.[3, 4]

I recommend that you use high-quality sea salt on your foods and add it to your water. Use it generously to your desired taste. Many people notice that increasing their salt intake makes a huge difference in their energy levels. Other sources of minerals include leafy greens, olives, avocados, sea vegetables, cucumbers, celery, pasture-raised animal products, and bone broth, so including these foods in your diet also augments your electrolyte intake.

Eating Too Many Carbs

This ketogenic diet mistake is straightforward. If you're taking in excess carbs, your body uses them for energy before it burns the fat. If you're starting your keto journey, you need to limit net carbs to approximately 20 to 30 grams or less per day and increase your intake of healthy fats for at least a month. This is what I call a *keto metabolic breakthrough*, and you can read more about it in Chapter 11.

After a month of restricting your carb intake, you can begin a "carb cycling" plan, where you consume a higher carb meal once a week or once a month depending upon what works best for your body. When you get to the stage of adding in carbs, use nutrient-dense sources such as sweet potatoes, carrots, beets, and your favorite low-glycemic fruits.

Overeating Protein

Many people on keto don't realize that it's a high-fat diet, and they mistakenly opt for lean cuts of meat rather than fattier cuts. It's always best to look for fatty cuts of meat or, if you prefer, you can add extra fat to your lean protein to make it fit into the keto template of 60 to 80 percent fat.

Eating too much protein can prevent some individuals from entering into a state of ketosis. The reason is that excess amino acids from overeating protein may be converted into glucose, and your body burns the glucose for energy instead of burning dietary fats.[5] Additionally, some people get a higher insulin response when they consume a higher protein diet.

A healthy protein goal is to consume approximately half your body weight in protein. For example, someone who weighs 160 pounds should eat around 80 grams of protein per day, although you need to adjust based on your activity level. If you're very inactive, you require less protein daily; if you exercise heavily, you may need more.

I've found that some people do better on a higher protein diet in which they consume 30 to 35 percent of their calories from protein. Others do better with much less protein—around 20 to 25 percent of calories from protein. Experiment to find what works best for you. Once you find your ideal amount of protein, be sure to fill in the extra calories with healthy fats.

GOALS THAT DETERMINE PROTEIN INTAKE

Weight loss

If you are looking to lose weight and you are staying active then you want to shoot for a protein range from 1.0–1.2 grams of protein per kg of body weight.

Example for a 160-pound person: 160/2.2 = 72.7 kg (1.0–1.2 g/kg = 73–87 g of protein daily)

Muscle building

If you are looking to build lean body tissue and are combining resistance training then you should aim for 1.2–2.0 grams of protein per kg of body weight.

Example for a 160-pound person: 160/2.2 = 72.7 kg (1.2–2.0 g/kg = 87–145 g of protein daily)

Extreme athletes

If you are a high level extreme athlete playing football, basketball, or other team or individual sport then you are going to want to be in the 1.4–2.0 g/kg range and possibly higher depending upon your overall activity.

Example for a 160-pound person: 160/2.2 = 72.7 kg (1.4–2.0 g/kg = 100–145 g of protein daily)

Sedentary individuals

If you are a sedentary individual that wants the benefits of ketosis and possibly weight loss then I recommend staying in the 0.8–1.0 grams of protein per kg of body weight.

Example for a 160-pound person: 160/2.2 = 72.7 kg (0.8–1.0 g/kg = 58–73 g of protein daily)

Having Too Much Stress and Getting Too Little Sleep

Stress and lack of adequate sleep are widespread issues in our society. These issues also can stall your progress. Consequently, for maximum results, you should begin a keto diet *after* you've taken steps to reduce your stress load for at least a month.

At the beginning of the keto journey, the adaptation process can be somewhat stressful on your body. If you're already stressed, adding more stress could prevent you from achieving ketosis, which is why I recommend that you reduce your stress level for some time *before* you begin living the keto lifestyle.

People who are under high amounts of stress tend to have rapidly fluctuating cortisol levels that disrupt blood sugar balance. If you're in this state and your blood sugar drops too low in your already-overworked system, it could set off a stress hormone cascade and bring on hypoglycemia, leaving you feeling chronically fatigued, and you might notice these other symptoms:

- Salt cravings
- Overly emotional
- Tired after exercising
- Brain fog
- Weight gain
- Trouble sleeping

- Frequent sickness
- Depression
- Anxiety
- Morning fatigue
- Lightheadedness
- Irritability

The good news is that after you become fat-adapted, you'll likely notice that you're more able to meet stressful daily demands.

Inadequate sleep is another factor that causes blood sugar dysregulation and may negatively affect your ability to achieve ketosis. If you're struggling to increase your energy, prioritize healthy sleeping habits, such as going to sleep earlier in the evening and keeping your room dark and cool. It's also a good idea to stay out of bright lights after dark and use a sleep mask over your eyes while you sleep. I discuss more about sleep habits in Chapter 13.

Not Going Enough

No one likes to talk about this subject, but you can't ignore constipation, and it may be preventing you from getting into ketosis. Constipation is all too common in today's society. When a person has constipation, excess waste backs up in the digestive system and causes an overgrowth of unwanted microbes. These microbes ferment the feces and produce endotoxins that drive up inflammation and stress on the body, which increases the production of stress hormones and further throws off your blood sugar balance.

Think about it like trash that sits and rots in your home. As it rots, it releases terrible odors. In the body, those odors are toxic, and they increase inflammation and stress hormones. The increased stress throws off your blood sugar level.

Constipation is improved by good hydration and good eating habits. The ultimate goal is to have a bowel movement within an hour of waking. Try starting the day off with the hydration strategies discussed earlier in this chapter. Two, or even three, bowel movements a day is a good sign that your body is functioning optimally.

Low stomach acid and poor bile flow are key factors in the development of constipation. In Chapter 6, I discuss some helpful strategies for improving the production of these digestive juices, so revisit that chapter if you need a refresher on those techniques.

THE IMPORTANCE OF HEALTHY BOWEL MOVEMENTS

Having good bowel habits may be one of the most important elements in your overall health journey. Prioritize having good bowel activity each and every day.

Healthy bowel movement habits:

- Happen one to four times daily.
- Move out all waste from previous meals within twenty-four hours.
- Best daily rhythm is early in the morning and/or shortly after meals.
- Reduce the microbial load on the body.
- Eliminate destructive endotoxins.
- Reduce inflammation throughout the body.
- Help calm the brain and nervous system.
- Enhance energy and mental clarity.
- Improve skin health and natural glow.
- Reduce chronic pain levels.

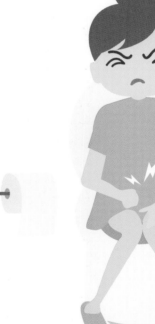

Exercising Too Much (or Not Enough)

It's not uncommon for people who are into fitness and health to overtrain their bodies. If you're working out intensely for an hour on more than five days a week, you may very well be overtaxing your system. Overtraining can cause a lot of issues with stress hormones that lead to blood sugar imbalances, cravings, and fatigue.

If you're in this situation, try backing down to three or four days a week of exercise and rest on the other days. Regular exercise should help you feel great and keto adapt more effectively, but you also probably need to reduce your intensity a bit when you first begin adapting into a keto lifestyle.

After you're keto adapted, your body can handle more stress, and it becomes more resilient. However, if the overall amount of stress in your life is high, you aren't sleeping well, and you're training really intensely, it could be too much pressure on your system. You may need to cut back if you're feeling fatigued or having trouble sleeping.

On the opposite end of the spectrum, you also should avoid a sedentary lifestyle. If you aren't moving much or engaging in any form of regular exercise, the result is that you'll have higher blood sugar levels, insulin resistance, and increased inflammation. Regular exercise helps upregulate a protein called *GLUT-4*, which pulls sugars from the bloodstream and stores it in muscles or the liver as glycogen. Having higher GLUT-4 activity allows your body to handle slightly more carbs while keeping you in a state of ketosis.[7]

Consistency and moderation are key. At a minimum, you should be striving for twenty minutes of low-intensity movement daily. This could entail taking a short walk and making sure you're standing up and moving around throughout the day. Doing so will help keep your tissues oxygenated and your lymph fluid stimulated by muscular contractions. If you're up for it, I highly recommend engaging in strength training exercises a few days a week because it helps your body put on lean body tissue, which improves your metabolism and mitochondrial health. The key is to find the right type and the right amount of exercise for you based on your age, the other stressors in your life, and your goals.

Eating Low-Quality Foods

A healing, sustainable keto lifestyle is not full of processed vegetable oils and meat products. You *can* achieve ketosis by eating only salami-wrapped mozzarella cheese from the gas station, but at what cost?

Keto is about more than weight loss, and although you can lose weight by eating processed forms of fat, why would you want to deprive your body of the other profound health benefits that go along with a ketogenic diet? When you consume a lot of conventionally raised animal products, fried foods, and refined vegetable oils, you end up consuming a lot of unhealthy fats and toxins. This is called *dirty keto*. Instead, I recommend *real food keto*, in which you strive to get the most nutrients and the fewest environmental toxins in your food.

On real food keto, you do your best to get organic produce and animal products whenever possible. Load up on healthy fats from foods such as coconut oil, avocados, olives, and raw nuts and seeds. Of course, be sure to eat lots of nutrient-dense vegetables and antioxidant-rich herbs and spices. These foods and flavors are not only delicious but they also enhance the benefits of a ketogenic lifestyle.

If you've done your detective work to investigate all these issues that can stand in the way of your progress and you're still stuck or confused, don't worry. I uncover lots more information that will help you with your keto metabolic breakthrough in the chapters to come, starting with how to address the side effects of the ketogenic diet.

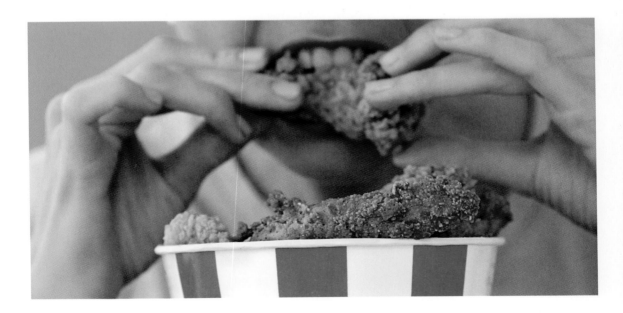

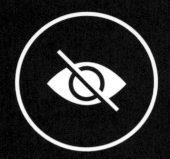

CHAPTER 8

THE HIDDEN CAUSES OF KETO SIDE EFFECTS

Even if you're brand-new to keto, there's a good chance you've heard about the common side effects that rear their ugly heads at the beginning of a ketogenic diet.

Am I really saying that eating fresh, healthy foods can cause unpleasant side effects?

The short answer is yes. The longer but more accurate answer is that you can mitigate and, in some cases, avoid side effects by following a few simple steps.

Although there are a variety of potential side effects that could manifest as you're becoming keto-adapted, all stem from three underlying issues:

- Hypoglycemia or low blood sugar
- Hypothalamic-pituitary-adrenal (HPA) axis dysfunction
- Electrolyte and mineral deficiencies

These three causes are seemingly different, but actually they're related. You've been operating in a sugar-burning mode for years. When you abruptly switch to using fats for fuel, your body must build the cellular "machinery" required to generate and use ketone bodies as its new and improved energy source. It makes sense, then, that your body is not able to generate enough ketones from day one to adequately fuel itself, which is why many people experience hypoglycemia during the first few days, or even weeks, of their new ketogenic lifestyle. Hypoglycemia then causes a disruption in cortisol signaling, which is what accounts for the HPA axis dysfunction (also called *adrenal fatigue*) that you may experience while becoming fat-adapted. The HPA axis dysfunction then leads to an increase in the secretion of minerals from the body in the urine.

In this chapter, I discuss these issues, their symptoms, and practical strategies for overcoming them. Once you understand the side effects, some extra thought and planning can help greatly diminish the signs of keto-adaptation.

Hypoglycemia (Low Blood Sugar)

During the keto-adaptation phase, people commonly report feeling brain fog, fatigue, dizziness, intense hunger, irritability, and depression. These are trademark symptoms of hypoglycemia, or low blood sugar, that is caused by the body's inability to use fat for fuel in an efficient manner. (Remember, your body has been in a sugar-burning mode for a long time.)

Although you should expect to experience hypoglycemia in the beginning, it should subside within a few weeks of beginning a ketogenic diet. Watch for the following signs and take steps to support your body during the transition.

Keto Flu

Keto flu is perhaps the most well-known keto side effect. It is what it sounds like—the onset of flu-like symptoms that manifest soon after a person begins a ketogenic diet. Typical symptoms include headache, nausea, fatigue, and runny nose. Keto flu is a classic indication of hypoglycemia that fortunately you can correct with the simple strategies I share later in this chapter.

WHAT IS KETO FLU AND HOW TO PREVENT IT

How long does it last?

1 week

Keto flu does not affect everyone, and symptoms can vary among those who do experience it. Often it lasts a week, but for some people it can last longer.

7 ways to prevent keto flu:

- Back off carbs slowly
- Increase your fat intake
- Increase your salt and mineral intake
- Hydrate well
- Get some exercise
- Reduce stress
- If all else falls, increase your carb intake

Symptoms

- Fatigue
- Headache
- Nausea
- Insomnia
- Irritability
- Upset stomach

Hydration

During the keto adaptation phase, you lose more hydration and electrolytes. It is key to drink lots of water and be sure to use extra salts to replace the electrolytes.

I recommend drinking a minimum of half your weight in ounces of water. The best time to drink a lot of water is first thing in the morning and in between meals.

Salts and trace mineral–rich foods

You should aim to add 2 teaspoons of high-quality salt to your food each day and add a pinch of salt to the water you drink to help your body to replace the electrolytes you lose as you keto adapt.

You should also look to consume a lot of trace mineral–rich foods such as bone broth, celery, cucumbers, wild-caught seafood, sea vegetables, pickles, olives, leafy and cruciferous veggies, and sauerkraut.

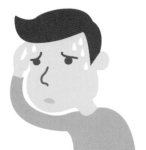

Sugar Cravings

Many people experience intense food cravings for sugary, starchy foods when they start keto. Such cravings challenge the limits of human willpower; however, they are *not* a sign of weakness. These cravings are merely a hypoglycemic response.

When your brain receives a signal that you're hypoglycemic, it initiates a "panic response" that signals to your body that you're undernourished (even if you consciously know you're not). At this point, your brain says to you, "WE NEED ENERGY NOW OR WE'RE GOING TO DIE!" Once you begin to produce sufficient ketones, this panic-fueled response lessens dramatically.

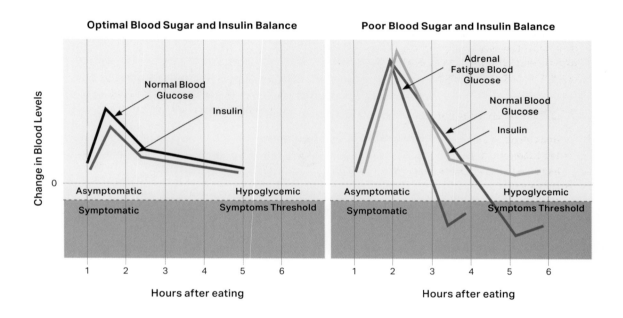

Dizziness and Drowsiness

Before becoming keto-adapted, you will likely experience a temporary energy deficiency. This is a short-term adaptation, but during this period you could experience drowsiness and a general lack of energy. You also may feel dizzy as you stand thanks to blood pressure dysregulation and improper cortisol response.

Reduced Strength and Performance

During keto-adaptation, your body is swiftly learning to use fat as fuel. Your muscles and brain contain tons of mitochondria that must learn to use ketones instead of glucose. As a result, you will likely feel a temporary but significant drop in physical strength. Luckily, once you become adapted, you should experience drastic improvements in strength and performance that surpass your previous sugar-adapted levels!

Hypoglycemia Mitigation Strategies

As you can see, many of the most commonly known keto side effects can be attributed to hypoglycemia. Here are my top strategies for addressing these issues and lessening the symptoms of hypoglycemia:

- **Eat every three to four hours.** Eating more frequently in the beginning stages of a ketogenic diet helps keep you satiated and keeps your blood sugar more balanced. After a week or two, you'll naturally be able to space out your meals to every four to five hours or longer and more seamlessly incorporate intermittent fasting into your lifestyle.

- **Drink mineral-rich beverages.** Instead of consuming only plain water, include some mineral-rich drinks between meals. Organic broths and electrolyte drinks are some examples. You also could put a pinch of sea salt in your water to add sodium and minerals that support your body during this transition.

- **Consume hydrating, mineral-rich foods.** Don't shy away from using mineral-rich salts and foods. Ideal snack foods include celery, cucumbers, and seaweed-based snacks such as seaweed chips.

- **Supplement with magnesium.** If you've followed these strategies and continue to experience the symptoms of hypoglycemia, add a magnesium supplement to your regimen. (You can read more about supplements I recommend in Chapter 15.)

- **Use exogenous ketones or C8 MCT oil.** Exogenous ketones and C8 MCT oil help train your body to use ketones for fuel before it becomes skilled at creating its own ketones. These supplements also soften the hypoglycemic response. I discuss exogenous ketones in greater detail later in this chapter.

HPA Axis Dysfunction (Adrenal Fatigue)

The HPA axis is a series of three glands (hypothalamus, pituitary, and adrenals) that are primarily responsible for regulating the stress response in your body. When something disrupts the communication patterns between these glands, it causes an abnormal or inaccurate response from your body to perceived stressors. This incorrect response is called *HPA axis dysfunction* or *adrenal fatigue.*

When you experience hypoglycemia, your brain's default response is, "We must be starving." This response not only causes sugar cravings but it also causes the adrenals to release cortisol. Cortisol signals the release of glucose (glycogen stores) to provide quick energy. Glycogen stores are swiftly burned up, hypoglycemia reoccurs, and the cycle continues.

HPA axis dysregulation promotes the onset of unpleasant symptoms while also exacerbating hypoglycemia-related issues. Following are some of the common side effects.

Sleep Problems

Due to the increased cortisol production that accompanies hypoglycemia and HPA axis dysfunction, you may experience sleep disruptions or even insomnia during the keto transition. Cortisol production is in direct opposition to the creation of melatonin (the sleep hormone). Although the cortisol response is helpful in emergencies, it's best to minimize this response as much as possible during keto-adaptation.

Heart Palpitations

During the early phases of keto-adaptation, you may notice heart palpitations, which can be attributed to all three causes (hypoglycemia, HPA axis dysfunction, and mineral imbalances). During HPA axis dysregulation, cortisol levels can climb. If they remain high, your body will develop cortisol resistance. As compensation, your body begins to secrete more adrenaline. Adrenaline magnifies the fight-or-flight response in your body, and high levels of adrenaline can cause heart palpitations and even panic attacks. Additionally, the loss of minerals can lead to a reduction in blood volume and pressure that may cause your heart to pump faster or irregularly.

HPA Axis Dysfunction Mitigation Strategies

I recommend that you proactively take steps to support the HPA axis as you transition to a keto lifestyle. Here are my top strategies to reduce side effects caused by HPA axis dysfunction:

- **Employ blood-sugar-balancing strategies.** Follow the hypoglycemia mitigation strategies outlined in the previous section. Hypoglycemia is one of the primary triggers of cortisol dysregulation, so you must address this first.

- **Begin magnesium supplementation.** Take a magnesium supplement. Magnesium L-threonate, in particular, is ideal because it can cross the blood-brain barrier, which means it can directly exert its calming effects on the hypothalamus and pituitary glands.

- **Use adaptogenic herbs.** Adaptogenic herbs can significantly benefit the HPA axis and help build your resistance to stress. By supporting the HPA axis and helping to regulate cortisol levels, adaptogens may help mitigate HPA axis–related side effects.

Electrolyte/Mineral Deficiencies

Electrolytes and minerals carry out essential roles in the body, including regulating hydration and supporting nerve conductivity. During keto-adaptation, you excrete an excess of minerals through the urine due to HPA axis dysregulation. The HPA axis is also responsible for regulating hydration levels through mineral retention and excretion. HPA axis dysregulation can also lead to hydration irregularities, and some common side effects result from these imbalances.

Increased Urination

The most obvious sign that your mineral balance is affected is an increase in urination, which serves as a positive sign that you're moving toward keto-adaptation. On a low-carb diet, insulin levels drop, which promotes the secretion of sodium in the urine. The sodium then pulls more water into the urinary system. Additionally, as your body burns through its glycogen stores during the initial stages of keto, the process releases water into the urinary system. While getting rid of extra water helps release toxins from the body, you need to take in extra fluids and electrolytes to avoid other related side effects.

Constipation

The consistency of your bowel movements is heavily influenced by its water content, which is likewise determined by your level of hydration. Constipation is a sign that you aren't maintaining mineral balance during keto-adaptation. Constipation may also be a side effect of changes in your microbiome. The precise makeup of gut bacteria is largely determined by what you eat. When you make drastic adjustments to your diet, your microbiome changes, which also can change your stools.

BRISTOL STOOL CHART

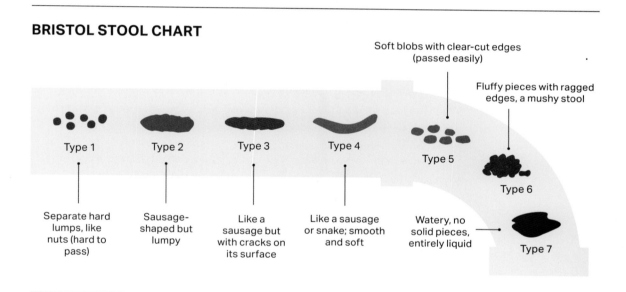

Soft blobs with clear-cut edges (passed easily)

Fluffy pieces with ragged edges, a mushy stool

Type 1 — Separate hard lumps, like nuts (hard to pass)

Type 2 — Sausage-shaped but lumpy

Type 3 — Like a sausage but with cracks on its surface

Type 4 — Like a sausage or snake; smooth and soft

Type 5

Type 6

Type 7 — Watery, no solid pieces, entirely liquid

Also consider that certain foods such as eggs, cheese, and nuts may contribute to constipation. If you're experiencing constipation, reduce your intake of these foods. Ideally, your stools should pass easily and resemble type 3 or 4 on the Bristol Stool Chart shown in the illustration.

Diarrhea

Changes in the microbiome can cause a variety of gut-related symptoms; constipation isn't the only result, although it is the most prevalent. Loose stools also are relatively common during the initial phases of a ketogenic diet. If you experience loose stools, consider taking a digestive aid such as psyllium husks, citrus pectin, or activated charcoal (two to three grams of charcoal every three hours until symptoms subside).

For some individuals, diarrhea is the result of low levels of stomach acid or a sluggish gallbladder. I discuss both these issues in detail in Chapter 14. Another possibility is a minor sensitivity to foods such as coffee, eggs, nuts, and cheese. Additionally, high doses of magnesium and vitamin C can cause diarrhea. Decrease your intake of these supplements until your stools become solid again. Excess mineral salt also can have a laxative effect, which is why it's best to increase salt intake gradually.

Muscle Cramps

A common keto side effect during the initial phase of transitioning into a keto lifestyle is muscle cramps, which are most likely due to mineral imbalances or inadequacies. Your body needs minerals for proper nerve impulse conductivity. When it doesn't get sufficient amounts, you may experience muscle cramps, which are essentially misconducted impulses brought on by inadequate hydration and mineral imbalance.

Mineral Imbalance Mitigation Strategies

Now you know more about the physiological changes that contribute to frequent urination, gut complications, muscle cramps, and heart palpitations. Fortunately, the strategies to overcome these challenges are simple. The following are my top suggestions for proper hydration and mineral balance:

- **Stay super hydrated.** Drink copious amounts of water, mineral-rich soups and broths, and other hydrating beverages.

- **Use high-quality salt.** Use a high-quality salt at all times. Mineral-rich salts replenish sodium levels and other trace minerals that are excreted more rapidly during keto-adaptation. Himalayan salt, Redmond Real Salt, and Celtic Sea Salt are the highest in trace minerals.

- **Consume mineral-rich foods.** Increase your intake of mineral-rich foods such as leafy greens, celery, cucumber, olives, avocados, vegetable broths, and seaweed.
- **Supplement with magnesium.** Magnesium helps balance electrolytes and hydration levels. It also can help ease constipation. Supplement with 200 to 500 milligrams of magnesium, two to three times per day. If diarrhea occurs, stop taking the supplements until your diarrhea resolves, and then resume taking magnesium at a lower dosage.

Precautions for Specific Conditions

Although a keto diet can be therapeutic for most people, you must take precautions to prevent severe side effects if you have two conditions: high blood pressure or diabetes. Being cautious is especially important if you use prescription medications.

High Blood Pressure

When you drastically decrease carbohydrate consumption, your blood pressure may drop naturally. Before starting a keto plan, discuss it with your physician and take steps to observe your body's response to the dietary changes. If you feel light-headed or dizzy or experience heart palpitations, a sharp decrease in blood pressure could be the culprit. Frequently monitor your blood pressure to assess your body's response to the adaptation phase.

Diabetes

When you eat fewer carbs and sugar, you need less insulin or blood-sugar-lowering medications to maintain blood sugar balance. Speak with your physician about this so your doctor can determine the proper changes for your medication dosage. If you experience symptoms such as fatigue, intense cravings, light-headedness, or heart palpitations, they may be signs your blood sugar has dropped too low. Use a blood glucose monitor to track your body's response to dietary changes and make sure your body is adapting appropriately.

Keto Breath

One of the often-discussed, unpleasant keto side effects is called *keto breath*. Although it's not entirely related to the three major causes I've discussed in this chapter, it is something that many people experience in the early stages of keto-adaptation.

When you begin producing ketones, you create them in several different forms. The ketone released through the breath is acetone, which has a distinct odor and causes the unpleasant breath commonly associated with keto. Fortunately, your body releases acetone in high amounts only during the initial stages of adaptation. It tapers off rather quickly—generally within one to two weeks.

If keto breath becomes an issue for you, brush your teeth more frequently and use natural breath fresheners throughout the day to help lessen the odor. It's also essential that you maintain proper hydration during this time because a dry mouth can exacerbate this side effect.

Other strategies for minimizing keto breath include oil pulling with coconut oil (swishing coconut oil in your mouth for five to ten minutes) and using a natural mouthwash made with essential oils rather than harsh chemicals. For a truly natural approach to fresh breath, try chewing on fennel seeds, rosemary, mint, or parsley.

The Keto Panacea: Exogenous Ketones

One of the best ways to get your body keto-adapted quickly and reduce the side effects of the keto-adaptation process is through the use of exogenous ketones, which are a supplemental form of ketones that are identical to the ketone bodies (beta-hydroxybutyrate or BHB) made by your body. By using an exogenous ketone supplement, you can help hasten your body's adaptation process because the supplements give your body a source of ketones that requires almost no processing. Exogenous ketones are useful not only for helping push you into ketosis but also as a quick energy source and performance enhancer.

HOW DO EXOGENOUS KETONES WORK?

Exogenous ketones increase the ketone (energy) levels in your body.

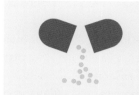

They provide ketones to teach the body how to adapt and remedy the symptoms of the keto flu.

They boost energy at any time of day (and are great for work or exercise).

They provide feelings of fullness in between meals or during a fast.

 Ketones can be used to improve fat loss, physical performance, mental focus, and longevity.

Most anyone who has struggled with keto side effects stands to benefit greatly from supplementing with exogenous ketones during the adaption phase and beyond. Additionally, exogenous ketones can be a powerful aid for people who have weak liver or gallbladder function or poor mitochondrial health.

Your Best Strategy: Be Proactive

When it comes to keto side effects, the best strategy is to expect to experience at least some of the symptoms I've discussed. However, proactively taking steps to be prepared for the possible side effects can go a long way to making your transition to keto-adaptation as straightforward as possible. As you start your keto journey, use this checklist to help you address the possible causes of the side effects.

Stay hydrated

Drink at least half of your body weight in ounces of water daily. Over time, you will desire more water, and eventually, you can drink as much as an ounce of clean water per pound of body weight (as in 160 pounds = 160 ounces). This quantity may seem like a lot, but your body performs best when it's well hydrated.

 ## Eat more salt

The right amount of salt varies slightly for everyone. In general, though, you should consume at least one to two teaspoons of salt daily by adding mineral-rich salt to your foods or your water throughout the day.

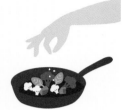

 ## Increase meal frequency

I typically don't recommend snacking, but during the keto-adaptation phase, eating every three to four hours eases the hypoglycemic stress on your body. In other words, you eat four to five small meals throughout the day. As you become adapted, fasting for longer periods will become much more manageable.

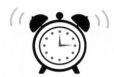

 ## Drink organic broths

Drinking broth is a great way to stay hydrated and take in minerals and amino acids. Also, broth makes a great snack between meals. Any broth will help provide minerals and electrolytes, but the best broths are made from organic, free-range or pasture-raised chicken or beef.

 ## Consume mineral-rich foods

Consuming mineral-rich foods helps maintain proper hydration and supports the HPA axis. Recommended foods include celery, olives, avocados, radishes, cucumber, seaweed, and fermented veggies such as pickles and sauerkraut.

 ## Eat fat with every meal

Every meal should have at least one source of healthy fat. Ideally, 60 to 80 percent of calories should come from fat for any given meal. The top sources are coconut fats, grass-fed butter or ghee, MCT oil, olives and olive oil, and avocados.

Take a magnesium supplement

Magnesium keeps your body running smoothly on the cellular level. When your body experiences blood sugar fluctuations, it uses magnesium quickly. For this reason, it's a good idea to supplement with a form of magnesium such as magnesium chloride, citrate, malate, glycinate, or threonate throughout the day, especially during keto-adaptation. Any of these forms of magnesium will work, but magnesium L-threonate works best at calming the stress response and improving mental clarity.

 ## Supplement with adaptogenic herbs

Adaptogenic herbs help your body to better adapt to stress. They help your body function at its optimal level during times of stress by modulating the production of stress hormones such as cortisol and adrenaline. Adaptogenic herbs include Panex ginseng, ashwagandha, Rhodiola, cordyceps, reishi mushroom, astragalus, holy basil, Siberian ginseng (Eleuthero root), and maca. Start with small doses and increase gradually. Some individuals respond to specific adaptogens better than others, so be sure to monitor how you feel. If you notice that an adaptogen induces cravings or makes you feel fatigued, the symptom indicates that you need to find an herb that is better suited to your body's needs.

 ## Use exogenous ketones

Finally, supplementing with exogenous ketones takes some stress off of your body and improves your ability to use ketones as a fuel source. Supplementation also enhances your body's ability to make ketones, which speeds the adaptation process. To get the most out of a ketone supplement, take it along with electrolytes and adaptogens to stabilize your blood sugar, improve your body's stress response, and support your brain.

The side effects of keto-adaptation do not have to define your keto diet experience. By being proactive and taking action steps before you experience symptoms, you're far more likely to stay the course and enjoy the experience of transitioning to your ketogenic lifestyle.

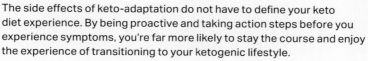

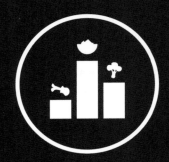

CHAPTER 9

THE TOP 25 KETOGENIC FOODS

Most of us grew up on a high-carbohydrate diet that was filled with foods such as bread, cereal, potatoes, burgers, fries, sugary desserts, soda, and more. As comforting as those foods may be, they're indulgences that are the very *antithesis* of health. Starchy, sugary foods are typically inexpensive, satisfy our cravings, and provide short bursts of energy—but that's where their usefulness ends.

To break the cycle of food addiction, feel better, and look better, you must eliminate the underlying source of your health problems. Eating lots of sugar and carbs disturbs your sleep, messes with your hormone levels, makes you cranky, and leaves you trapped in a cycle of chronic exhaustion.

So, say goodbye to the addictive foods that have kept you feeling less than your *best* self. On a ketogenic diet, the focus is on foods that support the pursuit of lower sugar and insulin levels so that you can effectively use fat for fuel.

In this chapter, I cover the top twenty-five foods that should be staples in every well-balanced ketogenic lifestyle. I selected these foods because they are the most nutritious and have the least amount of toxins. Some of these items are foods, some are beverages, some are herbs and spices that provide tremendous flavor to meals—and all of them are ideal choices as you begin to adapt to the keto way of life.

You may not have easy access to all of these foods. If you don't, that's okay. But aim to consume at least twelve to fifteen of these foods on a weekly basis, and incorporate multiple items into every meal. If you have a sensitivity or poor response to one or even a few of these, just stop eating those and try some of the others. There are plenty of foods you can enjoy!

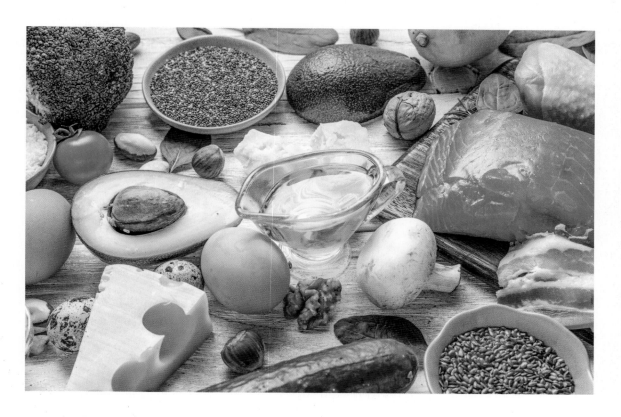

Lemons and Limes

Most citrus fruits are packed with sugar. Lemons and limes, however, are low in sugar and rich in anti-inflammatory nutrients such as citric acid, vitamin C, and bioflavonoids.

LEMON WATER BENEFITS

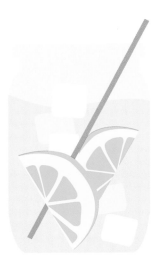

 Aids in Digestion and Detoxification

Because lemon juice's atomic structure is similar to the digestive juices in the stomach, it tricks the liver into producing bile, which helps keep food moving through your body and gastrointestinal tract smoothly. Lemon water also helps relieve indigestion or ease an upset stomach.

 Helps the Body Use Fat for Fuel

Regularly sipping on lemon water can help you lose those last pounds. That's because lemons contain pectin, a type of fiber commonly found in fruits. Pectin helps you feel full longer.

 Rejuvenates Skin and Body Healing

The antioxidants in lemon water fight damage caused by free radicals, keeping your skin looking fresh. It also helps the body produce collagen, which is essential in smoothing out lines in the face.

 Improves Mood and Energy

Skip the morning cup of coffee. Lemon water can boost energy levels without the caffeine crash. When negative-charged ions, like those found in lemons, enter your digestive tract, the result is an increase in energy levels.

 Improves Vitamin C Levels

Because your body doesn't make vitamin C on its own, it's important to get enough of it from the foods and drinks you ingest, like lemon water. Vitamin C stimulates white blood cell production, which is vital for your immune system to function properly, and also protects cells from oxidative damage.

Citric acid is a powerful ally; it helps combat the inflammatory effects of sugar, stabilize blood sugar levels, detoxify the gut, and alkalize the body. The citrate in lemons and limes also helps bind and remove oxalates from your body. Excess oxalates can cause kidney problems and joint pain.

There are many ways to incorporate these two powerhouse citrus fruits into your daily routine. Squeeze the juice of a lemon or lime onto your meat and veggies to help reduce your blood sugar and insulin responses after a meal. The juice also adds excellent taste to proteins such as fish and poultry (think lemon pepper chicken). Don't be shy—add a fresh squeeze to your water throughout the day and use it in food preparations such as marinades and dressings.

GIVE THESE RECIPES A TRY

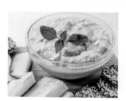

Creamy Lemony
Superfood Guacamole
(page 285)

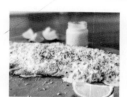

Coconut Lime
Seared Salmon
(page 313)

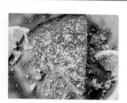

Coconut Custard
Lemon Pie
(page 329)

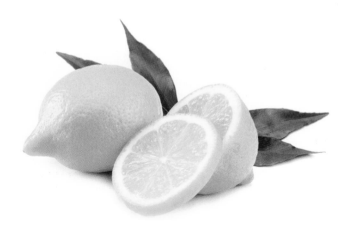

Herbs

Herbs contain some of the most potent antioxidants, and they pack a punch in terms of taste. Adding fresh or dried herbs to a dish can turn an ordinary, bland meal into a culinary treat. Herbs such as rosemary, sweet basil, and oregano contain polyphenols that enhance organic acid synthesis by improving the health of gut flora.[1] Organic acids are essential to bowel health and aid in nutrient absorption. These herbs destroy harmful bacteria and provide antioxidants, and their antifungal benefits help maintain a robust immune system.[2]

There are several categories of herbs that each serve distinct purposes. *Bitter herbs* such as ginger, turmeric, and parsley stimulate digestive function by supporting enzyme and bile secretion from the liver and gallbladder. As a result, food transit time increases, fats are better digested, and detoxification pathways get a boost.[3] *Carminative herbs* also support the digestive system, helping to improve bowel motility, reduce gas, and cultivate a healthy microbiome. Carminatives include herbs such as garlic, mint, ginger, turmeric, oregano, basil, thyme, rosemary, and cinnamon. These herbs add a pungent aroma to meals to stimulate the flow of digestive juices. Their natural oils also increase bile flow, so add these herbs to high-fat meals and enjoy the smells circulating the kitchen.[4]

GIVE THESE RECIPES A TRY

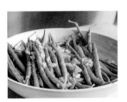

Garlic Herb Green Beans
(page 296)

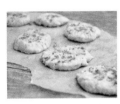

No-Bake Turmeric Cookies
(page 336)

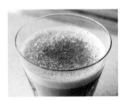

Cinnamon Coconut Smoothie
(page 344)

Unsweetened Coffee and Tea

Coffee and certain teas contain caffeine to give your metabolism a kick, and thankfully, they are a welcome part of a ketogenic lifestyle. Coffee contains chlorogenic acid that is anti-inflammatory and lowers blood sugar levels. Also, herbal teas provide plenty of benefits, from stimulating bile flow for a healthy liver to promoting detoxification.[5] When consumed in their natural, unsweetened form, coffee and tea can help improve energy levels, gut health, and brain function.

Some great herbal teas include green tea for energy in the morning, dandelion and ginger tea for digestive health, and chamomile or passionflower tea for relaxation in the evening. Brands like Traditional Medicinals or Yogi Tea, which offer organic tea blends, are probably available at your local grocery store. Another brand I recommend is Pique Teas, which you can find online at piquetea.com.

GIVE THESE RECIPES A TRY

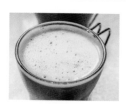

Fat-Burning Turmeric Coffee
(page 350)

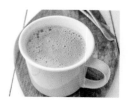

Matcha Tea
(page 348)

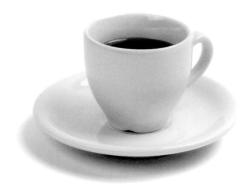

Low-Carb Vegetables

Veggies are always a good idea because the majority of them are low in carbs and excellent sources of vitamins, minerals, fiber, and antioxidants. Eating more vegetables is associated with a reduced risk of disease, primarily because of polyphenols, the beneficial chemicals found in veggies.[16] Avoid starchy, high-carb vegetables such as potatoes; instead, use low-carb substitutes such as cauliflower and zucchini noodles (sometimes called *zoodles*) in recipes that typically call for grain-based noodles and potatoes.

Cruciferous vegetables, including kale, broccoli, Brussels sprouts, cabbage, and cauliflower, have the lowest net carb count of all the veggies. They protect cells against oxidative stress and tissue damage.[7] Sprouts are low-carb options that are full of nutrients but often forgotten. Include broccoli, kale, and alfalfa sprouts in your diet for a healthy dose of glutathione-boosting agents, enzymes, and other phytonutrients.

GIVE THESE RECIPES A TRY

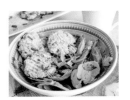

Keto Hash Browns
(page 272)

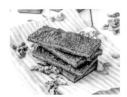

Grain-Free Kale Flatbread
(page 284)

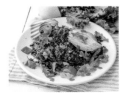

Naked Kale Burger Sauté
(page 310)

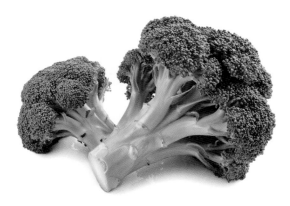

Nuts and Seeds

Nuts and seeds are keto superfoods. Walnuts, almonds, macadamia nuts, pumpkin seeds, and chia seeds are low-carb and full of healing omega-3 fatty acids, and they're a quick and powerful energy source. Thanks to their high fiber content, consuming small amounts of nuts and seeds before a meal can help curb your appetite and prevent excess calorie intake. However, it's best to avoid peanuts and peanut butter because peanuts are often high in mold toxins and omega-6 fats that can contribute to inflammation.

Nuts and seeds contain high concentrations of potent plant compounds that combat inflammation and support immune health. The healthy fats and antioxidants in nuts are shown to reduce inflammation, improve cardiovascular health, and prevent depression, Alzheimer's disease, and other cognitive conditions.[8]

GIVE THESE RECIPES A TRY

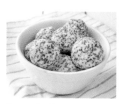

Protein Popping
Power Balls
(page 283)

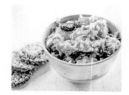

Cashew Artichoke
Dip
(page 288)

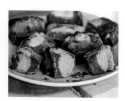

Frozen Coconut
Almond Butter Cups
(page 332)

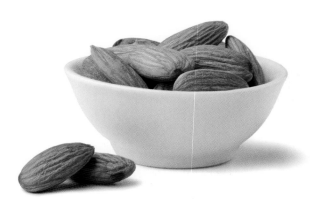

Avocados

The avocado is the quintessential ketogenic food because it's packed with healthy fat, fiber, vitamins, and minerals, but it contains only 2 grams of net carbs per cup. The nutrients and antioxidants in avocados have been clinically shown to promote healthy aging and weight loss.[9] Avocados are rich in potassium and magnesium, and researchers have linked them to an improvement in muscle strength and endurance in athletes who live a low-carb lifestyle.[10]

AMAZING HEALTH BENEFITS OF AVOCADO

1

Cardiovascular

Avocados contain beta-sitosterol, which lowers LDL (bad) cholesterol while raising HDL (good) cholesterol. They also protect against strokes and regulate blood pressure.

4

Muscle Development

Contains all nine of the essential amino acids (the building blocks of protein) that are required for proper protein synthesis and promote healthy, strong muscle.

2

Digestion and Metabolism

Vitamin A helps protect the epithelial cell lining in the GI tract, and high fiber content keeps you regular, preventing diarrhea and constipation.

5

Immunity

Avocados increase the strength of pathogen-fighting cells by aiding with nutrient absorption. They're a great source of glutathione, the "master" antioxidant.

3

Skin, Hair, and Nails

Avocados are packed with biotin, which helps protect cells from damage. Vitamins A and E help skin and nail tissues rebuild and keep hair shiny and lustrous. Avocados also include D-Mannoheptulose sugar that improves collagen formation.

6

Teeth and Bones

Avocados are rich in phosphorous, magnesium, and manganese, which help maintain bone health and reduce your risk for developing osteoporosis.

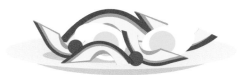

Nutrients were designed to work synergistically in nature. A study published in the *Journal of Nutrition* in March 2005 showed that adding avocados to salad increased absorption of the antioxidant compounds alpha-carotene, beta-carotene, and lutein by five to fifteen times the average amount of these carotenoids absorbed when avocado-free salad was eaten.[11]

I eat at least one avocado almost every day!

GIVE THESE RECIPES A TRY

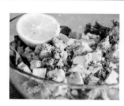

Super Avocado Salad
(page 319)

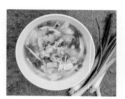

Chicken Avocado Chili
(page 302)

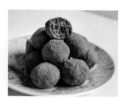

Chocolate Avocado Truffles
(page 325)

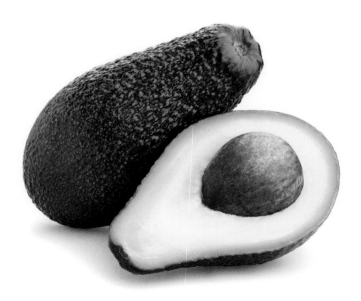

Berries

Berries are not technically ketogenic foods, but because of their low-glycemic impact and high nutrient density, I'm putting them on the list. The net carb count for 3.5 ounces of blackberries is only 5 grams. Raspberries and strawberries are a little higher at 6 grams, and the same serving size of blueberries contains 12 grams of net carbs.

Although you should limit your overall fruit intake to maintain ketosis, a small handful of berries can provide significant benefits. Berries are rich sources of phenolic compounds, which are shown to help reduce the risk of cardiovascular disease and cancer and incite anti-inflammatory responses that prevent tissue damage associated with high blood sugar and diabetes.[12,13]

GIVE THESE RECIPES A TRY

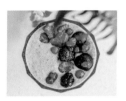

Sweet Raspberry Shake
(page 346)

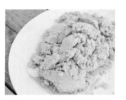

Chocolate Raspberry Cream
(page 322)

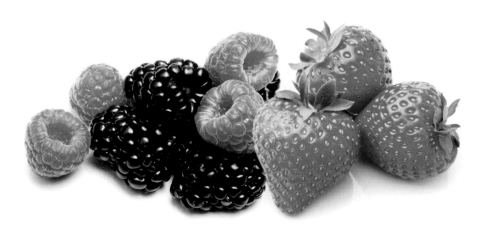

Eggs

Eggs are an excellent source of protein. Each egg contains just one net carb. Eating them can significantly improve satiety levels, and you can readily enjoy them on a ketogenic diet.

Despite their bad reputation, egg yolks are a critical part of the egg. Essential nutrients such as folate, B12, zinc, choline, and the fat-burning compound conjugated linoleic acid (CLA) are concentrated in the egg yolk. Research shows that eating the whole egg improves lipid profiles compared to eating only the egg white. Eggs and their yolks also alleviate symptoms of metabolic syndrome by improving insulin resistance and supporting weight loss.[14, 15] When possible, opt for organic, free-range eggs from a local farmer, and enjoy this keto-friendly food.

GIVE THESE RECIPES A TRY

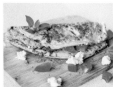
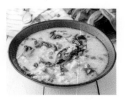

Tomato Basil Omelet
(page 270)

Egg Drop Soup
(page 317)

EGG FACTS

 Eggs are full of protein and healthy nutrients like iron, zinc, folate, and vitamins like A, D, and E.

 In the yolks is where you'll find half of an egg's protein and nutrients!

 Lutein in eggs helps keep your eyes and heart healthy.

 White and brown eggs have the same nutritional content.

 An egg a day is okay! Enjoy an egg every day without increasing your risk of heart disease.

Meat and Poultry

Organic grass-fed beef and pasture-raised poultry are must-have keto staples. Eating clean proteins helps limit your intake of toxins, hormones, and other harmful agents that accumulate in conventional meat products. Organic, pasture-raised beef and chicken contain omega-3 fatty acids that support brain function, promote heart health, and help maintain healthy blood sugar levels. Grass-fed meats are a rich source of CLA, which supports your immune system and boosts metabolic function.[16, 17] These proteins are excellent sources of B vitamins, zinc, and selenium, which is a trace element that acts as a powerful antioxidant that studies have linked to a reduction in inflammatory diseases.[18]

GIVE THESE RECIPES A TRY

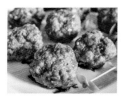

Turkey Sausage Balls
(page 271)

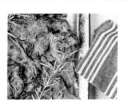

Lime Herb Lamb Chops
(page 308)

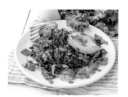

Naked Kale Burger Sauté
(page 310)

Fish

Wild-caught fish is a phenomenal source of the omega-3 fatty acids EPA and DHA. Research shows that eating fish three times a week is associated with successful weight management, thanks to the role of omega-3 in improving insulin resistance.[19] Consuming at least two servings of wild-caught (even farm-raised) fish per week is associated with a decrease in chronic diseases, including cancer and Alzheimer's.[20, 21]

Wild-caught fish such as salmon, mackerel, and sardines protect cardiovascular function, provide antioxidant protection to boost cellular health, and inhibit neurological degeneration.[22] A high-quality fish oil supplement is also an excellent way to benefit from all that fish has to offer.

GIVE THESE RECIPES A TRY

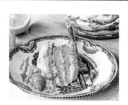

Savory Salmon
Pancakes
(page 274)

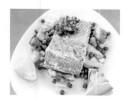

Super Salmon
Salad
(page 315)

HEALTH BENEFITS OF SALMON

1 Reduces risk of cancer and cardiovascular diseases

2 Aids in maintaining healthy skin and hair

3 Helps prevent macular degeneration and loss of vision

4 Helps maintain healthy insulin sensitivity in the body

5 Good source of vitamins, proteins, and minerals

6 Improves memory and efficiency of brain functions

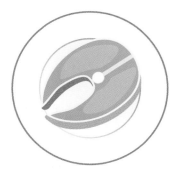

Seaweed

Seaweed is a nutritional powerhouse that reduces inflammation and repairs oxidative damage. It even helps to prevent inflammatory diseases such as cancer. Seaweed is rich in vitamin B6 and vitamin C, as well as the trace minerals phosphorus, potassium, zinc, iron, magnesium, selenium, and iodine. These provide immune system support, reduce blood pressure, curb cravings, and balance hormones.[23]

Seaweed contains other agents that provide a wide array of health benefits such as fatty acids and amino acids. These compounds help reduce inflammation and improve healthy aging and longevity.[24]

GIVE THESE RECIPES A TRY

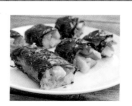

Smoked Salmon
Sushi Rolls
(page 278)

Grass-Fed Butter and Ghee

Although not everyone on a keto diet tolerates dairy well, full-fat dairy can provide significant benefits for those adhering to a keto lifestyle. Grass-fed sources of butter, cream, and ghee (clarified butter) are power-packed with nutrition. Surprisingly, research has shown that these full-fat products reduce the likelihood that a person will be overweight or obese.[25]

Full-fat, grass-fed cow's milk dairy is one of the world's most abundant sources of essential fatty acids and vitamins A, D, E, and K. These nutrients help reduce inflammation, increase metabolism, balance insulin levels, support gut health, and encourage detoxification pathways to operate more efficiently.[26, 27]

One of the benefits of consuming ghee is that those with dairy sensitivities tolerate it well because it contains no lactose, whey, or casein. Of course, if you have a life-threatening dairy allergy, you shouldn't use ghee. However, you can still enjoy the many delicious dairy substitutes made from coconuts and almonds.

GIVE THESE RECIPES A TRY

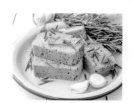

Garlic and
Rosemary Bread
(page 292)

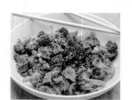

Beef and Buttered
Broccoli
(page 309)

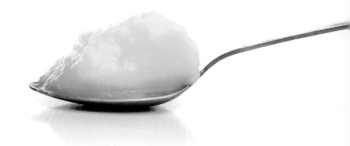

Coconut Milk and Coconut Milk Yogurt

Nondairy coconut milk and coconut milk yogurt are excellent sources of healthy fat. They contain medium-chain triglycerides (MCTs) that are known to help boost metabolism, energize the brain, and balance hormones.[28] The MCTs in coconut milk and coconut milk yogurt have been shown to protect against the formation of plaque in arteries and are associated with a reduced risk of heart attack and stroke.[29]

Organic, full-fat coconut milk is an ideal and satisfying addition to smoothies, stews, and ketogenic desserts. Also, unsweetened coconut milk yogurt is an option that's perfect for individuals with dairy intolerances. Just make sure you get the unsweetened version that is low in net carbs.

GIVE THESE RECIPES A TRY

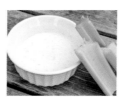

Ranch Dressing
(page 287)

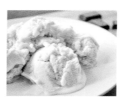

No-Churn Coconut Milk Ice Cream
(page 334)

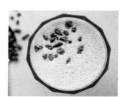

Chocolate Coconut Milkshake
(page 345)

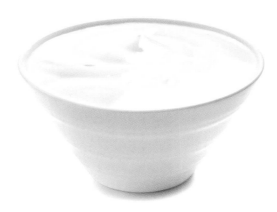

Dark Chocolate and Cocoa

You may be surprised (and happy) to hear this: Chocolate is on the keto menu! However, the type of chocolate matters. Dark chocolate is rich in antioxidant compounds and critical minerals such as magnesium. One ounce of chocolate made with 100 percent cacao powder contains just three grams of net carbs.

Unrefined cacao powder is often called a superfood because of its high concentration of flavanols and corresponding antioxidant effects. Raw cocoa is the world's best source of antioxidants, boasting forty times the number of antioxidants per milligram of blueberries.

Researchers have linked cocoa powder to improved heart and brain function because of its role in increasing circulation and reducing oxidative stress.[30] So, feel free to indulge in a little unsweetened dark chocolate.

GIVE THESE RECIPES A TRY

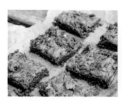

Keto Brownies
(page 328)

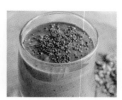

Chocolate Chia
Super Smoothie
(page 342)

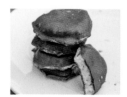

Peppermint Patties
(page 326)

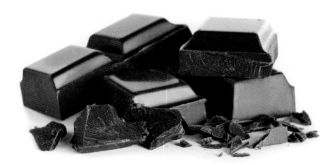

Cheese

Moderate amounts of organic cheese can be a significant part of a keto lifestyle for those who don't have an intolerance to dairy protein. Organic cheese from grass-fed animals contains CLAs that help drive metabolism, burn fat, and enhance immunity.

Cheese is a natural source of saturated fats, which, despite popular opinion, have been positively linked to improved cholesterol levels and decreased risk for cardiovascular-related disease.[31] Raw forms of cheese can even aid in digestion thanks to the presence of milk's natural enzymes, which serve to break down lactose and increase the availability of nutrients such as calcium, magnesium, vitamins A, D, and K2, and protein.

Some people find that they digest goat or sheep cheese better than cow cheese, so you may want to try one of those options.

GIVE THESE RECIPES A TRY

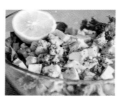

Super Avocado Salad
(page 319)

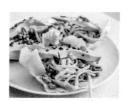

Taco Lettuce Wraps
(page 312)

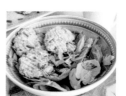

Keto Hash Browns
(page 272)

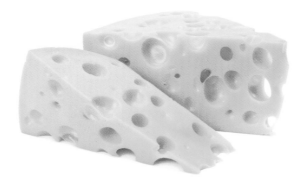

Cream Cheese, Sour Cream, and Cottage Cheese

Cream cheese, sour cream, and cottage cheese made without added sugar or sweeteners can be great allies in your keto journey. These foods can help stabilize blood sugar and insulin levels and provide protein to help control appetite and improve energy.[32, 33]

Cottage cheese contains a little more protein (14 grams) than the 9 grams of protein per ½ cup serving of cream cheese. Cream cheese has significantly more fat—41 grams—but it has only 3 net carbs in ½ cup, so it's an ideal keto food. Cottage cheese is high in protein but low in fat, so I recommend that you add other healthy fats to cottage cheese to make it a keto meal. Sour cream has 24 grams of fat, 5 net carbs, and 4 grams of protein in ½ cup, so it's also an excellent high-fat, low-carb food for a keto dieter.

As with any form of dairy, the best options of these foods are those sourced from grass-fed cows. Try a little dollop of cottage cheese, sour cream, or cream cheese with some of the recipes in this book.

GIVE THESE RECIPES A TRY

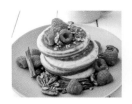

Cinnamon Pancakes
(page 269)

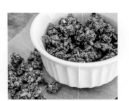

Chocolate Collagen Granola
(page 268)

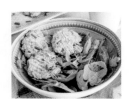

Keto Hash Browns
(page 272)

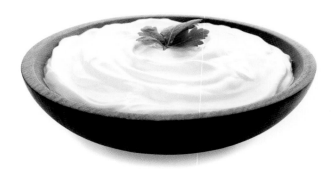

MCT Oil

Medium-chain triglycerides (also commonly referred to as MCTs or MCT oil) are fatty acids naturally found in coconut and palm oils. When appropriately used, MCTs have a remarkable ability to enhance ketone production and stabilize blood sugar.[34] The "medium" in the name refers to the length of the carbon chain (medium is classified as being between six and twelve carbons). MCTs include

- C6 (caproic acid)
- C8 (caprylic acid)
- C10 (capric acid)
- C12 (lauric acid)

Coconut oil is 50 percent lauric acid (C12); another 15 percent of coconut oil is C6, C8, and C10. Lauric acid is a beneficial fatty acid, but it metabolizes more slowly than the other MCTs and relies upon bile to be adequately digested (and is therefore not as ketogenic). C6 is the most common fatty acid to cause digestive problems, whereas C8 converts into ketones the fastest and most proficiently. Because C8 is the type that converts into ketones most efficiently, the most beneficial MCT oil or MCT oil powder supplements are comprised primarily of C8 and C10.

Many experts say that MCTs act like carbohydrates because they provide an immediate energy source. However, MCTs differ from carbohydrates in that they do not raise blood sugar or increase insulin levels. MCT oil can serve as a healthy substitute for heavy coffee and tea creamer, and it has many practical uses in cooking.

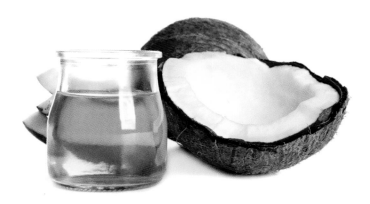

Approximate Fatty Acid Content of Some Commonly Used Oils in Food								
	Approximate grams per 100g of different chain length fatty acids							
Food	Short- and medium-chain triglycerides					Long-chain triglycerides		
	4	6	8	10	12	14	16	18+
Coconut oil	—	0.6	7.5	6	44	16	8.2	2.8
Coconut cream	—	0.1	1.4	1.1	8.4	3	1.1	1.2
Butter	3.2	2	1.2	2.5	2.6	7.4	22	34
Palm oil	—	0.2	3.3	3.7	47	16.4	8.1	14
Olive oil	—	—	—	—	—	—	12.5	83.5

GIVE THESE RECIPES A TRY

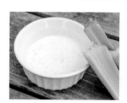

Ranch Dressing
(page 287)

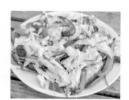

Chicken Fajita Salad
(page 306)

Coconut Oil

Coconut oil is perhaps the most well-known keto staple. Coconut oil provides many benefits, including helping to regulate blood sugar and hormone levels, boost thyroid function, fuel the body's metabolic demands, and provide healing support to cells, tissues, and organs.[35, 36] In one twelve-week study, obese patients who added coconut oil to their diets experienced a notable decrease in abdominal fat.[37]

Coconut oil is an affordable, effective way to burn fat and boost brain function. You can use it for cooking and in smoothies and hot beverages. Virgin coconut oil contains the highest concentration of MCTs that are converted easily into ketones.

GIVE THESE RECIPES A TRY

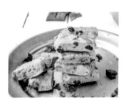

Protein Bars
(page 290)

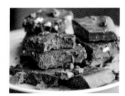

Chocolate Collagen Squares
(page 324)

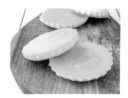

Turmeric Coconut Cream Cups
(page 330)

Olive Oil

Olive oil is a healthy fat that is yet another ketogenic powerhouse. It has long been a staple in Mediterranean diets, and its high concentration of oleic acid is linked to a reduction in cardiovascular disease.[38] Olive oil also contains vitamin E, which helps scavenge free radicals, support healthy blood flow, and improve blood sugar stability.[39, 40]

Unrefined extra-virgin olive oil contains the highest concentration of antioxidants. However, once the oil is heated or processed in any way, its beneficial compounds are easily destroyed. For this reason, it's best not to heat olive oil beyond low to medium-low heat. Olive oil is perhaps best used as a salad dressing base. I enjoy making fresh dressings with olive oil, lemon juice, and herbs.

GIVE THESE RECIPES A TRY

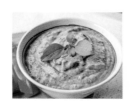

Avocado Pesto
(page 286)

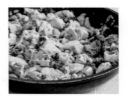

Chicken Lo Mein
(page 303)

OLIVES VS OLIVE OIL

The distinction between the fruit and the oil lies in the preparation and processing. There are pros and cons to both, but when consumed in recommended servings, they're both incredibly beneficial to your health.

Percentage of Fat	Olives		Olive Oil
	25%	VS	100%

Higher sodium	Lower sodium
Olives are cured or pickled in salt	Almost zero sodium
Beneficial polyphenol content is lower than olive oil, but polyphenols are still highly present in fruits harvested early and those that were irrigated properly.	Beneficial polyphenols are preserved in extra-virgin olive oil.

Olives are a great source of sodium, potassium, fiber, vitamin A, vitamin E, biotin, copper, calcium, and B vitamins.

Olives

Most of the carbohydrates found in olives are fiber, which means that a serving of olives (around seven olives) contains just one gram of net carbs. Eating olives can increase glutathione, which benefits the cardiovascular system and may help hinder cancer cell growth.[41]

The polyphenols hydroxytyrosol and oleuropein in olives are what give them their distinct taste and aroma. These compounds have a high absorption rate, which makes them readily available to the body.[42] Oleuropein has been shown to produce anti-inflammatory, anticancer, and antibacterial benefits.

GIVE THESE RECIPES A TRY

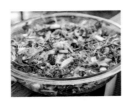

Super Sprout
Chicken Salad
(page 314)

Coconut Flakes, Flour, and Butter

Coconut flakes, flour, and butter are foundational ketogenic foods. The high amounts of fiber in these foods have been shown to decrease blood glucose levels and lower the risk for diabetes. The fiber in these products also can help prevent gut-related cancers.[43]

Unsweetened coconut flakes are a tasty way to help reduce triglyceride and LDL levels while increasing HDL levels.[44] It's easy to incorporate coconut flakes into your daily routine by adding them to trail mix, keto desserts, and smoothies, or even using them as an alternative to breadcrumbs. (Coconut flake–coated chicken is delicious.)

COCONUT FLOUR

 Baking with 100% coconut flour

Wheat in recipe	Coconut flour	Increase eggs	Increase liquids

1 cup = ⅓ cup + one egg + more

per ounce flour | water or coconut milk

 Using coconut flour in small doses

Recipe calls for	Add other grain flour	Add coconut flour	Increase liquids

2 cups = 1 cup + 1 cup + 1 cup

(other grain flour) | divide recipe | (add needed amount to equal original recipe) | (add same amount of liquid as coconut flour)

 Helpful tips & suggestions

- Eggs help bind. Use 1 egg per ounce of coconut flour (8 ounces in 1 cup).
- Don't want to use eggs? Use flax seeds.
  1 tablespoon flax seeds soaked in 3 tablespoon water = 1 egg
- Coconut flour is very absorbent. Add enough liquid to get batter to desired consistency.
- Use a liquid sweetener to help bind.
- Coconut flour is clumpy. Mix it with liquid ingredients and beat well.
- Use less coconut flour. Use ⅓ cup coconut flour to 1 cup other grain flour.
- Baking time is shorter with coconut flour. If a wheat flour recipe takes 30 to 50 minutes, a coconut flour recipe will take 18 to 20 minutes.
- Baking with coconut flour takes time. Be patient.

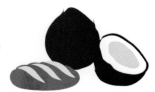

GIVE THESE RECIPES A TRY

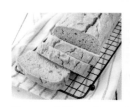

Coconut Flour Bread
(page 291)

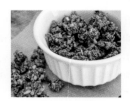

Chocolate Collagen Granola
(page 268)

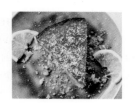

Coconut Custard Lemon Pie
(page 329)

Shirataki Noodles and Heart of Palm Noodles

Shirataki noodles are made from a fermentable dietary fiber known as *glucomannan*, which can hold up to fifty times its weight in water. Consequently, a serving of shirataki noodles has just one gram of net carbs! Studies suggest that people who eat 2 to 4 grams of these noodles every day are more likely to maintain a healthy weight, thanks to glucomannan's ability to increase satiety and promote digestion. Studies show that glucomannan also reduces the glycemic load of certain foods and supports healthy cholesterol levels.[45]

Individuals with type 2 diabetes can experience significant health benefits by eating shirataki noodles. Although glucose levels increased following a meal with glucomannan, insulin levels in people with type 2 diabetes were minimally affected.[46, 47] One popular brand of shirataki noodles available in stores and online is called Miracle noodles.

You also can try noodles made from hearts of palm. Hearts of palm are a nonstarchy vegetable cultivated from the inner bud of certain palm trees. They're rich in prebiotic fiber and trace minerals. Sliced hearts of palm make a tasty addition to salads and stir-fries. My family has come to *love* one particular brand of hearts of palm noodles: Palmini.

Hold the tomato sauce (because it's too high in carbs). Instead add some great olive oil or the Avocado Pesto (page 286), add some chicken or beef if you choose, and you have a terrific keto pasta meal!

Apple Cider Vinegar

Apple cider vinegar (ACV) is a powerful supplement loaded with incredible, living nutrients. The most healing form of ACV is raw and unpasteurized, with the "mother" intact. The mother is the fermented portion of the apple that contains a wealth of healthy bacteria and beneficial enzymes that help the body digest nutrients.

ACV is also a rich source of organic acids, which help with insulin response and decrease inflammation. Here's something that's good news for those keeping an eye on their blood sugar levels: ACV has been shown to help balance blood sugar when taken with meals. Research has shown that ACV can significantly reduce the glycemic index of a carbohydrate-rich meal.[48] So, be sure to add ACV to meats, vegetables, and other foods, or enjoy a drink made with ACV to get an extra helping of antioxidants and enzymes.

An added benefit to adding ACV to your meat and vegetable dishes is that the strong acids begin to break down the food before it goes in your mouth. This helps make the meal easier to digest and assimilate and takes stress off of your digestive system.

GIVE THESE RECIPES A TRY

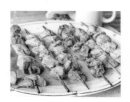

Golden Lime Chicken Kebabs
(page 304)

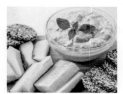

Creamy Lemony Superfood Guacamole
(page 285)

Organ Meats

Organ meats fit perfectly into the ketogenic diet model. They have high amounts of healthy fats, moderate protein levels, and very low carbohydrates. Organ meats from organic, pasture-raised animals are among the most nutritionally dense foods you can consume.

The most common and easy-to-find organ meat is liver. A common misconception is that the liver stores toxins and that consuming animal liver increases your body's toxic load. The liver functions to deactivate toxins, and then those toxins are transported from the liver and stored in our fat cells. So liver and other organ meats from organic, pasture-raised sources are low in toxins and very high in nutrients that support your body's ability to cleanse and heal. Liver and other organ meats also contain a concentrated amount of B vitamins and CoQ10, which is a coenzyme that is particularly beneficial for the brain and heart.

You can purchase beef liver from your local farmers who raise grass-fed cows or from online companies such as US Wellness Meats (https://grasslandbeef.com/). Try adding chicken liver to soups or stews. You can grind up beef liver and mix it with ground beef to mask the flavor of the liver, which some people find unappealing.

Bone Broth

Bone broth has become extremely popular over the last several years, but it has been used traditionally by cultures all over the world for much longer. Bone broth fits the ketogenic model by being high fat, moderate in protein, and extremely low in carbs. Bone broth is most often made from the bones of fish, chicken, turkey, beef, lamb, or venison. The secret behind bone broth's power is that the bones of these animals contain a wealth of nutrients that release after they've simmered in water for several hours. One of those nutrients is bone marrow, which helps provide the raw materials for healthy blood cells and immune development.

Other nutrients include gelatin, collagen, hyaluronic acid, chondroitin sulfate, potassium, calcium, magnesium, glycosaminoglycans, proline, glycine, and phosphorus. These nutrients are linked with benefits such as the healthy development of hair, skin, bones, joints, ligaments, and tendons.[49, 50, 51, 52]

GIVE THESE RECIPES A TRY

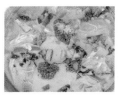

Coconut Curry Soup
(page 318)

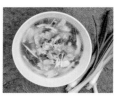

Chicken Avocado Chili
(page 302)

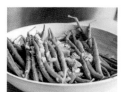

Garlic Herb Green Beans
(page 296)

THE INCREDIBLE TRUTH ABOUT
CARB AND CALORIE BACK-LOADING

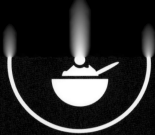

Carb back-loading is an innovative nutritional strategy that is showing promise for affecting energy production, fat-burning, and muscle-building and improving sleep quality. In this chapter, I explain the science behind this useful strategy and teach you how to apply calorie and carb back-loading to a ketogenic lifestyle.

The concept of carb back-loading is difficult to grasp because it sharply contradicts what we grew up believing about energy and eating. Most of us have learned that the morning is the best time to eat carbs to fuel the day, and, as our energy requirements decrease in the evening, we should eat fewer carbs. If we fail to adhere to these guidelines, we store the carbs we eat at night as fat.

Carb back-loading is essentially the opposite approach: You consume little to no net carbs during the day, and then you eat more carbohydrates in the evening. This strategy takes advantage of our natural morning physiology to stabilize blood sugar and stimulate fat-burning.

As a companion to carb back-loading, calorie back-loading is also a highly useful tool. The idea is to eat lightly during the daytime and reserve the majority of your daily calories for a large evening meal. For example, if you're eating 2,000 calories per day, you consume 600 to 800 of those calories during the day, and then you eat the remaining 1,200 to 1,400 calories during dinner.

Maintaining a caloric deficit throughout most of the day increases fat-burning processes and enhances ketone production. The substantial evening meal then stimulates your body's ability to use glucose as fuel and initiates thyroid hormone secretion, which activates cellular metabolism.

In this way, you're teaching your body to be metabolically flexible—meaning it's adept at using ketones as fuel earlier in the day and glucose later in the evening. In essence, you become a fat-burning powerhouse!

Back-Loading and Your Hormones

Carb back-loading works by optimizing your body's hormones to maximize fat-burning—more specifically, by controlling when insulin production takes place. When you're asleep, the production of the fat-storing hormone (insulin) shuts down, and the production of fat-burning hormones increases. In the morning, you naturally have elevated levels of powerful fat-incinerating hormones such as cortisol, noradrenaline, and human growth hormone (hGH), which is why that is prime fat-burning time!

However, when you eat carbs early in the morning and throughout the day, those beneficial hormone levels plummet, and insulin production once again elevates. Insulin signals the body to burn glucose as its primary fuel and store body fat. It also causes a cascade of unfortunate events such as increased hunger, cravings, fatigue, and brain fog.

The goal of carb and calorie back-loading is to stop this vicious cycle and to optimize fat-burning by suppressing insulin production until the evening. Following is what a typical day might look like when you practice carb and calorie back-loading:

- In the morning, you either fast while drinking calorie- and sugar-free liquids (water, tea, and coffee), or you consume a light meal that's high in protein and fat and contains minimal carbs. You also can eat fibrous foods such as nuts, seeds, and nonstarchy veggies. The goal is to consume only foods and liquids that do not elicit a glycemic response.

- At lunchtime, continue fasting or eat a small meal that is protein- and fat-rich; also avoid eating carbs (other than fiber). Again, nonstarchy veggies, nuts, and seeds are acceptable.

- For dinner, eat a large meal that contains nutrient-dense carbohydrates such as sweet potatoes, pumpkin, beets, carrots, berries, cassava, tapioca, and arrowroot flours.

Your body naturally stores sugar in a form called "glycogen" in your liver and muscles to use when needed, such as during periods of fasting, undereating, or exercising. Your body better tolerates carbohydrates in the evening because that is when glycogen stores are at their lowest. Because your body is seeking to fill these stores, eating these foods won't trigger fat storage. You can enhance the effects of this strategy even more if you exercise during the day.

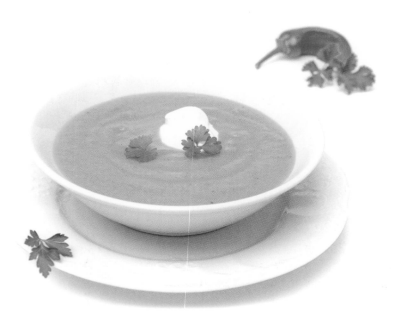

CARB AND CALORIE BACKLOADING BASICS

Step 1

Either fast or follow a low-calorie, keto-style nutrition plan during the day.

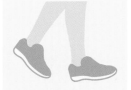

Step 2

Exercise with light cardio in the AM (could just be taking a long walk) and resistance training in the afternoon before your dinner feast.

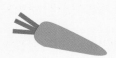

Step 3

Feast on healthy carbs, proteins, and fats from 5:00 to 7:00 PM.

Step 4

Stop eating at least three to four hours before bed to maximize fat-burning and muscle-building hormone release at night.

The training isn't necessary but will help improve fat burning and muscle development.

Insulin and Cortisol

In the morning, cortisol levels are at their peak, and your body is most sensitive to insulin.[1] Cortisol's main job is to liberate stored glycogen so your body can use it as fuel, and the heightened insulin sensitivity during the early hours makes this possible.[2] Once your body works through an adequate amount of glycogen, it begins burning fat. However, eating carbohydrates during this period of higher cortisol stops your body from burning up the glycogen and fat. You can keep this from happening by avoiding net carbs and excessive calories during the day.

Insulin and Thyroid Hormone

Would you be better off by never stimulating the production of insulin at all? Definitely not. Insulin is required for proper thyroid hormone activation and the conversion of inactive T4 into its active form, T3. Adequate T3 levels are what signal cells to produce energy by metabolizing both glucose and fat.[3]

However, keeping insulin levels elevated all day long also promotes fat storage and inflammation. So, the solution is to strategically stimulate insulin production—enough to support T3 activation but not enough to put the body into fat-storage mode. The added benefit of producing an isolated insulin response in the later hours is that your body can enjoy the fat-burning benefits of active T3 as you sleep!

Ultimately, it is the *continuous* insulin response that causes the most problems for many people because constant insulin surges disrupt blood sugar levels, cause hormone imbalance, and increase inflammation. Carb back-loading remedies this by promoting insulin production just once per day. Unless you're already highly insulin resistant, one insulin response per day is well tolerated and does not disrupt fat-burning physiology.

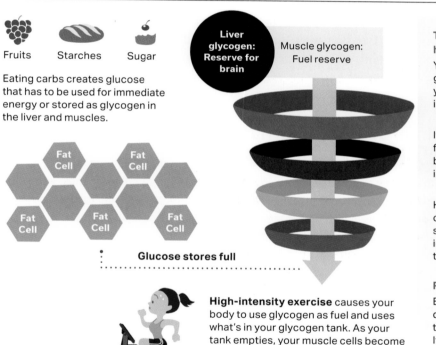

Fruits   Starches   Sugar

Eating carbs creates glucose that has to be used for immediate energy or stored as glycogen in the liver and muscles.

Liver glycogen: Reserve for brain

Muscle glycogen: Fuel reserve

Fat Cell   Fat Cell
Fat Cell   Fat Cell   Fat Cell

Glucose stores full

The capacity of the human glycogen tank
You hold around 100 grams of glycogen in your liver and 400 grams in your muscles.

If your glycogen tank is full, glucose pools in the blood, which increases insulin levels.

Higher insulin levels cause sugar to be stored as fat and increases inflammation throughout the body.

Result
Body fat and cellular damage increase throughout your body. If you continually create this reaction, you develop insulin resistance over time.

High-intensity exercise causes your body to use glycogen as fuel and uses what's in your glycogen tank. As your tank empties, your muscle cells become more insulin sensitive. As insulin levels drop, your body burns fat for fuel more efficiently.

Keto and Carb Back-Loading Cycles
A well-formulated ketogenic diet with an occasional carb back-loading cycle will continually deplete glycogen stores, stimulate fat-burning, and strategically increase glycogen stores to enhance physical and mental performance.

Benefits of Carb Back-Loading

The benefits of back-loading are well documented, and they're similar to some of the most significant benefits of following a ketogenic eating plan, making the two strategies extremely synergistic. Here are some of the benefits of practicing carb and calorie back-loading.

Improved Energy and Mental Clarity

Most people notice considerably enhanced levels of energy and mental clarity through strategically manipulating their calorie and carbohydrate intake because back-loading works to accentuate the benefits the stress hormones provide. Stress hormones such as cortisol and norepinephrine are designed to give you energy. Keeping carb and calorie intake restricted while the production of these hormones is at their highest amplifies their effects.

Improved Fat-Burning

Carb and calorie back-loading help the body burn fat all day *and* all night. During the day, back-loading pushes your body to use fat as its fuel. When you strategically produce insulin only at night, your body activates thyroid hormone for increased fat-burning during sleep.

Improved Exercise Performance

Back-loading helps optimize critical hormones involved in cellular energy production and muscle repair. As a result, many athletes who practice carb and calorie back-loading report feeling increased energy and strength during exercise.

Better Sleep

There's nothing like a large meal to make you sleepy. Unfortunately, plenty of people experience this during the day at work after eating a big breakfast or lunch. Instead, consume your most substantial meal that contains carbs in the evening to help minimize your body's production of cortisol and other stress hormones. This strategy also induces the production of serotonin. Serotonin helps you feel calm and satisfied, and it's the precursor to the well-known sleep hormone, melatonin.

The Research on Back-Loading

There's a growing body of research that supports the benefits of back-loading. For example, a 1997 controlled study compared the results for women who calorie front-loaded with women who calorie back-loaded to determine each strategy's overall effect on weight and fat loss over six weeks. The researchers reported that women who consumed 70 percent of their calories in the evening retained the most muscle and lost a higher percentage of body fat compared to the group who ate 70 percent of their calories before dinner.[4]

A more recent study from 2011 followed seventy Israeli police officers for six months. Half of the group followed a diet in which carb intake was spread evenly throughout the day, whereas the other half adhered to a carb back-loading strategy. The back-loading group experienced less hunger, more weight loss, and improved BMIs.[5] The study also examined inflammatory markers and the levels of fat-burning hormones such as leptin and adiponectin. All hormonal and inflammatory markers (including blood glucose and insulin levels) improved in the carb back-loading group.

Another study published in 2013 used seventy-eight obese police officers to determine the hormonal changes that would occur when half the group followed a carb and calorie back-loading plan. Results indicated that those who back-loaded experienced reduced hunger and cravings due to improved levels of leptin, ghrelin, and adiponectin.[6]

Three Steps to Accelerate Back-Loading Results

When I begin to transition patients from their traditional high-carb diet into a healing, ketogenic diet, I always use carb back-loading as a foundational part of the plan. Carb back-loading helps ease your body into keto adaption with minimal side effects. This approach allows you to gain all the beneficial effects of keto while still taking in carbs. One of the leading authorities on this approach is John Kiefer, who has broken the process down into these three simple steps in his book, *Carb Back-loading*.[7]

Step #1: Follow a Strict Keto Diet

For the first ten days, restrict daily carb intake to 20 to 30 net carbs. During this time, 65 to 75 percent of calories should come from fat, 20 to 30 percent from protein, and less than 5 percent from carbs. I recommend combining this with calorie back-loading by eating lightly during the day and enjoying a large dinner. This strategy works best when combined with regular exercise and especially resistance training.

Step #2: Perform a Carb Refeed

On day eleven, observe the same principles as you did the first ten days but work out in the late afternoon/evening and follow that workout with a large meal that contains plenty of carbs. On *refeed days* like this one, add 20 to 80 grams of carbs from nutrient-dense sources such as organic meats, whole fruit, sweet potatoes, carrots, cassava, and tapioca. If you're very lean and highly active, you can handle more carbs. If you're less active or overweight, keep your carbs on the lower end of the range.

Step #3: Repeat and Customize

Begin by carb cycling every ten days, as explained in the first two steps. In general, on days you don't engage in physical activity, you should keep carb intake extremely low. Experiment and find what works for you. Some people find they have the best results with a two- to three-day cycle, whereas others find they feel better when refeeding once every two to three weeks.

If you eat a carb-rich meal, and it takes you several weeks to get back into ketosis, adjust the carb count until you reduce your readaptation time to only a few days. Also, keep in mind that doing resistance training and high-intensity interval training just before your evening meal can reduce the impact of your carb intake.

CUSTOMIZE YOUR CARB CYCLING STRATEGY

Experiment and find the carb refeed cycle that works best for you:

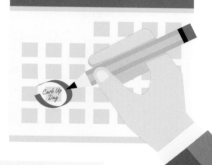

- Twice per week
- Once per week
- Once every 10 to 14 days
- Once per month

When you carb refeed, it's best to add carbs in later in the day to get the carb back-loading benefits.

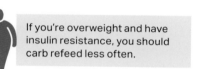 If you're overweight and have insulin resistance, you should carb refeed less often.

 If you're thin and highly active, you'll probably benefit from frequent carb refeeding cycles.

Traditional Carb Back-Loading Versus KMB Back-Loading

It's important to note that traditional carb back-loading and the back-loading I use in *Keto Metabolic Breakthrough* differ somewhat. Traditional back-loading requires consuming lots of carbs in the evening—as much as 100 to 200 grams. However, a target of 20 to 80 grams of carbs is much better because it minimizes inflammatory responses. Use this range to your advantage by setting your initial goal closer to 80 grams of carbs and scale back as you progress toward keto-adaptation. For athletes and those who engage in intense exercise, I recommend you stay in the upper limits of that range, from 60 to 80 grams of net carbs.

My version of this strategy also differs from traditional carb back-loading in that I advise choosing only nutrient-dense carbohydrates for your carb-heavy meals. It's common for those in the carb back-loading community to load up on processed junk foods such as pizza, cake, and ice cream on refeed days. However, I don't advise using this strategy because it can increase your exposure to environmental toxins, cause inflammation, and place undue stress on your gut and immune system.

Are Back-Loading and Ketosis Compatible?

You may be asking yourself, "But won't calorie and carb back-loading knock me out of ketosis?"

The answer to that is yes, it will—but it won't last long.

When you eat a large, carbohydrate-rich meal, your body produces insulin, and that insulin surge stops your body from producing ketones. However, because you'll be calorie and carb restricting for the next eighteen to twenty-four hours following this meal (as you will learn more about in the next chapter), insulin production will once again stop, and you'll begin burning fat and ketones for fuel.

Those who are highly active with plenty of lean body tissue can return to ketosis quickly after the large meal, whereas people who have insulin resistance require more time. For this reason, keto-adapted individuals who are very insulin resistant should stay under 10 grams of net carbs throughout the day and not exceed 20 to 30 grams of net carbs in their evening meal to lessen the amount of time required to get back into ketosis.

The goal of a ketogenic diet is to reach a state of nutritional ketosis, where your body is adapted to burning fat for fuel, and blood ketone levels remain between 0.5 and 3.0 mmol/L. In this state, your system works to preserve lean body tissue and uses fat as its primary fuel source.

When you achieve physiological ketosis, your body undergoes some significant changes. One of the most notable changes is how efficient the body becomes at preserving its stored glycogen. When you're not keto-adapted, your body has to burn through a good percentage of its stored glycogen before you begin burning fat.

However, in a state of ketosis, your body burns ketones and spares a large percentage of the glycogen. For example, if a workout would burn 300 grams of glycogen in a non-keto-adapted individual, it may only use 60 grams of glycogen in a keto-adapted individual (and instead use ketones for the bulk of the energy expenditure).

Therefore, you don't need to "fuel up" on carbs to be highly active, and your body will still be able to restore its glycogen at the end of the day with a single large meal containing carbs. My daily strategy is to consume 30 to 50 net carbs a day, and I eat the majority of those carbs in the evening between 5:00 p.m. and 7:00 p.m. I adjust my total net carb intake as needed depending upon my level of exercise intensity. You may need to experiment for a while before you discover what works best for you.

Every ten days or so, I may bump up my carbs and have 50 to 80 grams in my dinner. I find that my body is so metabolically flexible with this schedule that I am back in nutritional ketosis by midday the following day.

You'll have to experiment to determine the proper carb cycling strategy for your body and gauge how long it takes to get back into ketosis after having a higher carb meal. The less time it takes, the more metabolically flexible and insulin-sensitive your body is. Being able to bounce back into ketosis is a sign of robust metabolic health, and it's a great goal to strive for.

Daily exercise, quality sleep, a positive attitude, and intermittent fasting are all key strategies to implement to improve your metabolic flexibility and insulin sensitivity.

In Chapter 11, your journey begins in earnest as I break down exactly what you need to do to start working toward your keto metabolic breakthrough.

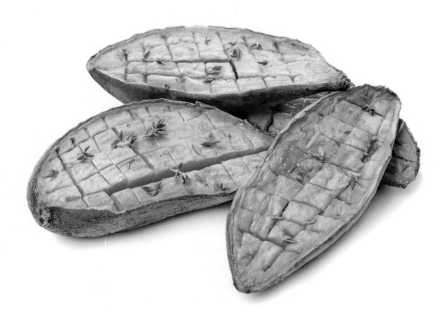

THE KETO METABOLIC BREAKTHROUGH

You should be proud of yourself. You've learned so much! You know the many far-reaching benefits of ketosis, the foods that promote a ketogenic state, and the challenges you may experience on your keto journey. In this chapter, I'm putting the pieces together to provide you with the path to success.

The goal is to get you keto-adapted in the safest, most sustainable way. Many people try to do too much too quickly, and they end up dealing with many of the side effects I discuss in Chapter 8. You can optimize your ability to burn fat by following strict guidelines for a set period. Those guidelines lead to what I like to call a *keto metabolic breakthrough*.

Based on your previous experience with keto and your current lifestyle, there are two potential paths for implementing a ketogenic diet:

- The keto novice path
- The keto veteran path

The primary difference between the novice and veteran paths is in the length of time it takes to transition from a higher carb diet.

I provide you with a detailed plan for both levels of experience and show you how to switch into a fat-burning state gently and effectively, regardless of your present state of health or knowledge of keto.

Before You Begin: Establish a Baseline

No matter whether you're a keto pro but need a structured plan to get you back on track or this is your first time attempting to transition into a keto lifestyle, the first step is the same: keeping a food journal. Start charting everything you eat, no matter how healthy or unhealthy your choices are, and calculate the totals for the following in grams:

- Total calories
- Total fat and calories from fat (1 gram of fat = 9 calories)
- Total protein and calories from protein (1 gram of protein = 4 calories)
- Total carbohydrates and calories from carbs (1 gram of carbs = 4 calories)
- Net carbohydrates (total carbs – fiber)

KETO PRO TIP

To make your life easier, you can use a food tracking app on your smartphone (such as MyFitnessPal or MyPlate). You enter the food you eat, and these apps do all the calculations for you.

Here's an example based on a 2,000-calorie diet:

Total calories	2,000 calories
Total fat	68 grams (612 calories)
Total protein	107 grams (428 calories)
Total carbs	280 grams
Fiber	40 grams (fiber doesn't have calories)
Net carbs	240 grams (960 calories)

Keeping track of your food and macros before you begin adjusting your diet helps you establish your baseline numbers and gives you a clear picture of how to approach your keto-adaptation path. Also, you'll be tracking your macros throughout your keto metabolic breakthrough and beyond, so it's just a good habit to start. Food tracking is an eye-opening experience for many people. Most people are shocked at how many calories and carbs they eat.

Once you get the hang of tracking what you eat and customize your keto journey the way I explain in this chapter, you won't need to track your macros. After a few months have passed, most people have found the foods and food plans that work best for them. Some people choose to continue to count macros, but my goal is to help you transition into a path that requires less effort.

The Keto Novice Path

If eating a high-fat, low-carb diet is new to you, then start here. People often want to jump right in when they first hear about all the benefits of ketosis or see social media posts about people who lose weight rapidly on keto. However, the "full throttle" approach is not a good idea. It's safer and more sustainable for you to transition gradually into a low-carb lifestyle. Your body has spent most of its time operating in sugar-burning mode; it has well-established metabolic machinery in place, and, as I've discussed, it takes time to adapt to a new form of fuel. Here's a practical carb-reduction guideline for a keto novice:

Reduce daily net carb intake by 40 to 50 grams per week.

So, using the earlier 2,000-calorie example, the net carb intake goal for the first week would still be reasonably high—around 200 grams. This method may seem more like a "slow-carb" approach than a "low-carb" one. Just remember that you're not in a race to see who can get into ketosis the fastest. My goal is to help you improve your health, lose weight, and reverse or prevent chronic illness. These are long-term goals that require a solid plan of action.

One additional benefit of taking this gradual approach to phasing out carbs is that you have the chance to use up all the nonketo foods in your refrigerator and pantry. Although some of those foods are probably not healthy, many people have a fixed food budget and prefer to use what they have rather than throw out food. If this describes you, then use these nonketo foods during the transition phase. Once that food is gone, don't buy or keep nonketo foods in the house. (I talk more about this in Chapter 12.)

Stage 1: Four-Week Transition Phase

After you have a baseline for your current caloric and net carb intake, it's time to start slowly reducing your consumption of carbs to minimize keto side effects and help you transition in the healthiest way possible. Here I describe how the next four weeks might look based on a 2,000-calorie diet.

WEEK 1

The net carb count from the example is 240 grams. The goal on the keto novice path is to reduce net carbs by 40 to 50 grams daily per week until you reach the target daily net carb intake and successfully enter ketosis. That means your goal for the first week is 190 to 200 grams of net carbs each day. During this time, it is beneficial to practice back-loading and eat most of those carbs in the evening rather than at breakfast or lunch. The remainder of your calories will come first from healthy fat and then protein. Remember, you're working toward the ultimate goal of taking in 65 to 75 percent of your calories from fat, 20 to 30 percent from protein, and 5 to 10 percent from carbs.

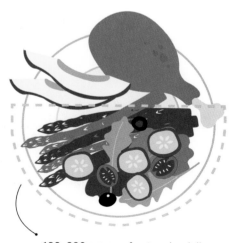

190–200 grams of net carbs daily

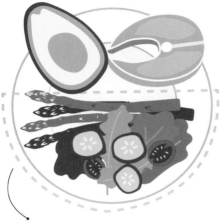

140–150 grams of net carbs daily

WEEK 2

Your net carb goal becomes 140 to 150 grams per day, with healthy fat becoming a more significant part of your diet. Again, using the carb and calorie back-loading principle, you should eat the majority of your carbs later in the day.

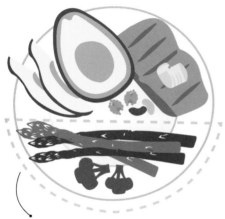

90–100 grams of net carbs daily

WEEK 3

Your total net carb intake becomes 90 to 100 grams per day, with the calorie deficit again being filled through healthy fats. And of course, the calorie and carb back-loading principle still applies.

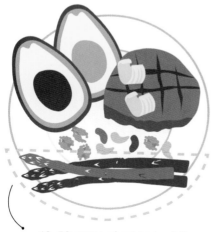

40–50 grams of net carbs daily

WEEK 4

Your goal is 40 to 50 grams of net carbs per day and more fat. Continue practicing back-loading. By this point, your body will most likely begin creating ketones.

Stage 2: Keto Phase

Your body is now primed and ready to dive deeply into ketosis for the next thirty days. For the next month, reduce your net carb intake to 20 to 50 grams per day or less. If you're a highly active individual, you may eat 30 to 50 grams of net carbs; if you're more sedentary, it's best to stay under 30 grams of net carbs.

During this period, regularly monitor your ketone levels to ensure you are, in fact, in nutritional ketosis. After spending thirty days in a ketogenic state, you can begin to experiment with carb cycling, which I describe later in this chapter.

The Keto Veteran Path

If you've successfully done a ketogenic diet in the past, your body is already equipped with the metabolic machinery it needs and will adapt more quickly and effectively than it would if you were trying it for the first time. You may have just come out of ketosis a few weeks ago and are looking to become fat-adapted again, or it may have been months or years since you were in ketosis. Either way, if you had success in the past, you can readily experience success again. However, it's best to ease back into things using the following formula:

Every week out of ketosis = One day of transition

So, let's say you were in ketosis before the holidays, but then you spent six weeks eating high-carb comfort foods. Six weeks equals a six-day transition back into eating 5 to 10 percent of your calories in the form of carbs. If it's been twelve weeks, give yourself twelve days, and so on. However, if it's been more than sixteen weeks since you followed a ketogenic diet, I recommend you follow the keto novice path to be on the safe side.

After you determine your transition length, divide the total number of days in half to create two phases to keto transition. If you have been off the plan for sixteen weeks and therefore need sixteen days of transition, that means each portion will be eight days long. If you require eleven days, stage 1 of the transition will be six days, and stage 2 will be five days.

Stage 1: Two-Part Transition Phase

After you have a baseline for your current caloric and net carb intake, it's time to reduce your consumption of carbs, except that you reduce them on a far more accelerated schedule than those who are keto novices. Here are the guidelines for the two parts:

- **Keto Transition Part I:** Reduce your net carb intake to 70 to 100 grams per day and practice carb back-loading.

- **Keto Transition Part II:** Decrease your net carbs to 50 to 70 grams per day and practice carb back-loading.

Stage 2: Keto Phase

Stage 2 is the same for veterans as it is for novices. For the next thirty days, reduce your net carb intake to 20 to 50 grams per day. If you're a highly active individual, you may have 30 to 50 grams of net carbs; if you're more sedentary, it's best to stay under 30 grams of net carbs.

During this period, regularly monitor your ketone levels to ensure you are, in fact, in nutritional ketosis. After spending thirty days in a ketogenic state, you can begin to experiment with carb cycling, which I describe next.

Where Carb Cycling Fits into the Picture

Once you've experienced a few weeks in nutritional ketosis, you're ready to try carb cycling. Carb cycling is a method where you periodically and strategically eat more carbs to take advantage of the many benefits of carb back-loading I discuss in Chapter 10. Following a ketogenic diet but also practicing carb cycling is often referred to as a cyclical ketogenic diet, and it's a strategy that many long-term keto dieters implement—including me.

Please note that carb cycling is not for everyone. People with specific conditions should maintain ketosis for long periods to gain the benefits desired. Following are some of the issues that don't pair well with carb cycling:

- Significant insulin resistance

- Morbid obesity

- Seizure disorders

- Neurodegenerative conditions

- Brain tumors or other cancers that respond well to ketosis

Additionally, if you feel great in ketosis, you don't need to carb cycle. I recommend carb cycling only if you have been in ketosis for at least a few weeks and are starting to experience a reduction in keto benefits, such as if you experience the following issues or conditions:

- Energy level decrease that persists for several days

- Weight-loss plateau that lasts for at least a week

- Lingering hypothyroid symptoms such as hair loss, feeling cold, and brain fog

- Frequent insomnia

- Reduced physical performance (decrease in strength, speed, or endurance)

Remember that carb cycling may be beneficial for individuals dealing with these symptoms only after they have unquestionably been in ketosis for a few weeks. Also, keep in mind that the preceding symptoms are common keto side effects that you may experience in the early stages of your keto journey, so don't rush to carb cycle if you're still in the transition phase of becoming keto-adapted. However, if you have been keto-adapted for several weeks and the side effects haven't subsided, it's time to consider carb cycling.

There are several other reasons you may want to follow a cyclical ketogenic diet. Maybe you want more freedom and variety in your diet. It's also common for athletes to use this keto diet variation because they want to increase their muscle mass or training endurance. Many athletes find that a 5:2 ratio (where they spend five days of every week following a strict keto plan and then eat more carbs once or twice a week) can be beneficial for improving overall performance. Other athletes need more carb back-loading days, and some need fewer.

When you apply carb cycling, I recommend you use the carb back-loading strategies I discuss in Chapter 10. To fit the plan to your needs, experiment to find the appropriate amount of carbs that make you feel your best, and work to consume those carbs later in the day.

For the majority of people, I recommend starting with a 10:1 ratio, where you spend ten days following a strict keto plan and then enjoy a single day of carb back-loading. From there, you can adjust the carb levels to find what works for you.

It's helpful to track your ketone levels through blood or breath and compare those with how you're feeling. Ultimately, however, the biggest key is to listen to your body. The same carb cycling schedule that works wonders for your best friend may completely derail your progress. We're all unique—and that's a good thing!

Over time, you will know how you feel when you're in ketosis and how you feel when you're out of ketosis for too long. When you develop a kinesthetic understanding of how your body responds to foods and various states, the lifestyle approach to keto becomes so much easier and, frankly, a lot of fun.

Where Intermittent Fasting Fits into the Picture

You will notice that each week on both the novice and veteran paths, I recommended calorie and carb back-loading. If you want to accelerate results, you may take this idea a step further and start practicing intermittent fasting.

Intermittent fasting, or time-restricted eating, is not for everyone, but if you can tolerate it, it's an incredible tool. As I discuss in Chapter 2, intermittent fasting is lengthening the window of time between meals. The practice trains your body to tap into its fat stores and helps improve your metabolism.

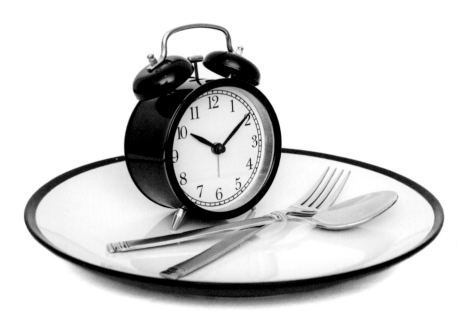

The term "fasting" can be intimidating, but if you think about it, you fast every night while you sleep. With intermittent fasting, you're just increasing the time between your dinner on one day and your first meal the next day.

Start with a twelve-hour window and slowly increase it as your body becomes accustomed to the practice. Consume water and other calorie- and sugar-free beverages such as tea and coffee during the fast. For the best results, avoid putting coffee creamer or anything with calories into your body during the window.

Lots of keto followers find they feel best when they consume just one or two meals in a time window, such as 12:00 p.m. to 6:00 p.m. This means that for eighteen hours a day, your body is fasting! It may sound difficult to go eighteen hours without eating, but it becomes much easier with practice. Some like to use intermittent fasting during the week and take the weekend off, whereas others feel better practicing it seven days a week.

It may take some time to build your metabolic muscles and adhere to an intermittent fasting schedule, but once you do, you'll be amazed at how energetic and mentally alert you feel—and how easily you get back into ketosis after a carb-rich meal.

7 WAYS TO DO DAILY INTERMITTENT FASTING

1 **Simple fast:** 12 hours

2 **Brunch fast:** 14 hours

3 **Crescendo fast:** 16 hours, 2 days per week

4 **Cycle fast:** 16 hours, 3 days per week

5 **Strong fast:** 16 to 18 hours daily

6 **Warrior fast:** 19 to 21 hours daily

7 **1-day fast:** Full 24-hour fast each week

Meet Heidi

Eating well is hard. It is perhaps one of the hardest challenges we face in our modern society. I have met patient after patient who shares this struggle; believe me, you are not alone.

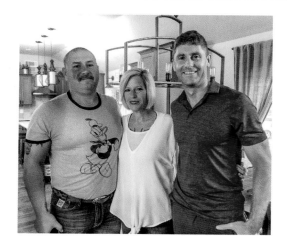

One such person is Heidi. She was depressed, significantly overweight, and in pain. Heidi had fallen off of every single fad diet bandwagon that came along for years on end. Eventually, she battled with psoriasis, arthritis, and chronic pain so severe that it often prevented her from getting out of bed. Acid reflux kept her up at night, and she had zero energy for anything.

My keto challenge caught her attention, but she wasn't ready. She recognized the need for a change, but comfort food is *really* comforting and also *really* difficult to kick. It took Heidi two months to convince herself even to try the plan!

Once she got started, she quickly realized just how badly she was addicted to sugar and carbs. We followed the keto novice approach and slowly started reducing her net carb intake. By week 2, the scale started showing some real progress. Also, her skin began to clear, her inflammation cooled, and her brain fog lifted.

After one month, Heidi transitioned into a full keto diet and felt incredible. Once she discovered the fat-burning foods that worked best for her, the results were undeniable. After a few months, Heidi began to go for walks around her neighborhood. A year later—and 130 pounds gone from her frame—she walks five days a week, has abundant energy, and loves life!

Many of us can relate to Heidi's journey. We all struggle with letting go of something, even though we know that when we do, it will be so freeing. The keys are patience and persistence. Stay the course, realize that making the change takes a marathoner's mentality rather than a sprinter's mindset, and know that the benefits of being in fat-burning mode are real and attainable!

In the next chapter, I discuss the mindset needed for success and go over the must-have essentials you should have in your kitchen to make keto a healthy and sustainable lifestyle.

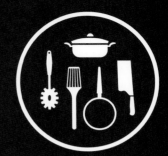

CHAPTER 12

THE KETO METABOLIC KITCHEN MAKEOVER

Let's face it—making lifestyle changes is *not easy*. You've probably been eating the same way for a long time, and old habits can be hard to shake.

The key to making the changes I describe in this book a permanent part of your lifestyle is through consistent practice. Healthy lifestyle habits are a skill set that you must carefully hone and practice as you would any other skill. You must also intentionally create an environment where you can more easily adhere to healthy lifestyle principles so that they become automatic habits rather than forced or unnatural additions to your day.

The challenge is that we have to handle a lot of daily demands in our work, home, and social lives. Consequently, we often feel that we don't have much energy left to develop another set of skills. However, learning to apply a keto lifestyle will help your energy and mental clarity, and that will improve your work life, family life, and social activities.

As you read, remember that expectations are vitally important to your keto metabolic breakthrough. Understand that you don't have to master everything at once. If it helps, think of this book and its principles like a college course. You would never think of taking the final exam on day one—that would just set you up for failure!

It takes time to absorb the material, apply it to your life, set up routines that support the changes, and troubleshoot challenges. If it takes you three to six months to experience the keto metabolic breakthrough effect fully, that is okay and normal!

In this chapter, I cover the importance of lightening the stress load you place on yourself, explain how to set yourself up for success, and give you strategies for overcoming cravings. I also provide a useful guide for what to keep on hand in your kitchen to support long-term success.

The Success Equation

Everyone learns, applies, and masters principles at a different rate depending upon three things:

- Level of motivation
- Level of knowledge on the topic
- Level of stress and pressure in life

The following "success equation" shows you how these three pieces of the puzzle interact:

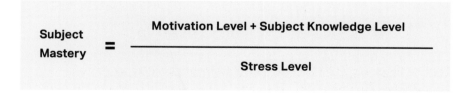

$$\text{Subject Mastery} = \frac{\text{Motivation Level} + \text{Subject Knowledge Level}}{\text{Stress Level}}$$

Assuming that the three pieces of the formula are measured on a scale from 1 to 10 (with 1 being very little to none and 10 being the highest possible level), the ideal level of mastery on a subject such as keto is a 2 or higher. A mastery ratio of at least 2 enables you to move in a positive direction and make tangible progress. In other words, your level of motivation and knowledge about keto should be twice as much as your level of stress.

For example, let's say you would consider yourself to be highly motivated, and your amount of knowledge concerning keto is about half what it should be, but you have a high-stress job, multiple demands at home, and an extremely active social life. A numeric representation of this might look like this:

Motivation level = 8/10

Keto knowledge level = 5/10

Stress level = 10/10

Mastery of keto = (8 + 5) / 10 = 1.3

At 1.3, your mastery ratio is too low to expect sustainable results. Once you finish this book, you will undoubtedly know more about ketosis and overall health, but increasing your knowledge alone will not reduce your stressors and demands in life.

If you feel your stress and pressure level is consistently near a level 10, one of the first things you need to do as you begin is an honest examination of your priorities. In the interest of your health, you may need to put a few of your less critical obligations on the back burner or ask your family for more help. You may also need to temporarily scale back your social engagements if your social life revolves around carb-rich restaurant foods and alcohol.

All the knowledge and motivation in the world can't compensate for being chronically overstressed and frequently placing yourself in the path of temptation. Use the tips in this chapter to help lower your stress level, and don't be afraid to ask for help from your close friends and loved ones.

The Three Ps of Nutrition and Lifestyle Success

Three action steps are critical to helping make things easier for you and lowering the stressors and demands as you work toward your keto metabolic breakthrough. I call them the *Three Ps*, and they are the foundational principles required to make any significant health-related lifestyle change sustainable:

- Plan ahead

- Prepare your meals

- Protect your home

We often tend to go on autopilot with meal planning and preparation, but a successful transition into keto requires conscious thought and action, and that's what the Three Ps are all about.

Plan Ahead

If you wake up in the morning and have no idea what you'll be eating that day, there's no doubt that you'll choose your meals with a focus on convenience and routine rather than health. It's too easy to get distracted by work, family, and social obligations during the day. When this happens, food cravings, indulgences, and bad habits naturally influence your food decisions.

The solution for this is to get organized: You plan what you're going to eat for the entire day during the previous day. Even better, plan the week before! For example, on the weekend, you can plan what you will eat throughout the entire week and shop accordingly. This process eases anxiety and lessens the chance that you'll make an impulsive decision that will derail your progress.

KETO PRO TIP

You don't need a fancy list of meals and exhaustive recipe lists. My most successful patients and their families find they do best when they use the same six to ten recipes each week. If you can find a handful of meals you enjoy that fit keto nutritional principles, you are going to do well in your new lifestyle.

Prepare Your Meals

Now that you have taken the time to create a meal plan, the next step is to schedule time to prepare the food. If you have a busy schedule, you can make your favorite keto recipes in bulk and freeze or refrigerate multiple servings to reheat throughout the week. Many of my clients prepare food just twice a week (on Sunday and Wednesday, for example).

If food preparation seems overwhelming, find simple recipes and meals that don't take long to make. Make enough grilled chicken breast for several salads, then eat a serving each day with fresh spinach, avocado slices, and olive oil. You also can prepare enough food at dinner to have for lunch the following day. For example, make two servings of grass-fed burgers with steamed broccoli smothered in olive oil and herbs. Then set aside the extra meal for the following day!

KETO PRO TIP

Some local restaurants may be able to cater to your demands (using olive oil for salads, grass-fed butter with beef, no bread, and so on) if you contact them in advance and let them know you want to eat with them regularly.

Protect Your Home

Your home is your sacred space, and it's vitally important to protect it and keep it pure. The moment you walk out of your home, you'll find a world of temptation waiting to take you off course. You may not be able to control the food that your coworkers eat or what your friends order at a restaurant, but you can protect your home from food choices that could derail your success.

Protecting your home is much easier if your family is on board with your decision to make different lifestyle choices. If your family is not participating, you must sit them down and have a conversation about what you're doing and why you're doing it and ask for their support.

KETO PRO TIP

Have a designated part of the pantry that is your safe keto space, and when you go into the pantry, focus your eyes only on the keto-friendly area.

Strategies for Curbing Sugar Cravings

Sugar cravings are tricky. They can be hard to beat, and overcoming them doesn't mean they'll be gone permanently. Once again, the key is consistency. Make a habit of practicing these ten strategies to break free from sugar cravings:

- **Eat more healthy fat.** When you cut back on sugar and carbs, you must include more healthy fats in your diet. Healthy fats will improve your satiety levels, curb hunger, and reduce cravings between and after meals.

- **Hydrate your body.** When you're dehydrated, your body may experience hunger and sugar cravings as a result. So, drink up! Take in a minimum of half your body weight in ounces of water daily. I like to drink 16 to 32 ounces in the morning upon rising and 16 to 32 ounces between each meal. Unless you want to pee all night long, reduce your water intake after dinner to 8 to 16 ounces.

- **Consume salts.** Minerals are vital to energy, and mineral depletion can lead to increased cravings for sugar and carbs. Stress and sugar can deplete your minerals too quickly. You can help replenish your body's mineral levels by consuming a pinch of salt every few hours. Doing so may also reduce cravings and improve energy and mental clarity. Be sure to use high-quality sea salt or, even better, Himalayan salt, Redmond Real Salt, or Celtic Sea Salt.

- **Take apple cider vinegar (ACV).** Drinking water with ACV has been shown to improve blood sugar stability. You can drink 8 ounces of water with 1 to 2 tablespoons of ACV each morning or between meals. It's also beneficial to add ACV to meat or vegetable dishes to improve digestion and reduce post-meal cravings.

- **Use lemon/lime juice.** Lemon and lime juice can have a similar effect to ACV on digestion and help reduce cravings and promote healthy digestion.

- **Use some stevia.** Stevia is an all-natural sweetener that comes in liquid and powder form. If you're having intense sugar cravings, you can squirt a drop of stevia in your mouth or add some to water with ACV or lemon or lime juice to make a refreshing drink. Not only does this trick help satisfy your cravings but it improves your hydration and blood sugar/

insulin levels. Some of the recipes in this book include stevia in the ingredient list.

- **Go for a walk.** Getting your body moving by taking a walk or doing some light exercise can help stop cravings and improve neurotransmitter balance.

- **Prioritize sleep.** The better you sleep, the better your hormone balance and neurotransmitter production. A good night's sleep also significantly reduces hunger and cravings throughout the day.

- **Get daily sun exposure.** If the sun is shining, go outside and get fifteen or more minutes of sun exposure. Sun exposure helps improve your circadian rhythms, reduces stress hormones, improves sleep quality, and reduces cravings.

- **Practice prayer and meditation.** Emotional and habitual eating are habits that take effort and conscious thought to break. If you think you may be unknowingly feeding a sugar craving to get the neurological high you feel when you eat sweets, I recommend taking thirty minutes each day to find a quiet place, practice deep breathing, and pray or meditate over your mind/emotions and addictions. This time presents you with a valuable 30,000-foot view of your life that can help change your perspective on your daily needs.

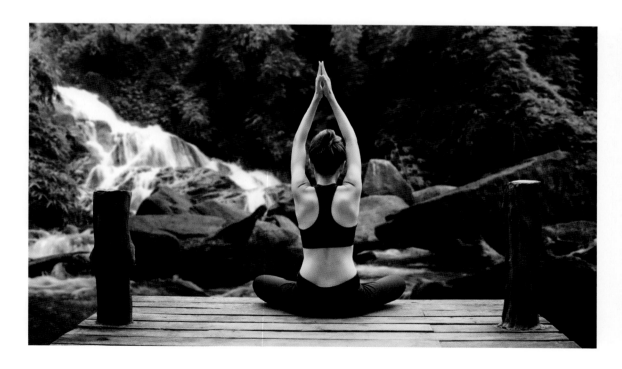

Keto Refrigerator Essentials

When it comes to long-term success, nothing keeps you on the road to victory more than having your kitchen stocked only with the best ingredients. The following foods are what I keep on hand in my refrigerator and freezer, and I advise you to use some or all of these as well. The list isn't exhaustive, but it's a great start!

Vegetables and Fruits	Proteins
Asparagus	Eggs*
Avocado	Precooked chicken*
Bell pepper	Smoked salmon
Broccoli	**Dairy**
Brussels sprouts	Cream cheese*
Cauliflower	Grass-fed butter
Celery	Mayonnaise
Cucumber	Raw dairy products*
Green beans	Sour cream*
Lemons/lemon juice	**Beef and Poultry**
Limes	Other healthy meat sources such as grass-fed hot dogs, sausages, or chicken/turkey breakfast sausages
Onion	
Parsley	
Salad greens	*Organic and pasture-raised
Freezer Foods	
Berries	
Veggies such as broccoli and cauliflower	
Wild-caught fish	

Put onions in the refrigerator only after you have peeled and cut into them. The same goes for avocado.

If the avocado is ripe, put it in the refrigerator to slow down the ripening process so it won't spoil.

Keto Pantry Essentials

Your pantry is just as crucial as your fridge—in fact, it may be even more so! The pantry is notorious for being filled with processed, shelf-stable inflammatory foods. As you give your kitchen a makeover, use this list of healing staples to stock your pantry:

Small Meals	Fats
Canned sardines (in water)	Avocado oil
Canned tuna and wild salmon	Avocado oil dressing
Nut butters	Extra-virgin olive oil
Organic olives	Ghee
Organic pickles	MCT oil
Raw, sprouted, or dry-roasted nuts and seeds (no peanuts)	Virgin coconut oil

Liquids/Drinks	Coconut-Based Food
Bone broth	Coconut aminos
Chicken, beef, or vegetable broth	Coconut butter
Coffee	Coconut flakes
Herbal teas	Coconut flour
Keto protein powder (for smoothies)	Coconut flour wraps
	Coconut milk

Condiments and Baking Staples	
Almond flour	Organic mustard
Apple cider vinegar	Raw cacao or cocoa
Baking powder	Sea salt and dried herbs
Baking soda	Stevia
Maple syrup	Unsweetened or stevia-sweetened dark chocolate
Monk fruit	

BONE BROTH

Bone broth is different from regular chicken or beef broth. Bone broth is made with the bones of chicken or beef, and it is much richer in vital nutrients than the broth made from the meat of the animals. Bone broth contains unique amino acids called glycosaminoglycans, which are great for our joints, skin, and intestinal lining. Also, bone broth contains bone marrow and a high amount of minerals such as magnesium, calcium, and potassium that are great for our immune system. I recommend using bone broth from grass-fed beef or organic, pasture-raised chickens. The brand my family and I use is Kettle and Fire, and you can purchase it online or in many grocery stores.

In general, I'm not a fan of snacking because it tends to elevate insulin, destroy metabolic flexibility, and negatively affect our ability to burn fat. However, there are times when you need a quick snack or a meal on the go. Here are some meal-replacement options you can have on hand to grab when you're traveling, working late, or running out the door for a meeting or errand:

- Almonds, macadamia nuts, pecans, or walnuts
- Beef or turkey jerky (without sugar)
- Flax crackers
- Kale chips
- Keto or collagen protein bars
- Nut butter packets you can squeeze directly into your mouth
- Seaweed snacks
- Sprouted seed crackers
- Trail mix with nuts and coconut flakes

Shopping Strategies

Before you head to the grocery store, you need a good plan so that you buy only the best foods to keep at home and use in recipes. Use this list to keep yourself on task and avoid getting overwhelmed when you get to the grocery store:

- **Create a shopping list.** Write down the foods you need before you go to the store. As you add the items to your cart, check them off. Your brain enjoys the sense of accomplishment that comes from checking things off a list.
- **Never shop hungry.** Every experienced grocery shopper knows it's a bad idea to go shopping on an empty stomach. You're far more likely to indulge in rich foods that you know you don't need, so fill up before you go food shopping.
- **Begin on the perimeter.** The outside edges of the grocery store are where the produce, meat, and other fresh items live. So, shop along the perimeter and fill your cart with perishable goods before you go down any of the middle aisles.

- **Avoid the bakery and carb-heavy aisles.** You won't find anything on the cereal and chip aisles or at the bakery department that fits into the diet of a keto shopper. If you need something in these aisles (such as unsweetened chocolate bars or seed-based crackers), consider buying them online.

- **Shop online.** Many online retailers offer healthy, nonperishable items. Amazon, Thrive Market, and Vitacost are some examples. These virtual stores often provide more variety and steeper discounts than you can find in your local grocery or health food store.

The achievement you experience in your keto metabolic breakthrough depends on the Success Equation, the Three Ps, and how well you protect what comes into your home. If you make changes in your life that enable your mastery ratio to be a 2 or higher, apply the Three Ps, stock your kitchen with the foods I've suggested, and follow my meal planning strategies, you'll have the best foundation on your health journey. And in the next chapter, I share the most powerful factors that will affect your success with the keto lifestyle.

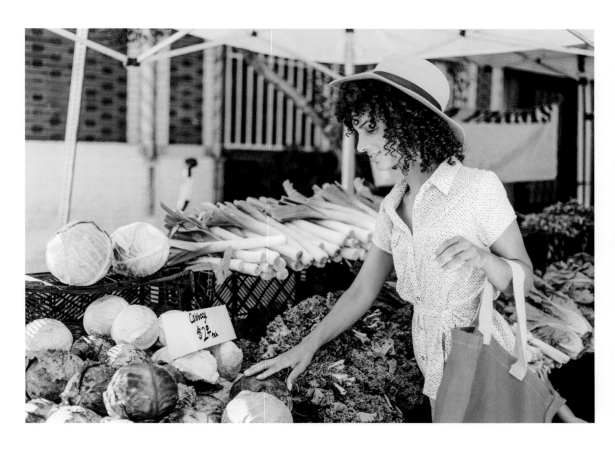

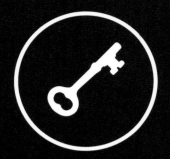

CHAPTER 13

THE MOST POWERFUL KETO SUCCESS FACTORS

When people hear about the "miraculous" effects of a ketogenic diet, they tend to jump in with unrealistic expectations. Although some people do burn off excess body fat quickly and safely, others don't experience such positive and speedy success—and that can be immensely frustrating.

The keto metabolic breakthrough is a powerful strategy to burn fat, look better, and feel better. However, as with any plan, you may hit roadblocks along the way. When that happens, you need to investigate underlying issues and use specific strategies and action steps to keep you moving in the right direction.

Everyone responds to weight loss and dietary changes differently, which is why it's essential to understand what factors influence your ability to burn fat. In this chapter, I uncover why some people have a more difficult time losing weight on a ketogenic diet than others, and I offer ways you can overcome roadblocks you encounter.

I also provide a quiz at the end of this chapter to help you better understand where your roadblocks may occur so you can identify the strategies that may be most helpful for you.

Realistic Goals Lead to Success

If you need to lose weight, you probably already have in mind a specific number of pounds that you hope to lose. The thing to remember is that everyone has a different weight toward which their body tends to gravitate. If you have already lost weight but have now reached a plateau, consider whether your current weight may be a healthy weight for you.

It's not uncommon for people to be so obsessed with weight loss that it becomes a chronic stressor in their lives. As frustrating as it can be to experience slow progress, as long as you're making the right choices and following the process laid out in this book, trust that your body knows what it's doing. It has an innate wisdom that will guide you toward your ideal weight.

Also, consider how long you've followed your current lifestyle before starting the switch to a ketogenic lifestyle. Keto is an excellent weight-loss strategy, but if you've been eating lots of carbs and sugar your entire life, don't expect to lose all of the weight overnight. Just stick with the plan and take pride in knowing you're nourishing your body with the right nutrients. The benefits will come as your metabolism changes. It's a process!

You might have heard some radical claims about the speed at which keto works. Perhaps you have a friend who lost 20 or 30 pounds in thirty days. You shouldn't expect those same results; they're not realistic. I define "successful weight-loss progression" at roughly 4 to 5 pounds per month. If you're 100 pounds overweight and lose 5 pounds per month, you need twenty months to get to your ideal weight. This pace is both normal and healthy.

Some people may respond quickly to the changes and lose 50 pounds in the first few months, but at some point, those people will hit a plateau. In this case, it's best not to look at each month's progress. Instead, consider the average; if you lose 10 pounds the first month and 2 pounds the second month, you're losing an average of 6 pounds a month. That is fantastic! As long as you're averaging 4 to 5 pounds of weight loss per month, you're on the right track.

Not Being in Ketosis

Are you in ketosis? It's a simple but essential question. If you're eating plenty of fat but not measuring your ketone levels daily, you can't say whether you're consistently in ketosis. If you haven't already purchased a ketone meter and started measuring, now is the time. The ideal methods for measuring ketone levels are either a blood ketone monitor or a breath acetone measuring device:

- **Measuring via blood:** A blood ketone monitor provides the most accurate measure of ketone levels. While nutritional ketosis is defined as having 0.5 to 3.0 mmol/L on a blood ketone meter, most people experience notable weight loss at ketone levels over 1.0 mmol/L.

- **Measuring via breath:** Breath analysis eliminates the need to continually purchase blood test strips and is more convenient (and less painful) than measuring via blood.

If your ketone levels are elevated and your blood sugar is stable, then you can eliminate this as a potential weight-loss roadblock. You can read more about determining whether you're in ketosis in Chapter 4.

KETO PRO TIP

If you've been following a keto diet for some time but are still struggling with cravings, feeling tired, or having brain fog throughout the day, you *are not* in nutritional ketosis. Test as often as you can until you are fully aware of how your body feels when you're in ketosis.

Not Eating Enough

One of the most common mistakes that could keep you from losing weight on a ketogenic diet is not taking in enough calories. Research has mostly debunked the old idea that weight loss is all about consuming fewer calories. Calories still matter, but it's not quite as simple as saying, "When you eat fewer calories, you lose weight."

Your ability to burn fat has more to do with hormone balance and mitochondrial health than it does with your calorie consumption. Balanced hormones come from making the right dietary choices, and you can enhance mitochondrial health with the weight-loss hacks I discuss in this chapter.

Although fasting and calorie restriction can be useful tools at certain times in your keto journey, restricting calories for long periods can slow your metabolism. If you're not eating enough, your body will eventually go into starvation mode. If you've been practicing calorie restriction, increase your overall caloric intake in the form of healthy fats, and see how the change affects your weight-loss efforts. Check your ketones throughout the day and monitor your fat-burning state and how you respond to meals. Testing regularly throughout the day following meals is the only way to see how specific meals affect your ability to stay in fat-burning mode.

KETO PRO TIP

If you intentionally follow a calorie-restricted diet and are still struggling to lose weight, you may not be eating enough overall calories. Temporary calorie restriction can be beneficial, such as doing a one-day fast every week. Just make sure you eat healthy keto foods until you are satiated (but not overly full) on the other six days.

The following are possible symptoms of undereating:

- Hunger and cravings just a few hours after eating

- Ongoing, persistent hunger and cravings

- Too much weight loss

- Fatigue a few hours after meals

- Brain fog a few hours after meals

- Relief of fatigue after eating

These symptoms also can be related to blood sugar and hormonal imbalances, so they don't always mean you're undereating. If you experience these symptoms but don't find relief by upping your caloric intake, undereating is likely not the cause of the problem.

Eating Too Many Calories

This issue may seem like a contradiction to the last factor, but it's true: You can eat too little and also too much. When you regularly consume lots of healthy fats, your body learns how to regulate hunger levels efficiently. However, you don't have license to stuff your face with whatever keto foods you desire all day long every day. Instead of working to take in a specific number of calories, work to find the range that meets your body's needs.

The source of the calories also matters. If your weight loss stalls, perhaps you're taking in too many calories from carbs and proteins and not enough from fats. When you go keto, stick to the following macronutrient ratios:

- Healthy fats are 60 to 80 percent of daily calories.

- Clean protein sources are 20 to 30 percent of daily calories.

- *Net carbs* (total carbs minus fiber) are roughly 5 percent of daily calories.

If you feel you might benefit from tracking what you eat and the macronutrients in each food, apps such as the CRON-O-Meter (a popular dietary tracking tool) can be beneficial. Such devices can help you determine your daily caloric needs on a ketogenic diet. See the "Resources" section at the end of the book for some suggestions of apps you can try.

KETO PRO TIP

If you feel tired and bloated after a meal, you're probably overeating. Try slowly reducing portion sizes until you no longer feel fatigued and bloated after eating.

Aside from stalled weight loss (or even weight gain), you may experience the following symptoms if you're overeating:

- Bloating after meals

- Indigestion after meals

- Nausea after meals

- Physical fatigue shortly after meals

- Mental fatigue shortly after meals

These symptoms also can be related to underlying digestive and hormonal imbalances, so they don't always mean you're overeating. If you reduce your portions and find that you're still suffering from these symptoms, the cause is likely not that you're eating too much.

Having a Hidden Food Sensitivity

Food allergies can be pretty scary. We all know people who have an allergy to peanuts or dairy and have extreme—even life-threatening—bodily reactions if they accidentally consume that food.

Food *sensitivities*, on the other hand, are small inflammatory responses to certain foods, and they're far more common than you may realize. For many, common ingredients such as gluten, dairy, soy, peanuts, shellfish, or eggs can cause unpleasant reactions such as bloating, fatigue, headaches, and the inability to lose weight.

Regularly consuming foods to which your body is sensitive can inflame the gut and cause complications. These hidden sensitivities are often at the root of conditions such as leaky gut syndrome, and the result can be a host of autoimmune-like symptoms.[1]

If you eat a small- to medium-sized meal, and soon after you feel tired and experience bloating, joint pain, eczema, acne breakouts, fatigue, or mood changes, it's possible you have a food sensitivity. Once you suspect you may have some food sensitivities, you can have testing done to confirm or rule out food groups. You can learn more about clinical lab tests that determine your immune response to foods by visiting www.DrJockers.com and searching for *food sensitivities*.

Often, testing is not even required to ascertain whether you have a sensitivity to a particular food. Just pay attention to how your body responds when you eat certain things.

KETO PRO TIP

Try removing one suspect food group at a time to see whether you notice a difference after a few weeks of not eating that food. Experiment with cutting out dairy, eggs, coffee, chocolate, nuts, and seeds.

FOOD SENSITIVITIES VS FOOD ALLERGIES

Food Sensitivities		Food Allergies
	Age	
Any age		Developed from **Infancy**
45% of the population suffer from food sensitivity.		2% of adults and 6–8% of children have an allergy.
	Reaction	
Delayed reaction occurs up to **72 hours** after eating the offending food.		Reaction occurs within **2 hours** of eating the offending food.
Results in bloating, joint pain, IBS, tiredness, eczema, low mood, headache, weight gain		Affects skin, digestion, airways
Is it deadly? No.		Is it deadly? Even trace amounts of foods trigger severe **life-threatening** reactions.

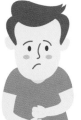
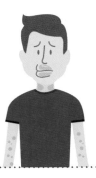

Which foods?

Most common sensitivities

 Wheat/ gluten

 Milk/ dairy

 Corn

 Eggs

Sugar

Most common types of allergies

 Peanuts

 Tree nuts

Eggs

 Milk

Fish/ shellfish

How many? Can be multiple	**Self-assessment** Pulse testing can be effective. Delayed onset of symptoms can make this tricky.	**How many?** Rarely more than one or two foods	**Self-assessment** The immediate reaction is easier to identify.

Having Leptin Resistance

Leptin is a hormone that stimulates feelings of fullness after a meal. If you are leptin resistant, your fat-burning pursuits will be hampered. Factors such as inadequate sleep, exposure to toxins, chronic stress, binge eating, and long-term caloric restriction can contribute to leptin resistance.[2]

People with leptin resistance often struggle with frequent hunger and cravings, especially at night. Also, they are often very carb sensitive and will gain weight quickly when eating carbs. People with leptin resistance are often insulin resistant as well; they or someone in their family may have been diagnosed with prediabetes or diabetes.

One of the biggest lifestyle factors involved in leptin resistance is poor sleep from either staying up too late or getting poor-quality sleep. It's important to prioritize an early bedtime before 11:00 p.m. and make sure your room is dark and cool (typically 65 to 70 degrees) without loud noises or other intrusions that could wake you. It's also wise to be evaluated for sleep apnea and have that addressed if it's an issue.

Fortunately, following a ketogenic diet and focusing on good sleep habits can help reset leptin receptors and get your body back into fat-burning mode. For most people, resetting takes anywhere from six to eight weeks. That means if you are in the early stages of keto and frustrated because you haven't lost much weight, be patient and give your body a few more weeks to reset.

KETO PRO TIP

If you're in ketosis, but your weight-loss efforts have stalled, leptin resistance may be the culprit. Practicing intermittent fasting, prioritizing good sleep and taking polyphenolic herbs (which are in matcha tea, organic coffee, and turmeric) regularly in addition to following a keto diet can help your body heal its leptin receptors.

Having Thyroid Issues

If you have thyroid problems, you may have a difficult time adapting to a ketogenic diet. An estimated 27 million Americans have some form of thyroid dysfunction. Up to 60 percent of those people are unaware of their condition.

One thyroid condition known as *hypothyroidism* is generally traditionally thought of as the thyroid not producing enough hormones. However, this isn't the full story. Thyroid hormones can be imbalanced due to issues with the liver and gut or because of high stress. The liver and gut microbiome play a key role in the expression of active T3. Also, when you have chronic stress, your body produces an inactive form of T3 called *reverse T3*. These factors have nothing to do with the thyroid gland itself, but they affect the ability of the thyroid hormone to do its job and turn on the energy production within every cell of the body.

HYPOTHYROID SYMPTOMS

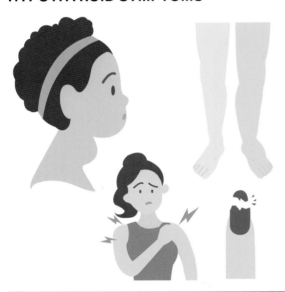

- Decreased libido
- Goiter
- Slow heart rate
- Fatigue
- Fluid retention
- Elevated liver enzymes
- Depression
- Poor memory
- Brittle nails and dry skin and hair
- Low body temperature and cold sensitivity
- High cholesterol
- Hoarseness
- Headaches and muscle aches
- Weight gain
- Tingling sensation in hands
- Constipation

Women are five to eight times more likely than men to develop thyroid issues, and 80 percent of hypothyroid conditions in this country are thought to be autoimmune-related.[3] People who struggle with an inactive thyroid or thyroid hormone imbalance tend to experience low energy, weight gain, mood imbalances, brain fog, and lower vitality. If you have these symptoms, you may have an underlying thyroid condition.

One problem that exacerbates the issue is that conventional medicine uses outdated reference ranges for thyroid lab testing. If you have any of the symptoms I listed and have hit a plateau in your weight loss, have gained weight, or are struggling with your energy on a keto diet, then I recommend that you get more thorough thyroid testing done. In particular, I recommend testing for the following hormones and comparing them to the optimal ranges listed here.

Test	Description	Standard Lab Range	Optimal Range
TSH (thyroid-stimulating hormone)	A hormone produced by the pituitary gland that tells the thyroid gland to produce thyroid hormone.	0.45–5.0 uIU/ml	0.45–1.8 uIU/ml
T4 (Thyroxine)	The primary hormone produced by the thyroid gland. It's an inactive hormone and must be converted by liver enzymes and gut bacteria into active T3.	4.5–12 mcg/dL	6–12 mcg/dL
Free T3 (Triiodothyronine)	Some of the T3 is bound in the body and therefore becomes unusable. The free portion of the T3 is essential because it's what activates cellular metabolism. This number is perhaps the most important on thyroid labs.	2.0–4.4 pg/ml	3.0–4.0 pg/ml
Reverse T3	An inactive form of T3 that cannot be used by the cells of the body. Chronic stress is known to increase RT3 levels.	9.2–24.1 ng/dL	Under 20 ng/dL
Thyroglobulin (TG) antibodies	The protein portion of the thyroid hormone that is needed to bind to T4. Those with autoimmune thyroid problems tend to make antibodies to this protein, so when TG antibodies are high, T4 levels aren't within an optimal range.	0–0.9 IU/ml	0–0.5 IU/ml
Thyroid peroxidase (TPO) antibodies	An essential enzyme that converts iodide ions to iodine atoms to be connected onto the tyrosine portions of the TG protein. People with autoimmune thyroid conditions make antibodies to this enzyme.	0–34 IU/ml	<20 IU/ml

Some people in the functional medicine community have the idea that following a ketogenic diet is harmful to the thyroid. Research doesn't support this idea. There is some evidence that following a ketogenic diet may lower T3 levels. This reduced T3 production is not unique to ketosis. This result occurs for people on both calorie-restrictive and protein-restrictive diets.[4] The evidence seems to indicate that lowered T3 is a physiological adaptation that allows for a deeper state of ketosis and preserves muscle mass.[5, 6]

If you have a thyroid condition, you must monitor how you feel on a day-to-day basis to determine how you're responding to a ketogenic diet. Your T3 levels may be slightly depressed, but if you feel great, you don't have reason to be concerned. This drop in T3 allows for deeper ketosis and preservation of muscle mass. Also, low T3 levels are associated with a longer life span.[7]

Having Healthy T3 Levels

In Chapter 6, I discuss how effectively keto reduces inflammation and improves mitochondrial health, which then enhances thyroid hormone and adrenal function. That said, it's still possible that someone with a preexisting thyroid or adrenal issue may struggle on a ketogenic diet.

If you start keto and don't lose weight, or you experience an increase in hypothyroid-like symptoms, it's possible you had low free T3 levels and were unaware of this condition. Successful T4-to-T3 conversion depends upon several different micronutrients, including iodine, selenium, and zinc, which is why I typically recommend supplementation for those with existing conditions. I also often recommend a bovine-based thyroid and pituitary glandular supplement to help support optimal thyroid levels. (Read more on this in Chapter 15.)

Having Adrenal Health Issues

As I discuss earlier in the book, your body perceives and adapts to stressors via the HPA axis. When you experience chronic stress, it creates a change in the HPA axis that reduces your body's ability to adapt to new stressors. This condition is commonly called *adrenal fatigue*, although it's more of a sensory issue. This cycle of stress and poor adaptation can lead to many unpleasant problems, such as chronic inflammation, weight gain, and accelerated aging.[8]

Two of the biggest drivers of HPA axis dysfunction are blood sugar imbalance and inflammation. Fortunately, living a ketogenic lifestyle is a powerful way to improve blood sugar stability and reduce inflammation. However, it takes a mindful approach, particularly if you have known (or even undiagnosed) adrenal issues.

Sympathetic Versus Parasympathetic Tone

When it comes to how you approach your health, one of the most important considerations is how much stress you allow into your life. When your body experiences stress, it increases your *sympathetic tone,* which is a part of the nervous system that controls fight-or-flight mode. In this mode, all of your body's noncritical functions shut down, which enables you to focus on getting you out of harm's way. This response is a healthy and natural defense mechanism, but when it goes on for an extended period, it creates a state of *sympathetic dominance.*

On the other hand, when you habitually relax, play, laugh, enjoy family time, breathe deeply, and engage in gratitude exercises and prayer, you stimulate the *parasympathetic tone,* which is the part of the nervous system that enhances healing and repair mechanisms. Strive to be in a state of parasympathetic dominance if you want to heal and repair effectively from the daily stressors of life.[9]

To experience the long-term benefits of nutritional ketosis, you need healthy adrenal function. I recommend a handful of strategies for supporting your HPA axis and adrenal hormones. For many people, incorporating a mix of these strategies into their daily routines may be the key to breaking through a plateau:

- **Don't fast (at first).** If you suffer from HPA axis dysfunction or adrenal fatigue, I recommend that you eat breakfast within an hour of waking and consume a keto-style meal or snack every three to five hours. As your body becomes fat-adapted, you'll notice reduced hunger and be able to extend the time between meals.

- **Stay hydrated.** Water is critical for balancing stress hormone production. A state of dehydration naturally stimulates stress hormones. Drinking water is one of the best ways to dampen the stress response and put you back into a state of rest and repair. Start each day with 16 to 32 ounces of water and then consume a minimum of 8 ounces of water every two to three hours away from meals. Your goal should be to drink a minimum of half your body weight in ounces of water each day.

- **Take deep breaths.** The average person takes twelve to eighteen breaths per minute. These short, shallow breaths stimulate a stressful state. Take time each day to breathe deeply and allow the rest and peace that comes with this practice to wash over you. Taking four to six breaths a minute for five minutes each day can stimulate the parasympathetic nervous system and improve your HPA axis function.

- **Dry brush your skin.** The Ayurvedic practice known as *dry brushing* boosts circulation and also boosts lymph flow and detoxification. Take a soft-bristle brush and gently stroke from your extremities toward your heart. This practice helps to stimulate endorphins and other feel-good chemicals.

- **Ground your body.** You're always surrounded by unhealthy electromagnetic frequencies (EMFs). These EMFs increase stress within your body and alter neurotransmitter function. The earth emits natural EMFs that act as antioxidants and help to reduce EMF-based stress. Unfortunately, rubber shoe soles block our ability to absorb these healing frequencies. By walking barefoot on grass, dirt, sand, or even concrete, you can absorb natural EMFs from the ground that balance your electrical rhythms. This is called *grounding*. Nature is full of healing properties, so pack a lunch and eat it outside on the ground or take a walk in the woods.

- **Reduce caffeine and sugar intake.** Caffeine energizes you by stimulating your adrenals to pump out more stress hormone. If your body is already in a state of adrenal fatigue, consuming caffeine overtaxes your body and causes adrenal exhaustion. Sugar also causes your adrenals to work harder to maintain blood sugar balance. So consider removing both from your diet if you're interested in repairing your adrenals.

- **Use essential oils.** Essential oils are the lifeblood of plants. Some oils that help with adrenal fatigue include lavender, vanilla, rose, lemon balm, chamomile, rosemary, and frankincense. You can diffuse them, apply them topically with a carrier oil, or add a drop or two of therapeutic-grade oils to your meals.

- **Get more sleep.** Getting at least eight hours of sleep each night is an essential key to health and healing. Keep your bedroom dark and cool and put your phone on airplane mode to reduce EMF exposure. If possible, I also recommend taking a short nap in the early afternoon to reduce stress hormones and allow for a short recharge.

- **Get moving.** In this case, "moving" doesn't mean that you have to do a high-intensity exercise. You just need to engage in any sort of low-intensity movement without having specific physique-related goals. A sedentary lifestyle creates stress on your body, and light movement creates anti-inflammatory, healing effects, especially for your adrenals. Move as much as possible during the day, and never sit for too long. Aside from enhancing adrenal function, movement has a number of other benefits, including improving circulation, enhancing tissue oxygenation, reducing stress and tension, and improving mood and happiness.

- **Take care of your spine.** Stress on the upper cervical spine can cause an increase in sympathetic tone and stress hormone production. Over time, the result can be poor tissue healing and adrenal fatigue.[10] Chiropractic adjustments can correct neck subluxations and significantly reduce stress on your body.[11] Other spine-related issues include forward head posture and loss of a healthy curve in the neck, both of which put pressure on the nervous system and lead to an increase in sympathetic tone. Do your best to work on improving your posture.

- **Get a massage.** A massage can reduce muscle tension, increase blood and lymph flow, help promote tissue healing, and stimulate feel-good endorphins. All of these benefits help to relax the HPA axis. If you're interested in a less expensive option, you could always consider trading shoulder massages with your spouse. There are also several self-massage tools on the market, such as a foam roller, that can provide some relief.

- **Listen to calming music.** Listening to classical, meditation, or worship music can be extremely therapeutic. These forms of music are soothing and also known to boost endorphins and stimulate the formation of serotonin. Also, listening to calming music can help uplift your spirits and enhance tissue repair.

- **Practice positive visualization.** Visualization is powerful. See yourself healthy and full of life while you breathe deeply and focus on the present moment. What you think about and envision, you genuinely do become. Begin to move toward healing by envisioning yourself well! This practice will help reduce stress and promote the healing process.

- **Play more.** Mammals are biologically programmed to play. Just watch your children and pets—they prioritize rest and play above everything else. Adults should take a cue from this by engaging in some hobbies, playing with pets or kids, and just having fun!

- **Schedule downtime.** Schedule time to relax and read an enjoyable book or watch an uplifting movie. Steer clear of horror movies, loud music, media that challenges your value system, and negative people. Create an environment that uplifts, encourages, and empowers you.

- **Put your phone away.** Research has shown that using your cell phone increases the stress response and inflammatory processes.[12] Use it less often. When you must talk on the phone, use the speaker phone or Bluetooth headphones, and keep the phone as far away from your body as possible.

- **Reduce chronic infections and heal your gut**. One of the leading causes of adrenal fatigue is leaky gut syndrome and infections caused by *H. pylori,* parasites, and bacterial and yeast overgrowths. A functional medicine practitioner can perform lab tests to help you determine whether you suffer from any of these conditions. My team at DrJockers.com uses the GI-MAP test from Diagnostic Solutions to look for infections, and then we recommend specific protocols to address them.

- **Eliminate food sensitivities.** Identify any food sensitivities through either a lab test or biofeedback test. If you're sensitive to a particular food, remove it from your diet for ninety days. I typically start adrenal-fatigued patients on an elimination diet by removing the most common food irritants, including gluten, grains, dairy, eggs, sugars, corn, peanuts, soy, coffee, chocolate, nuts, and seeds. After two weeks on an elimination diet, we begin to add foods one at a time to see if they cause stress or inflammation. The goal is to find the foods that are most tolerable while your body heals.

- **Consume adequate salts.** Minerals are essential to the production and utilization of stress hormones. Using the highest quality salts on your foods throughout the day is a great strategy to boost mineral content. My favorite salt types include Himalayan salt, Redmond Real Salt, and Celtic Sea Salt. In addition to salts, consuming celery, cucumbers, fermented vegetables (pickles and sauerkraut), and sea vegetables (seaweeds) can improve your mineral levels and stress hormone production and utilization.

- **Laugh more.** People say that laughter is the best medicine, and this is true when it comes to the adrenals. Laughing helps to stimulate endorphins and other feel-good neuropeptides that reduce your stress response and enhance healing. Chuckling about your daily activities and light joking with friends can be highly therapeutic.

- **Go outside.** Sun exposure not only helps to boost vitamin D levels but it also improves the ability of mitochondria to produce energy for healing and repair, which takes some of the stress off the adrenals and allows them to heal.[13] Our bodies also absorb biophotons, which are light particles from the sun that create reactions in our cells that promote DNA repair and synthesis.

- **Relax in the bath.** Epsom salt baths are relaxing and rejuvenating. The salts provide magnesium and sulfates to help support adrenal health and liver detox. Take a nightly thirty-minute soak with lavender and chamomile oils in the water. Dim the lights and play some worship or classical music and focus on taking deep breaths. This nightly ritual is *extremely* restorative and will help you sleep better and feel rejuvenated.

- **Meditate and pray daily.** Meditation and prayer help to calm the mind and bring about a state of peace and tranquility. In 1 Peter, God tells us to cast all of our anxieties onto Him—and we need that respite from our troubles and stresses now more than ever. Researchers studied individuals with active religious and spiritual lifestyle habits and found they have significantly better mental health and adapt more quickly to health issues.[14] Take time each day to thank God and give Him your struggles. You don't have to take the weight of the world on your shoulders.

- **Stretch your body.** Light stretching or a yoga class can be one of the most beneficial things for those dealing with adrenal fatigue. Gentle movements and stretches, coupled with breathing exercises, help calm the adrenals and improve parasympathetic tone. If you have severe issues with your HPA axis, do not engage in an intense yoga session with demanding positions or a hot yoga class because those varieties of yoga can be too draining on your adrenals.

- **Start a gratitude journal.** We often spend a lot of time focused on our frustrations. Taking time each day to journal about what you're most grateful for can be an essential daily activity. You can incorporate journaling into your breathing, meditation, and prayer practices. Writing in a journal helps relax your mind, increase endorphins, and reduce stress hormone production.

Using Specialized Stress Hacks

There are always going to be some people who are the exception to the rules. These people are the individuals who are doing it all, but they're still not getting the results they desire, or they're looking to take things to the next level. For these people, six additional strategies can help boost metabolism and enhance fat-burning while on a ketogenic diet.

High-Intensity Interval Training

High-intensity interval training, or HIIT, is a short-duration workout that involves rapid bursts of exercise involving large groups of muscles. Engaging in this type of activity improves mitochondrial function and stimulates a process called *mitochondrial biogenesis,* or the growth of new mitochondria. This process significantly increases your body's ability to burn fat.[15] Two to four HIIT-style workouts a week could be a great way to break past a weight-loss plateau or to start incorporating more exercise into your life.

Resistance Training

Resistance training, such as lifting weights, requires placing a large amount of stress on targeted muscle groups. While cardio gives the appearance of "burning off" more calories during a workout compared to resistance training, building muscle is a great way to increase your resting metabolism—which then keeps you burning fat long after your workout.[16] Studies have shown that lifting weights increases your metabolism for several hours immediately following your workout.[17]

KETO PRO TIP

To take the benefits to the next level, you can combine resistance and HIIT training with fasting. For example, I like to finish dinner at 6:00 p.m. and fast (but drink lots of hydrating beverages) until 12:00 p.m. to 2:00 p.m. the next day. Then I work out and consume a fat-burning meal afterward.

BENEFITS AND GUIDELINES FOR FASTED EXERCISE

There are great benefits and certain guidelines to follow when doing high-intensity training, such as sprints, or resistance training after 14+ hours of intermittent fasting.

Fasted exercise benefits include

- Improving fat-burning
- Increasing growth hormone production
- Mitochondrial biogenesis
- Improving ketone production
- Improving muscle growth and development

Guidelines for fasted exercise:

- Be sure you are well-hydrated
- Only do short, high-intensity workouts (no more than 30 minutes)
- Consume high-quality protein or BCAAs directly after workout
- For muscle-building, use BCAAs preworkout

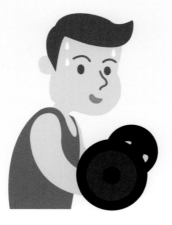

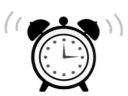

If you use the branched-chain amino acids (BCAAs) post-workout, you can wait until you get hungry before having your first meal even if that's a few hours later. The delay in eating will allow time for higher growth hormone production.

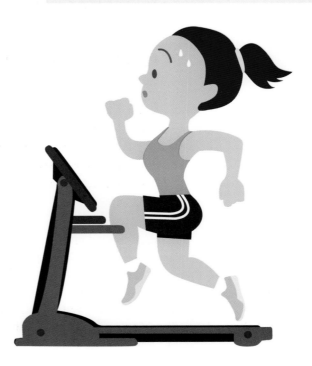

Intermittent Fasting

Intermittent fasting (IF) is the practice of confining your meals to a small window of time, so you go longer between meals than you typically have. The easiest way to make the most out of IF is to make your window from dinner to lunch or dinner the following day. In other words, consume no calories from the time you finish dinner the previous night until mid or late afternoon the next day.

Different styles of intermittent fasting are great for optimizing insulin sensitivity, reducing inflammation, and increasing growth hormone in the body. If you've never attempted IF, start with a twelve-hour window—for example, finish dinner at 6:00 p.m. and don't eat again until at least 6:00 a.m. the next morning.

Every two weeks, increase your fasting window by two hours, progressing up to fourteen and eventually sixteen hours of fasting each day. Some people do well when they extend beyond sixteen hours and fast up to eighteen hours. Listen to your body, see how you feel, and choose the fasting window that works the best for your lifestyle.

One strategy I often employ is a feast-famine weekly cycle in which I do daily eighteen- to twenty-hour fasts five days a week. One or two days a week, I do a twenty-four-hour fast, meaning I consume only one meal. (For example, I eat dinner on Saturday and fast until dinner on Sunday.) Then one day a week, I have a "feast day" when I consume a more substantial amount of food with higher protein and carb counts. You could try this cycle, although I don't recommend this method for anyone who is very insulin resistant.

Here are a couple of other fasting strategies:

- **Forty-hour fast once per week:** Fasting from dinner Saturday until lunch on Monday, for example.

- **Alternate-day fasting:** Eating two to three meals on one day and then fasting the following day. Continue to cycle eating days and fasting days.

You can experiment with these fasting strategies and see which one helps you break through your plateau.

BENEFITS OF FEAST-FAMINE CYCLING

- Regulates cell growth and cleansing pathways
- Creates hormonal optimization
- Improves lean body tissue development
- Stimulates fat-burning
- Balances inflammation and immune activity
- Enhances mental and emotional well-being

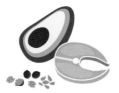

Going through phases of feasting on nutrient-dense foods and periods of intermittent and extended fasting improves your metabolic flexibility and energy efficiency and makes you an incredibly strong and resilient human being.

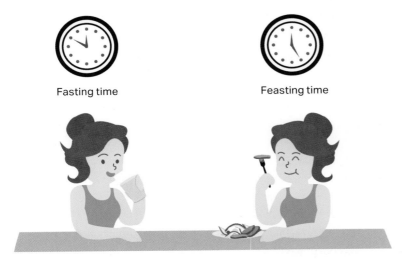

Fasting time

Feasting time

Times of fasting

Cell cleansing and healing is favored over growth, building, and reproduction.

Times of feasting

Growth, building, and reproduction is favored over cell cleansing and healing.

Carbohydrate Cycling

Although following a strictly ketogenic diet can be powerful for a month or two to get your body adapted to fat-burning, periodically eating more carbs is essential. It's the cycling in and out of ketosis that seems to provide the maximum benefit for people when it comes to a healthy metabolism. When you carb cycle, you choose one meal (or one day) out of the week or every ten days and increase your carb intake. Smart carb choices include sweet potatoes, beets, carrots, pumpkin, cassava, tapioca, and your favorite fruits.

Cold Exposure

Your body produces heat by releasing it from the mitochondria as needed. Exposing your body to cold stimulates this process, which also speeds up your metabolism and increases your ability to burn fat. To start, turn your shower as cold as it can go for thirty seconds just before you get out. Even better, flex and pump your arms and legs to drive blood flow as the cold water hits you to increase the activation of heat shock proteins and endorphins that help you more effectively burn fat.

Over time, you'll get more comfortable with the cold water, and you may even look forward to how good you feel after your cold plunge. You may also want to increase the time, perhaps even building to a 100 percent cold shower if you like the way it makes you feel. After you're well adapted to the cold, partaking in ice baths a few times per week can take things to the next level. Exposing your body to extreme temperature changes is excellent for boosting metabolism.

Sauna Therapy

Another way to expose your body to temp changes is through sauna therapy. What started as an intuitive and enjoyable practice many years ago is now a trendy but powerful health strategy. Lots of my clients have found using the sauna to be a highly effective weight-loss hack. Several studies on regular sauna use have identified different mechanisms by which it stimulates fat loss. Sweating helps to detoxify the body and rid you of harmful toxins that can cause hormone imbalance and contribute to weight gain.[18] Try getting in a fifteen- to thirty-minute sauna session three to five times per week to see how it affects your weight-loss goals.

Quiz Time!

The ketogenic diet is a powerful weight-loss strategy that offers far superior results to low-fat or low-calorie diets in terms of overall health.[19, 20] However, not everyone experiences dramatic weight loss right away. Some people have issues that they must address, such as thyroid or adrenal issues, or they make common ketogenic diet mistakes that could hold them back from experiencing the results they seek.

If you're struggling on keto or have plateaued, now is the time to take the Keto Plateau Quiz. Once you take the quiz and tally your results, review the chapter to select the strategies you'll implement. I don't recommend applying all of the weight-loss hacks at once. That approach wouldn't be realistic or sustainable. Instead, try adding one or two that seem the most appealing and observe how your body responds.

Implementing the tips in this chapter can help you break through and experience the results you desire. If you still struggle to achieve your goals, consider whether your weight-loss goals are realistic. It may be a good idea to look for a health coach who can help you troubleshoot the challenges you're facing.

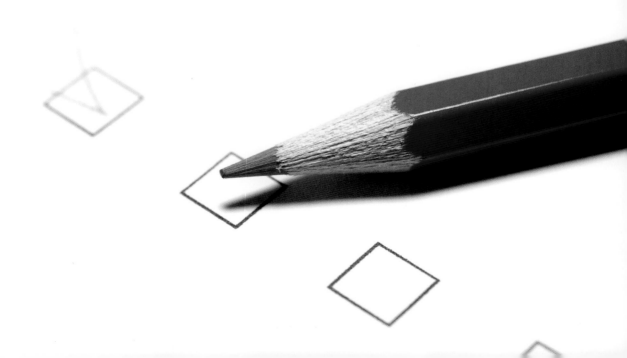

KETO METABOLIC PLATEAU QUIZ

If you've been following ketogenic diet nutrition principles for a few months and still aren't feeling well or seem to be stuck at a weight-loss plateau, use this quiz to help you uncover the source (or sources) of your struggle.

This quiz covers eight potential roadblocks. Answer each question set and discover what may be holding you back from experiencing the amazing effects of a ketogenic lifestyle.

Potential Roadblock #1: Am I in Ketosis?

When you're in nutritional ketosis, you shouldn't experience cravings, should rarely feel hungry, and should have plenty of energy and mental clarity. Answer these questions and total your score:

1. Do you struggle with carb cravings throughout the day or night?

○	○	○	○
Never	**Sometimes**	**Often**	**All the time**
0 points	*1 point*	*2 points*	*3 points*

2. Do you feel mentally sluggish and fatigued?

○	○	○	○
Never	**Sometimes**	**Often**	**All the time**
0 points	*1 point*	*2 points*	*3 points*

3. Do you feel hungry throughout the day?

○	○	○	○
Never	**Sometimes**	**Often**	**All the time**
0 points	*1 point*	*2 points*	*3 points*

Total Score: _____

If you scored a 4 or higher, you most likely are NOT in ketosis. If you don't already have one, purchase a blood or breath ketone meter to measure your ketones, and go back to the basics to ensure you're not eating too many carbs. It may help you to track your macros for a few weeks.

Potential Roadblock #2: Am I Eating Enough?

Due to the appetite-suppressing effects of ketones and the desire to cut calories to lose weight, some people undereat for a prolonged period, which can impact metabolism in a negative manner. Answer these questions and total your score:

1. Do you purposely limit the amount of food you consume to hit a calorie goal?

○	○	○	○
Never	**Sometimes**	**Often**	**All the time**
0 points	*1 point*	*2 points*	*3 points*

2. How many meals do you consume each day?

○	○	○	○
4+ meals	**3 meals**	**2 meals**	**0–1 meal**
0 points	*1 point*	*2 points*	*3 points*

3. Do you eat until you feel satiated and full?

○	○	○	○
All the time	**Often**	**Sometimes**	**Never**
0 points	*1 point*	*2 points*	*3 points*

4. How many calories do you typically consume each day?

○	○	○	○
More than 2,500	**2,000–2,500**	**1,500–2,000**	**Less than 1,500**
0 points	*1 point*	*2 points*	*3 points*

5. How often do you exercise each week?

○	○	○	○
0–1 time	**2 times**	**3 times**	**4+ times**
0 points	*1 point*	*2 points*	*3 points*

Total Score: _____

If you scored a 10 or higher, you may be eating too little. Try adding another 100 to 200 calories a day to your diet and see how you feel. Always measure your ketones to ensure you are in nutritional ketosis.

Because a keto diet is high in fat, and fat is energy dense, it can be fairly easy to overeat. Answer these questions and total your score to see whether you're overeating:

1. Do you have a very large appetite?

○	○	○	○
Never	**Sometimes**	**Often**	**All the time**
0 points	*1 point*	*2 points*	*3 points*

2. Do you burp or have indigestion after meals?

○	○	○	○
Never	**Sometimes**	**Often**	**All the time**
0 points	*1 point*	*2 points*	*3 points*

3. Are you tired and sluggish after your meals?

○	○	○	○
Never	**Sometimes**	**Often**	**All the time**
0 points	*1 point*	*2 points*	*3 points*

4. How often do you exercise each week?

○	○	○	○
4+ times	**3 times**	**2 times**	**0–1 time**
0 points	*1 point*	*2 points*	*3 points*

5. How intense are your workouts?

○	○	○	○
Very hard	**Hard**	**Moderate**	**Light**
0 points	*1 point*	*2 points*	*3 points*

6. How many total meals and snacks do you normally consume each day?

○	○	○	○
1	**2**	**3**	**4+**
0 points	*1 point*	*2 points*	*3 points*

7. How long is your daily intermittent fasting window (the time between your last meal on one day and your first meal the following day)?

○	○	○	○
19+ hours	**16–18 hours**	**13–15 hours**	**10–12 hours**
0 points	*1 point*	*2 points*	*3 points*

Total Score: _____

If you scored 12 or more, you are likely overeating. Reduce your daily caloric intake and see if that helps you start to lose weight and/or experience an increase in energy and overall vitality. Check your ketone levels to make sure you're in nutritional ketosis.

Potential Roadblock #4: Do I Have Overstressed Adrenals?

Chronic, unrelenting stress can block you from getting into ketosis and experiencing the fat-burning benefits that come with this lifestyle. Answer these questions and total your score to see if your adrenals may be overstressed:

1. Do you feel like you're under a high amount of stress?

○	○	○	○
Never	**Sometimes**	**Often**	**All the time**
0 points	*1 point*	*2 points*	*3 points*

2. Do you struggle with carb cravings throughout the day or at night?

○	○	○	○
Never	**Sometimes**	**Often**	**All the time**
0 points	*1 point*	*2 points*	*3 points*

3. Do you have trouble staying asleep at night?

○	○	○	○
Never	**Sometimes**	**Often**	**All the time**
0 points	*1 point*	*2 points*	*3 points*

4. Do you struggle with depression, headaches, anxiety, lack of focus, or irritability?

○	○	○	○
Never	**Sometimes**	**Often**	**All the time**
0 points	*1 point*	*2 points*	*3 points*

5. Do you feel like you need a daily nap in order to function?

○	○	○	○
Never	**Sometimes**	**Often**	**All the time**
0 points	*1 point*	*2 points*	*3 points*

6. Do you feel like you gain weight when you're under stress?

○	○	○	○
Never	**Sometimes**	**Often**	**All the time**
0 points	*1 point*	*2 points*	*3 points*

7. Do you have trouble getting out of the bed in the morning?

○	○	○	○
Never	**Sometimes**	**Often**	**All the time**
0 points	*1 point*	*2 points*	*3 points*

Total Score: _____

If you scored a 14 or higher, you are most likely dealing with overtaxed adrenals. Be sure to follow the strategies in this chapter for improving adrenal function. Retake the quiz after a week or two of implementing some of those ideas to check whether your score improves.

Potential Roadblock #5: Do I Have a Food Sensitivity?

Food sensitivities are tricky because they don't always cause an immediate reaction. The inflammation is gradual, so most people never link the symptoms to particular foods. If you have a food sensitivity, it may hold you back from achieving the benefits that come with nutritional ketosis. Answer these questions and total your score to see if this may be your issue:

1. Do you feel bloated and tired after meals?

○	○	○	○
Never	**Sometimes**	**Often**	**All the time**
0 points	*1 point*	*2 points*	*3 points*

2. Do you have to clear your throat a lot during the day?

○	○	○	○
Never	**Sometimes**	**Often**	**All the time**
0 points	*1 point*	*2 points*	*3 points*

3. Do you have eczema, acne, rosacea, or psoriasis?

○	○	○	○
No	**Very mild**	**Mild**	**Moderate to severe**
0 points	*1 point*	*2 points*	*3 points*

4. Do you suffer from chronic pain?

○	○	○	○
Never	**Sometimes**	**Often**	**All the time**
0 points	*1 point*	*2 points*	*3 points*

5. Do you struggle with depression, headaches, anxiety, lack of focus, or irritability?

○	○	○	○
Never	**Sometimes**	**Often**	**All the time**
0 points	*1 point*	*2 points*	*3 points*

Total Score: _____

If you scored an 8 or higher, you probably have a food sensitivity. Remove all four of the most common allergen groups (nuts, eggs, shellfish, and dairy from your diet) for two weeks and see if you feel better and your score improves. If so, add in one group at a time and give yourself several days to see if any of the foods make you feel worse.

Some people have significant issues with sensitivity to the fat-burning hormone leptin and the fat-storage hormone insulin. Answer these questions to see if you are one of them:

1. Have you or a family member ever been diagnosed with prediabetes or diabetes?

No one	Family only	Only me	Both family and me
◯	◯	◯	◯
0 points	1 point	2 points	3 points

2. Do you gain weight when you consume carbohydrate-rich foods?

Never	Sometimes	Often	All the time
◯	◯	◯	◯
0 points	1 point	2 points	3 points

3. Do you rarely feel satiated when you're eating a meal and therefore tend to overeat?

Never	Sometimes	Often	All the time
◯	◯	◯	◯
0 points	1 point	2 points	3 points

4. Have you had trouble losing weight your entire life?

Never	Sometimes	Often	All the time
◯	◯	◯	◯
0 points	1 point	2 points	3 points

5. Do you tend to stay up late at night (past 11:00 p.m.) when you're able to?

Never	Sometimes	Often	All the time
◯	◯	◯	◯
0 points	1 point	2 points	3 points

6. Do you feel tired after meals?

○ **Never**
0 points

○ **Sometimes**
1 point

○ **Often**
2 points

○ **All the time**
3 points

Total Score: _____

If you scored a 10 or higher, you likely have a degree of insulin/leptin resistance. Following a keto diet and prioritizing healthy lifestyle activities such as exercise, good sleep, and stress management will help you overcome this and break through your plateau.

Potential Roadblock #7: Do I Have Healthy Thyroid Activity?

Hypothyroidism is one of the most underdiagnosed conditions in the world. Therefore, you may be dealing with low thyroid hormone activity and not even know it. An underactive thyroid can make you feel fatigued and cause a weight-loss plateau (or even weight gain, in some cases) when you begin a keto diet. Answer these questions and total your score to see if you may be dealing with an underactive thyroid:

1. Do you feel cold often, even when it isn't necessarily cold outside or in the house?

○ **Never**
0 points

○ **Sometimes**
1 point

○ **Often**
2 points

○ **All the time**
3 points

2. Are you losing the hair on your head or along the outer third of your eyebrows?

○ **No hair loss**
0 points

○ **Mild**
1 point

○ **Moderate**
2 points

○ **Severe**
3 points

3. How often do you move your bowels in a two-day period (without laxatives)?

○ **5+ times**
0 points

○ **3–4 times**
1 point

○ **2–3 times**
2 points

○ **0–1 time**
3 points

4. How many days a week do you feel constipated (without laxatives)?

○ **0 days**
0 points

○ **1–2 days**
1 point

○ **3–4 days**
2 points

○ **Most of the time**
3 points

5. Do you have to strain to move your bowels (without laxatives)?

○ **Never**
0 points

○ **Sometimes**
1 point

○ **Often**
2 points

○ **All the time**
3 points

6. Does your skin feel dry and flaky?

○ **Never**
0 points

○ **Sometimes**
1 point

○ **Often**
2 points

○ **All the time**
3 points

7. Do you feel lethargic and mentally sluggish?

○ **Never**
0 points

○ **Sometimes**
1 point

○ **Often**
2 points

○ **All the time**
3 points

8. Do you feel like you need a daily nap to function?

○ **Never**
0 points

○ **Sometimes**
1 point

○ **Often**
2 points

○ **All the time**
3 points

9. Do you struggle with depression or a lack of motivation?

○ **Never**
0 points

○ **Sometimes**
1 point

○ **Often**
2 points

○ **All the time**
3 points

10. Do you feel like you gain weight easily?

○ **Never**
0 points

○ **Sometimes**
1 point

○ **Often**
2 points

○ **All the time**
3 points

Total Score: _____

If you scored a 20 or higher then you're probably dealing with a thyroid issue. Be sure to follow the strategies in Chapter 6 for improving thyroid function, and use the strategies in Chapters 13 through 15 to improve your thyroid hormone levels. Also, I recommend that you see your physician and functional health practitioner to get labs to confirm your thyroid health.

Potential Roadblock #8: Am I Stressing My Body Enough?

Many people read about the keto diet and think that the nutrition plan by itself will help them accomplish all their goals. However, if you're not stressing your body with exercise, then you may not reach the goals you would like. Answer these questions to see if you're active and engaged enough. If you tested high on the overstressed adrenals or low thyroid questions, then you don't need to take the test because you don't want to add more stress to your system.

1. How often do you exercise each week?

○	○	○	○
4+ times	**3 times**	**2 times**	**0–1 time**
0 points	*1 point*	*2 points*	*3 points*

2. If you work out, how intense are your workouts?

○	○	○	○
Very hard	**Hard**	**Moderate**	**Light**
0 points	*1 point*	*2 points*	*3 points*

3. How often do you engage in weight lifting or resistance training each week?

○	○	○	○
3+ times	**2 times**	**1 time**	**Never**
0 points	*1 point*	*2 points*	*3 points*

4. Do you engage in light activity each day, such as taking a twenty-minute walk?

○	○	○	○
Always	**Most days**	**Occasionally**	**Rarely or never**
0 points	*1 point*	*2 points*	*3 points*

5. Do you use a sauna or take either a cold-water bath or shower?

○	○	○	○
Every day	**Most days**	**Occasionally**	**Never**
0 points	*1 point*	*2 points*	*3 points*

6. How long is your intermittent fasting window (the time between your last meal of one day and your first meal the following day)?

○	○	○	○
19+ hours	**16–18 hours**	**13–15 hours**	**10–12 hours**
0 points	*1 point*	*2 points*	*3 points*

Total Score: _____

If you scored a 12 or higher, your body needs to be stressed more through intermittent fasting, resistance training, and the application of a heat or cold therapy to enhance fat-burning.

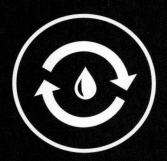

CHAPTER 14

ENHANCING FAT DIGESTION

Whether you're carefully following a ketogenic diet or merely trying to lower your overall carb intake, increasing the amount of healthy fat in your diet is always a good idea. The problem is that the less-than-ideal lifestyle habits you've been practicing up until now may be causing some problematic fat-digestion issues.

If you have been faithfully executing the steps of the keto metabolic breakthrough plan, but you're still feeling tired or sluggish or you're struggling to lose weight, abnormal fat metabolism may be a significant contributing factor. In this chapter, I examine the common causes and symptoms of lipid malabsorption, as well as some strategies for improving fat metabolism.

Why Fat Digestion Is So Important

Healthy fat metabolism is critical for your health and the success of a ketogenic diet. Fats help to transport certain nutrients, balance blood sugar, optimize hormones, promote satiety, and provide a fuel source once you are keto-adapted.

Lots of people overeat every day, but many of them are not getting enough healthy fat. And a poor diet only compounds the issue: The more carbs and sugars you eat, the harder your body has to work to digest fat properly. However, once you start eating a diet full of healthy fats and focus on removing needless carbs in the form of grains and sugar, you can take active steps to support the digestion of fats.

Improper digestion of fats can contribute to many issues, such as low energy levels and energy crashes, food cravings, constipation, and poor nutrient absorption. Other symptoms of poor fat digestion include

- Gastrointestinal (GI) issues such as nausea, vomiting, abdominal pain, gas, and bloating

- Headaches and migraines

- Inability to lose weight

- Skin issues such as itchiness, discoloration, and rashes

- More severe complications such as hypothyroidism, chemical sensitivities, and fibromyalgia

As you can see, fat malabsorption is a serious matter. If you're struggling to digest fats, you must resolve this problem.

Underlying Causes of Fat Malabsorption

If you've been following a strict ketogenic diet for a few months but you're experiencing several of the symptoms I've outlined, your problems may be due to one or more of the following six reasons.

Chronic Stress

In times of distress, digestion is no longer a priority for your body—and that spells disaster for those who are chronically stressed. Your digestive processes work best when your body is relaxed.

As a high-functioning, high-energy individual, I know it's not always possible to eat in a fully relaxed state, and that's one reason I fast in the mornings and consume mostly liquid meals (such as keto smoothies) during the day. I eat my most substantial meal when I'm in my most relaxed state, which is in the evening. So, to lessen the effects of stress on your digestive tract, actively find ways to reduce your stress load, and enjoy your biggest meal of the day when you feel the most at ease.

Poor Diet

Another cause of improper fat digestion is a poor diet. Processed fats and carbs cause inflammation, particularly in the gut. It just makes everything your body already has to do so much harder. This is why it is so important to stick with real foods, healthy produce, and grass-fed and organic animal products. Be sure to check out Chapter 12 for the full list of foods that should be at the center of your keto diet.

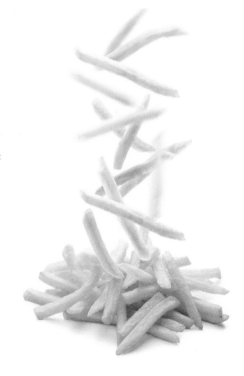

Low Stomach Acid Levels

Optimal stomach acid (HCl) production is critical for digestion. Symptoms of low HCl production include heartburn, bloating, skin problems, hair loss, and fatigue.

SYMPTOMS OF LOW STOMACH ACID

Heartburn or GERD	Bloating and cramping	Constipation or diarrhea
Lots of food sensitivities	Acne and/or eczema	Dry skin or hair
Asthma and allergies	Anemia and weakness	Hair loss in women
Indigestion or burping after meals	Gas within an hour after eating	Chronic intestinal infections
Undigested food in stools	Chronic fatigue	Weak or cracked nails
Protein and mineral deficiencies	Osteoporosis	Any autoimmune disorder

Low stomach acid levels lead to a vicious cycle of improper digestion, malnutrition, and gut microbial imbalance.[1, 2] This imbalance leads to more significant issues, such as leaky gut syndrome and autoimmunity.[3] If you have a history of antibiotic use, bacterial infections, chronic stress, or heartburn medication use, or if you've been eating a carb-rich diet, there is a strong possibility you don't have adequate HCl production. In the "Support Stomach Acid Levels" section later in this chapter, I suggest some ways you can address this issue.

The Baking Soda Stomach Acid Test

This quick and inexpensive stomach acid test works by creating a unique chemical reaction that takes place when you mix the OH− ions of the baking soda with the hydrogen that's in stomach acid (HCl). The result is carbon dioxide gas production, which should cause you to burp within a specific amount of time.

This test has many variables that can cause false positives or negatives. Therefore, to get as accurate a result as possible, perform this test on three consecutive mornings and determine the average of the three tests. You should test in the morning before you've had anything to eat or drink. The results can vary, depending upon how you interpret what you experience. The test is also simple enough to perform every month so that you can note any changes or improvements.

Follow these steps in the morning before you've had anything else to eat or drink:

1. Mix ¼ teaspoon of baking soda in 4 to 6 ounces of cold water.

2. Drink the solution all at once.

3. Start a timer and note how long it takes for you to burp and how often you burp. Track your burps for five minutes. Do not confuse an actual reaction with the small burps that come from swallowing air as you drink the solution.

If you have not burped significantly within five minutes, it's a sign that you're producing insufficient stomach acid. If you experienced early and repeated burping, you may be producing too much stomach acid.

Sluggish Bile Flow

Many people have obvious gallbladder issues that inhibit fat digestion. For example, if you have had your gallbladder removed, you will have trouble digesting fats, and support may be necessary via supplementation. Read more about bile-healthy foods and ways you can use supplements later in this chapter.

FOUR MAJOR FUNCTIONS OF BILE

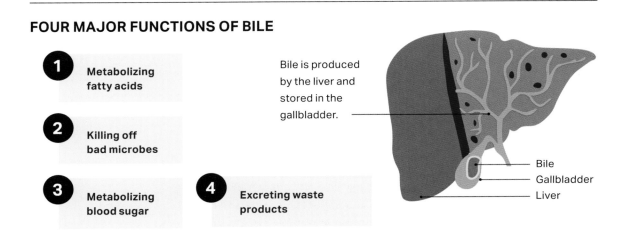

1 Metabolizing fatty acids

2 Killing off bad microbes

3 Metabolizing blood sugar

4 Excreting waste products

Bile is produced by the liver and stored in the gallbladder.

— Bile
— Gallbladder
— Liver

Underactive Thyroid

Fat metabolism issues and poor thyroid function go hand in hand because of the critical role played by thyroid hormones in liver detoxification.[4] Impeded liver detoxification affects bile production—and therefore, fat digestion. Hypothyroidism not only adversely affects the ability to digest fats but also your overall ability to burn fat.

Gut Dysbiosis

Imbalanced levels of good and harmful bacteria in the gut can create inflammatory conditions. Over time, this imbalance becomes an internal stressor that inhibits stomach acid production and slows bile secretion. Having the right kinds of gut bacteria can also play a role in successfully recycling bile (yes, your body reuses bile). Low HCl and bile secretion can exacerbate microbiome imbalances.[5]

Eight Steps to Improve Fat Metabolism

Now that I've established the importance of good fat digestion, it's time for me to share some strategies for improving it. If you're having trouble digesting fats, follow these eight steps.

Step 1: Remove Inflammatory Fats

Unhealthy fats negatively affect your metabolism and digestion. Fats such as canola, soybean, cottonseed, corn, safflower, and peanut oil often are heavily processed and have inflammatory effects. Instead, choose organic and pasture-raised animal products and base your diet around the nutrient-dense foods I discuss in Chapter 9.

In my experience, the clients I've met who have gallbladder problems often struggle to consume eggs, onions, pork products, cheese, and nuts. I suggest that my clients with fat malabsorption remove these foods from their diets for a week or two. Most of the time, people feel better after eliminating these items. They typically don't have to give them up forever. After a few months, without these foods, the bile sludge clears up, and the people can digest their foods better.

If you eliminate these foods and decide to add them back to your diet after you feel better, only add one item each week to see if that food triggers unwanted symptoms. If you feel like you tolerate it well, then you can include it as part of your diet, but I suggest keeping it to three or fewer servings per week.

Step 2: Use MCT and SCT Oils

Long-chain fats in foods like avocados, nuts and seeds, olives, and meat require more energy to digest.[6] They depend on the efficient production and use of bile to be emulsified, and they need pancreatic lipase to be absorbed and assimilated. If you have trouble digesting fats, eat types of fat that are easier to metabolize, such as MCT and SCT oil. MCT and SCT oils don't depend upon bile or pancreatic lipase for digestion and assimilation.

Although small amounts of MCTs are in coconut oil, using a refined MCT oil is better. SCT oil is a newer product derived from butter that provides similar benefits to MCT oil and is extremely easy to digest (www.sctoil.com). SCT has the added benefit of containing beneficial nutrients found in grass-fed butter, such as CLA, butyrate, and vitamins A and K2.

Step 3: Eat Bile-Healthy Foods

To improve fat absorption, you must stimulate bile flow. Optimal bile flow supports fat digestion, blood sugar balance, balanced bacterial growth in the gut, and healthy cholesterol levels. The best foods for bile production include the following:

Apple cider vinegar	Fermented veggies and drinks (kombucha)
Artichokes	Ginger
Asparagus	Lemons and limes
Celery	Milk thistle
Cilantro	Mint
Dandelion	Parsley

As you can see, many of these foods are bitter. I always tell my clients, "Bitter is good for the liver," because it has such a positive impact on bile flow. So, make an effort to consume more bitter herbs with your meals.

Step 4: Support Stomach Acid Levels

Stomach acid production is critical for digestion and overall gut health. If you have any of the symptoms I discussed earlier in this chapter, you will more than likely need to support stomach acid production actively. The easiest way to do this is to avoid drinking a lot of fluid for at least thirty minutes before meals and about an hour afterward.

I also recommend drinking 1 or 2 tablespoons of apple cider vinegar in 4 ounces of water about fifteen minutes before your meal; apple cider vinegar stimulates stomach acid and bile production. Consuming fermented foods like pickles and sauerkraut can also help with stomach acid and bile flow. You may also use an HCl supplement as you work to improve your body's ability to make the proper amount of stomach acid.

Another helpful strategy is to eat protein-rich foods first because they will drop to the bottom of your stomach where the most concentrated acids are to help break them down. You need more acid to digest protein in meat than you do for digesting vegetables. When you eat the protein first, it has more time to sit in the strongest acids, which breaks down the protein bonds more effectively. (See page 94 in Chapter 6 for some other suggestions of ways to support stomach acid levels.)

Step 5: Hydrate Early and Often

Water is life. When you're chronically dehydrated, your bile can become thick and sludgy, which slows down the flow of bile tremendously. Try to drink 16 to 32 ounces of water within the first hour of waking up and then 16 to 32 ounces of water between each meal during the day. Drinking plenty of water also keeps your bowels moving and prevents the buildup of waste and overgrowth of unwanted bacteria.

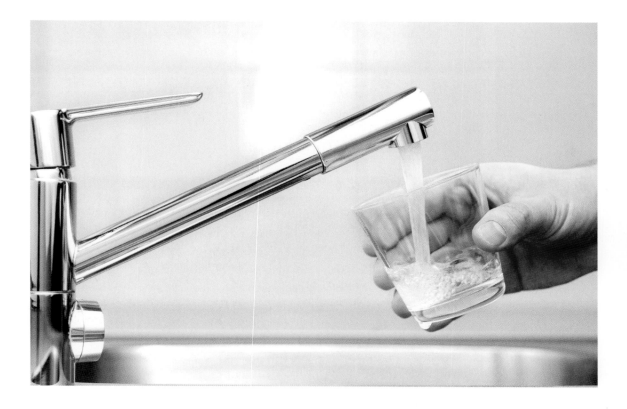

Step 6: Supplement with Ox Bile

If you have gallbladder issues or have had yours removed, your liver can only do so much to make up for lost gallbladder function. In most cases, additional support is beneficial. Ox bile is a supplemental form of the bile that your body produces. The best ox bile supplements contain both ox bile and HCl for the most comprehensive fat-digestion support. It's especially important to supplement with ox bile if you eat a large meal with lots of long-chain fats because your liver may struggle to make enough bile to metabolize it all.

Step 7: Support Your System with Bile Salts

Bile salts are compounds created by the liver that contribute to the fat emulsification effects of bile. The liver produces a large family of bile salts through complex biochemical interactions—and we now know that the amino acids methionine, choline, and taurine are essential for this process. Therefore, if you have digestive issues, you may not be absorbing enough of these critical amino acids from food. Fortunately, you can buy supplements of these amino acids. I have one in my online store called Bile Flow Support that also contains bitter herbs that stimulate the flow of bile.

You also can get sunflower lecithin, which comes as a powder. Put 2 to 3 tablespoons in a smoothie or protein shake each day to add more choline to your diet and thin out the bile. Another compound that can help with bile flow is called TUDCA, which is a conjugate form of the amino acid taurine.

Step 8: Clear the Sludge

Prolonged periods of poor diet, exposure to toxins, and chronic dehydration often cause bile to become thick and sludgy. As a result, your digestion can be severely inhibited, and eventually the dysfunction can progress into gallstones or pancreatitis.[7] The traditional solution for this is gallbladder removal. However, no one wants to have an organ removed unless it's necessary, and you should do everything you can to avoid this eventuality.

If you have been formally diagnosed with biliary sludge or you want to optimize bile flow, the thirty-day sludge-clearing protocol in the sidebar may be beneficial; it's designed to stimulate bile flow as it binds up toxins to prevent adverse side effects. You must stay properly hydrated while you follow this protocol, so drink a minimum of half your body weight in ounces of water daily.

Sludge-Clearing Protocol

Follow this protocol for thirty days. Make sure to stay hydrated, eat bitter foods, and consume medium- and short-chain fats, and you should experience encouraging results.

1. Take 500 to 1,000 milligrams of activated charcoal one hour before meals to help bind toxic biliary sludge. If you weigh less than 125 pounds or suffer from chronic constipation, take just 500 milligrams.

2. Take two capsules of a bile salt supplement (choline and taurine) or herbal bitters such as dandelion and ginger twice daily immediately after meals to help improve bile flow.

3. Take 200 to 400 milligrams of a magnesium supplement one to two hours after meals to help promote bowel elimination. This step is especially important if you have chronic constipation. Start with 200 milligrams. If you still aren't moving your bowels well, then go up to 400 or 600 milligrams to get things moving.

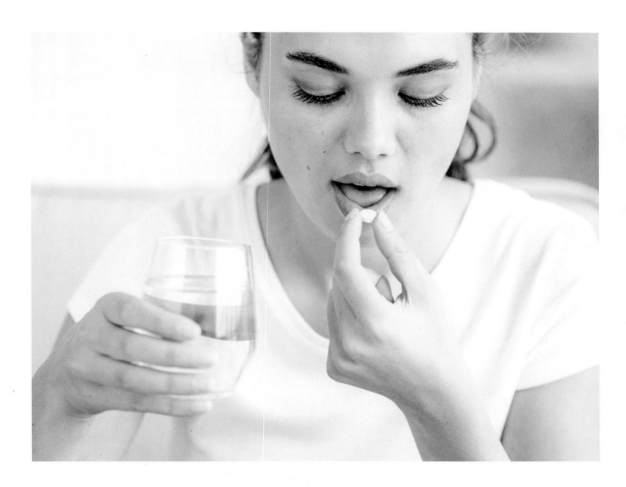

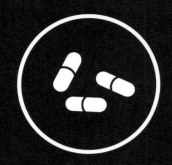

CHAPTER 15

SUPPLEMENTS FOR FUELING
YOUR KETO JOURNEY

By now, you should have a better understanding of the benefits of ketosis and be familiar with the nutrition strategies that will help you get your body keto-adapted safely and effectively. You should also understand the challenges that come with the process and the specific health issues that could derail your goals.

In this chapter, I discuss the supplements that support your body during the adaptation process and beyond. As much as I believe in each of these supplements, I also consider the most crucial aspect of living a keto-charged life to be the changes you make to your diet and lifestyle habits. Supplements are designed to be just what their name suggests—supplemental to the changes required to maintain a healthy ketogenic diet.

Some people choose to use supplements from the start to supercharge their results; others want to see how they progress without supplementation. Neither approach is wrong. Just know that you accomplish 80 to 90 percent of your health improvements through nutrition and lifestyle alterations, and supplements can help you with the last 10 to 20 percent.

If you're generally healthy but looking to optimize your health, the nutrition and lifestyle strategies I've discussed will probably be all you need. However, if you struggle with specific chronic health issues, supplements can be extraordinarily helpful. As a general rule, the longer you've been suffering from chronic health problems, the higher your chances of seeing noticeable improvements through implementing lifestyle changes *and* taking supplements.

These supplements are not meant to treat or cure any disease but are intended only to support a healthy lifestyle. Discuss supplement usage and dosages with your doctor, especially if you are taking any prescription medications.

MCT Oil

Medium-chain triglycerides (MCTs) are unique fatty acids found naturally in coconut and palm oils—and you may recall they made my list of the top twenty-five ketogenic foods in Chapter 9. That's because MCTs have a remarkable ability to stabilize blood sugar and enhance ketone body production. You may also remember that the term "medium" refers to the length of the fatty acid chain.[1] Medium-chain fatty acids contain between six and twelve carbon chains and include the following:

- C6 (caproic acid)
- C8 (caprylic acid)
- C10 (capric acid)
- C12 (lauric acid)

MCTs have a slightly lower caloric load (8.3 calories per gram) than most fatty acids, which have 9 calories per gram.[2] The majority of long-chain fatty acids also depend upon bile salt emulsification to be metabolized and absorbed. Fortunately, MCT oil is easily absorbed and used, even by people who have pancreatitis, cystic fibrosis, and Crohn's disease.[3] The sole exception is lauric acid, which depends upon bile and enzymes to be metabolized.

How to Buy MCT Oil

MCT oils and powders are widely available in health food stores and online. Read labels and avoid any brands containing lauric acid (C12) because you can get it by consuming coconut oil; also, C12 is harder to digest. Here are the best types of MCT products:

- C8 MCT provides the fastest surge in ketones with the least metabolic burden on the body. MCT oils made only with C8 will cost significantly more than other varieties.

- C8 and C10 MCT is a combination that will elevate ketones and give you all the benefits that MCTs have to offer. It's typically more expensive than coconut oil but less expensive than a C8-only variety.

A third approach is to purchase products that contain MCT fats as one of their key ingredients—for example, protein powders and coffees. Just be aware that it's harder to ascertain the quality of the MCTs used in such products if the source or type of the MCT is not listed.

The type of MCT oil I use most commonly is the C8-only caprylic acid because it offers potent ketogenic effects. It also has antimicrobial and immune-supportive benefits. Due to its potent ability to form instant ketones, you can use it in the same ways you would use exogenous ketones, which I will explain later in this chapter.

CAPRYLIC ACID (C8 MCT) BENEFITS

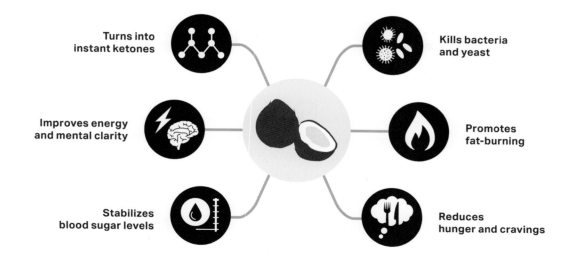

- Turns into instant ketones
- Kills bacteria and yeast
- Improves energy and mental clarity
- Promotes fat-burning
- Stabilizes blood sugar levels
- Reduces hunger and cravings

Taking too much MCT oil too quickly may cause nausea, sore throat, and diarrhea. Begin with 1 teaspoon daily and gradually increase by ½ teaspoon (up to 6 teaspoons) as long as you have no unpleasant symptoms. If you notice unwanted symptoms, stop taking MCTs for a full day. When you resume, decrease your dosage by ½ teaspoon.

If your system is prone to becoming upset easily, begin with just ½ teaspoon daily for the first week. If you experience any adverse symptoms, stop using MCT oil. If you don't experience any symptoms, add ½ teaspoon each week until you find your ideal amount.

Some people find that cheaply made brands cause more symptoms, whereas higher-priced brands tend to be more tolerable and effective. As it usually is in life, you get what you pay for.

How to Use MCT Oil

You can add MCT oil to lots of drinks, including tea, coffee, and green juices. Use it as a salad dressing or add a spoonful to meat and veggie dishes. MCT oil powder is excellent in smoothies and "fat bomb" style recipes. Just remember to work your way up as your tolerance increases.

SCT Oil

Short-chain triglyceride (SCT) oil has similar benefits to MCT oil. As the name implies, SCTs have shorter chains—between two and five carbons. The most common and well-studied SCT is butyrate (or butyric acid), which is found primarily in butter or the clarified form of butter called ghee.

This short-chain fatty acid is also naturally occurring in the body. As you pass prebiotic fiber through the digestive tract, your gut bacteria use this fiber as fuel to produce butyrate as a by-product. Over time, however, toxic overload and poor diet adversely affect gut health and your ability to produce enough butyrate, which is why butyrate supplementation may help with the following:

- Promoting intestinal barrier function
- Potentially aiding in healing leaky gut
- Boosting metabolism and fat-burning
- Helping balance the microbiome
- Boosting brain function
- Supporting mitochondrial health[4, 5]

These benefits make butyrate a critical consideration for anyone who battles inflammatory bowel conditions, intestinal cancers, neurological disorders, and metabolic disorders such as diabetes and obesity. Additionally, SCT oil contains fat-soluble nutrients such as Vitamin A retinol, Vitamin D, E, and K2. It also serves as a rich source of choline, which is a crucial nutrient for neurological tissue and bile production.

SCT Oil Versus MCT Oil

Both MCT and SCT fats are keto-friendly and do not depend upon enzymes to be metabolized. However, they do have some notable differences:

- MCT oil is derived from coconut or palm oil, whereas SCT oil is derived from grass-fed butter.
- MCT oil comes in either oil or powder form, whereas SCT is creamy and more like butter.
- MCT oil is purified to contain only the fatty acids themselves, but SCT oil contains fat-soluble vitamins and other helpful compounds.

- SCT oil is made from dairy, but it's purified to be free of whey, casein, and lactose, which are the dairy components that cause sensitivities and allergies.

How to Use SCT Oil

You can use SCT oil in the same ways you would use ghee or butter—in coffee or tea, on a slice of keto bread, or melted on meat and vegetables. You also can cook with it on low to medium-low heat. I recommend beginning with a teaspoon daily and increasing your intake from there.

DIFFERENT FATTY ACID LENGTHS

Butyric C4:0

Short-chain fatty acids

(2–5 carbons)

Food Sources:

Found naturally in dairy products (butter, cheese, and cow's milk) and human breast milk and also produced by gut bacteria when they ferment fiber sources.

Benefits:

Turn easily into ketones without the need for bile emulsification and very little pancreatic lipase. Also, very helpful for the gut microbiome.

Caprylic C8:0

Medium-chain fatty acids

(6–12 carbons)

Food Sources:

Diary products, coconut oil, coconut fats, and human breast milk

Benefits:

Convert into ketones for cellular energy quickly without the need for bile emulsification (other than 12 C - lauric acid, which does need bile). Antimicrobial and antiyeast activity. C8 and C10 are quick ketone elevators; C8 is the fastest.

Cons:

Can be challenging on the digestive tract and cause nausea, acid reflux, and diarrhea if the individual takes too much too quickly.

Palmitic C16:0

Long-chain fatty acids

(13+ carbons)

Food Sources:

Animal meats, dairy, eggs, coconut and palm oils, nuts, seeds, avocados, olives, and other plant- and animal- based fats.

Benefits:

Often come with fat-soluble vitamins (A, D, E, K1, and K2). Slow conversions to ketones in the body.

Cons:

Take a lot of digestive juices to metabolize in the form of bile emulsification and salivary and pancreatic lipase. Possible lipid rafts for endotoxins produced by bad gut microbes to increase inflammation if fatty acids are not properly metabolized.

Exogenous Ketones

Typically, your body must digest fats, carry them to the liver, convert them into ketones, and then transport them to the cells for energy. Exogenous ketones side-step this process and instead provide direct fuel as you consume them.

You can use exogenous ketones to supply your body with a source of ketones that require almost no processing by your gut and liver. Consequently, the supplement is ideal, not only to help you get into ketosis but also as a quick energy source and performance enhancer.

Ketones also have a protein-sparing effect, meaning that when ketones are circulating in the bloodstream, your body uses protein more efficiently. Many high-performance athletes use exogenous ketones to support their training and performance and to recover more effectively.

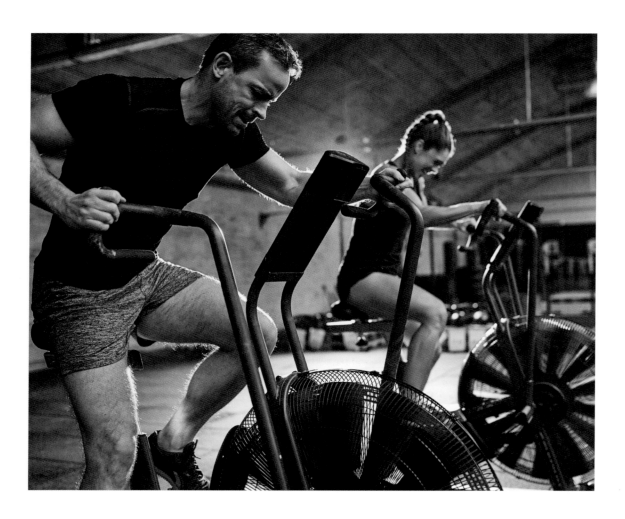

How to Use Exogenous Ketones

The majority of the research on exogenous ketones focuses on their impact on the brain and neurological health, including how ketones affect seizure activity, anxiety, migraines, cognition, and more. Based on this research, my personal use, and the testimonies of my patients, exogenous ketones are ideal for supporting the following conditions and goals:

- Neurodegenerative diseases
- Seizure disorders
- Anxiety and OCD-related disorders
- Headaches and migraines
- Hypoglycemia
- Fasting and intermittent fasting support
- Overcoming keto flu
- Faster keto-adaptation
- Improved short-term cognitive performance
- Improved exercise performance

How to Buy Exogenous Ketones

Exogenous ketones are a combination of the BHB ketone and electrolytes. Ketones taste unpleasant on their own, so manufacturers usually mix them with sweetening agents to make them more appealing. Look for ketones that are sweetened with monk fruit or stevia.

When to Take Exogenous Ketones

According to my friend and top keto researcher Dr. Dominic D'Agostino, exogenous ketones are most effective when taken in combination with MCT fats. Taking exogenous ketones without MCTs causes a rapid ketone spike that fades within an hour or less. When taken with MCTs, however, the ketone spike can last up to three hours.

Timing is the key to getting the most out of supplementation. For example, if you want to get keto-adapted while reducing unwanted side effects, use exogenous ketones in the morning to extend your fasting window by one to three hours.

If you have trouble with energy crashes between meals due to hypoglycemia, use exogenous ketones three to four hours after your last meal to help your body deal with lower blood sugar levels more effectively.

Depending on your health goals, I recommend the timing strategies outlined in the following table:

Health Goal	When to Take
Improve exercise performance	About ten to thirty minutes before your workout
Improve brain performance	About ten to thirty minutes before your mental performance
Enhance fat burning	As a replacement for a meal (in the form of an exogenous ketone drink)
Reduce anxiety	Take at the onset of anxiety symptoms or ten to thirty minutes before an activity that would typically cause anxiety
Reverse mental decline	As a meal replacement or as an aid to extending your fasting window when you feel tired or mentally fatigued
Reduce seizures	At the onset of any noticeable seizure activity or daily as a preventative measure
Reduce headaches/migraines	At the first signs of headache and/or before any action that may provoke a headache
Shorten stress recovery time	About ten to thirty minutes before a stressful activity or immediately after a stressful event
Prevent jet lag from travel	About ten minutes before you want more energy and better mental clarity while traveling; also to help reduce the impact of jet lag on mental recovery

Exogenous Ketones Myths

People seem to either love exogenous ketones or hate them, and some half-truths have been promoted as a result. Here are two of the myths I want to dispel:

- *Exogenous ketones block the body's ability to produce ketones.* Because exogenous ketones are a ready fuel source, consuming them fuels your body and temporarily inhibits the breakdown of body fat. However, this happens only briefly, and the use of exogenous ketones helps your body become more efficient at producing endogenous ketones from your body fat.

- *You can eat whatever you want and remain in ketosis.* This statement is another half-truth. Indeed, if you take enough of the exogenous ketones, your ketone levels will be within the nutritional ketosis range. However, your body is not creating these ketones from its fat stores, and you'll still have high blood sugar and insulin levels.

It's interesting to note that if you consume a high-carb diet, there is a benefit to having ketones in your bloodstream. They may reduce the amount of insulin your body produces and slightly reduce the amount of inflammation and oxidative stress that typically accompanies a poor diet.

I recommend that you use ketones to improve your overall performance and experience during your keto metabolic breakthrough. If you enjoy the way using them makes you feel, continue them after you become keto-adapted to help you achieve your goals.

Electrolytes

Electrolytes are substances that can be used to conduct electricity when dissolved in water. You need electrolytes to survive because they play a role in every metabolic process within your body.

There are five critical electrolytes used to produce cellular energy and conduct nerve impulses to all your organ systems and skeletal muscle systems:

- Sodium (Na+)
- Chloride (Cl–)
- Potassium (K+)
- Magnesium (Mg+)
- Calcium (Ca+)

Electrolyte levels change along with the fluid volume of your body. Dehydration, overhydration, and significant dietary changes are factors that affect the electrolyte levels in your body. You lose electrolytes when you sweat, bleed, and experience diarrhea or vomiting.

Your kidneys and several specific hormones regulate the concentration of each electrolyte. One such hormone is insulin, whose main electrolyte activity is to increase sodium retention. So, when insulin is higher, you retain more water.

How Keto Impacts Electrolyte Balance

As you transition into a ketogenic diet, your insulin levels naturally fall, and therefore, your body excretes more sodium and more fluid. This is one reason you need to take in more electrolytes—and especially sodium—while on a ketogenic diet. You can easily get more sodium by adding salt to your foods and consuming natural sodium- and mineral-rich foods. Many of the foods listed in Chapter 9 are full of trace minerals and electrolytes. Including those foods in your diet should provide for your electrolyte needs.

In some cases, taking supplemental electrolyte powders can be helpful. This is especially the case if you exercise heavily or compete in athletics because you will be sweating out the electrolytes.

Taking an Electrolyte Powder

A suitable electrolyte powder should contain 75 to 300 milligrams of potassium, sodium, calcium, and magnesium per serving. Don't overdo it; if you take in too many electrolytes, you may have loose bowels. Check to ensure your electrolyte powder doesn't contain added sugar or artificial sweeteners such as aspartame or sucralose. If you can't find an unsweetened powder, try to find one with stevia, monk fruit, or non-GMO erythritol. (Read more about sweeteners in Chapter 16.)

Herbal Adaptogens

Adaptogenic compounds are a unique array of compounds used in ancient and natural medicine. They're known to help the body adapt to stress. Popular adaptogenic herbs include Panex ginseng, ashwagandha, rhodiola, cordyceps, astragalus, holy basil, Siberian ginseng (Eleuthero root), and maca.

Adaptogenic herbs help the body function at its optimal level during times of stress. The herbs accomplish this by modulating the production of stress hormones such as cortisol and adrenaline.[6, 7]

As with most other supplements, start with small doses and gradually increase. I suggest you use adaptogenic herbs in the morning and mid-afternoon. You may notice an increase in energy and mental clarity after taking them, so if you take them at night, they could cause insomnia.

A few notable exceptions to this are reishi mushroom, magnolia officinalis, lavender, chamomile, passionflower, lemon balm, and ashwagandha, which are all known to have relaxing effects and can be taken in the evening. You can use these items in teas or essential oils and, in some cases, in the extract form.

Some people find they respond better to certain adaptogens more than others, so monitor how you feel as well as your level of ketosis. If you notice a certain herb induces cravings or makes you feel fatigued, you're probably having a stress response to the herb itself. The following table outlines how I recommend using adaptogens.

Adaptogen	Starting Dose	Max Dose
Ashwagandha	200–400 mg, one dose per day	400–800 mg, two doses per day
Astragalus	500 mg, one dose per day	500–1,000 mg, two doses per day
Cordyceps	300–500 mg, one dose per day	500–800 mg, two doses per day
Holy basil	300 mg, one dose per day	300–600 mg, two doses per day
Lemon balm	100–250 mg, one dose per day	500 mg, two doses per day
Maca	1.5 g, one dose per day	1.5–3.0 g, two doses per day
Panex ginseng	200 mg, one dose per day	400 mg, two doses per day
Reishi mushroom	250–500 mg, one or two doses per day	500–1,000 mg, two doses per day
Rhodiola	100 mg, one dose per day	100–200 mg, two doses per day
Siberian ginseng	100 mg, one dose per day	200 mg, two doses per day

There are many other adaptogens available that I have not mentioned here. If you have great results with the adaptogens I've suggested, feel free to research others. Just remember to start slowly and gradually work your way up if you feel good with a lower dosage.

KETO PRO TIP

Some people practice what is called "adaptogen rotation." They take one to five of these herbs every day for ten days. Then they switch to a different one to five adaptogens for the next ten days, and so on. The rotation isn't necessary, but some individuals feel they receive more benefits from using adaptogens in this manner.

TOP 8 BENEFITS OF USING ADAPTOGENIC HERBS AND MUSHROOMS

Adaptogens help the body build metabolic reserves to adapt to the stressors of life. Stress pulls our body away from metabolic homeostasis, and adaptogens help bring our physiology back to a state of balance. They improve our physical, mental, and emotional strength and endurance. Here are the many benefits of using adaptogens.

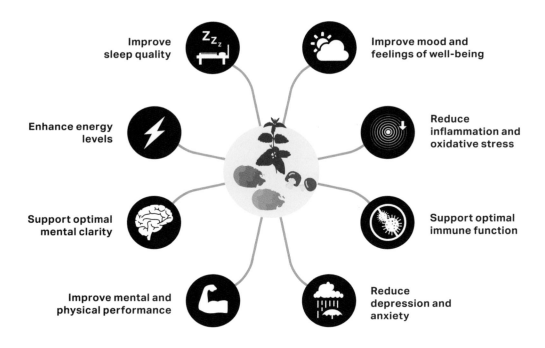

Improve sleep quality

Improve mood and feelings of well-being

Enhance energy levels

Reduce inflammation and oxidative stress

Support optimal mental clarity

Support optimal immune function

Improve mental and physical performance

Reduce depression and anxiety

Digestive Support

Digestive issues are relatively common during the transition to a keto lifestyle. An increase in healthy fat requires more bile production and more of the fat-digesting enzyme, lipase.

The supplements you may need to support your gut during this time include digestive enzymes, probiotics, betaine HCl, bile salts, and ox bile, all of which I have mentioned elsewhere in this book. However, here's a summary.

Digestive Enzymes

The key enzymes to take during your keto transition are the fat-digesting enzyme lipase and the protein-digesting enzymes protease and peptidase. A common myth is that using enzymes inhibits your body's ability to produce digestive enzymes, and you'll become dependent upon supplemental enzymes. *Stress*, not supplementation, is the antagonist to proper digestion. Digestive enzymes work to break down food compounds, making them less irritating to your gut and less stressful on your body. This actually enhances your ability to produce digestive juices and reduces overall gut inflammation while improving nutrient absorption.

Some benefits of digestive enzymes include

- Reducing stress on the digestive system
- Reducing inflammation in the gut
- Improving digestion
- Increasing nutrient assimilation
- Supporting healthy microbiome balance
- Reducing food sensitivities and allergies
- Improving the body's immune response
- Improving cellular energy production
- Reducing autoimmune reactions
- Improving skin and tissue healing

Stomach Acid

At rest, the gastric juices of your stomach are typically between a 3.0 and a 3.5 on the pH scale. However, stomach acid pH levels must be between 1.8 and 2.2 to digest dense protein (such as steak) effectively. This jump is quite substantial, so, in some cases, you need a high level of stomach acid production for proper digestion.

Therefore, if you eat a steak and afterward feel tired and have heartburn, gas, and bloating, it's a sign that you're not producing adequate stomach acid. Other indications include chronic iron, zinc, and B12 deficiencies, weak fingernails, and food sensitivities.

If you have these symptoms, I recommend that you do the baking soda-stomach acid test from Chapter 14. If the results reveal that you're not producing enough stomach acid, follow the steps I cover in Chapter 6 to support stomach acid levels.

If you regularly experience digestive issues, I suggest drinking 1 to 2 tablespoons of apple cider vinegar in a few ounces of water about fifteen minutes before you eat. If you don't notice a significant improvement, and you failed the baking soda test, try the Betaine HCl Challenge:

1. Purchase a bottle of Betaine HCl with pepsin (which costs about $20).

2. Eat a high-protein meal of at least six ounces of meat (veggies are okay, too).

3. In the middle of the meal (never before the meal), take one capsule of Betaine HCl.

4. Finish the meal and determine which of these four outcomes you experience:

   o **You don't notice anything.** If you don't feel any difference, you probably have low stomach acid levels.

   o **You notice your usual indigestion and heartburn**. If you usually have indigestion, and you have the same experience after taking the Betaine HCl, you have low stomach acid and didn't use enough HCl. I recommend trying the test at another meal and using a higher dosage.

   o **You notice unusual indigestion and heartburn.** If you feel burning, hotness, or heaviness in your chest, you have adequate stomach acid levels. It's also possible that you have a hiatal hernia.

In either case, I recommend digestive enzymes over stomach acid support.

- ○ **You notice burning in your stomach but not your chest**. If you feel burning in your abdomen and not your chest, you have a weak stomach lining and possibly an ulcer. If this is the case, you shouldn't take Betaine HCl until you've healed the ulcer. Use digestive enzymes only.

Do this test a few times to ensure accuracy. There are three reasons why you might get incorrect results:

- **You didn't eat enough protein.** The body doesn't need much HCl to digest low-protein meals. Therefore, the supplement may have caused too much of an increase. Be sure to have 6 ounces of meat in your meal.
- **You took the capsule before the meal.** Taking HCl before you eat will almost always cause indigestion. It's best to take it in the middle of your meal.
- **You have esophageal sphincter dysfunction or a hernia.** Hiatal hernias and weak contractile activity of the esophageal sphincter can cause indigestion. If you suspect you may have one of these conditions, have a doctor examine you to rule these out before doing the test.

How to Dose HCl

Supplemental Betaine HCl has made a massive difference in so many of my patients' lives. You can find HCl in dosage ranges of 300 to 500 milligrams per capsule, often combined with 100 to 200 milligrams of pepsin (a digestive enzyme). Always take Betaine HCl halfway through the meal or at the end of the meal. Never take it before you eat.

If you have a history of gastritis or stomach/intestinal ulcers, do not use Betaine HCl because it can exacerbate these issues. Instead, use digestive enzymes and gut-supportive nutrients such as L-glutamine, aloe vera, MSM, zinc carnosine, ginger, and a form of licorice root called DGL.

Additionally, if you regularly take an NSAID such as ibuprofen or aspirin, do not take HCl. Regular use of NSAID medications make you much more at risk for a weak stomach lining and the development of stomach or intestinal ulcers.

There are two protocols for taking HCl regularly, depending on whether you have acid reflux:

- **If You Don't Have Acid Reflux:** Take one capsule during or after the meal and see if you notice a mild burning sensation in your stomach or chest. When you notice this with a single capsule of HCl, you're producing enough on your own. If you don't notice a burning sensation, you're not producing enough HCl. In this case, continue to increase your dosage until you induce indigestion. Then reduce the dosage to the level you were using just before you experienced those symptoms.

- **If You Have Acid Reflux:** Before your next meal, don't take any antacids or acid reflux meds. Then take one HCl capsule during or directly after the meal. If you continue to have indigestion, increase your dosage. Continue this process until you find the amount you need so that you don't have heartburn. Use this dosage until your indigestion returns. When the indigestion returns, it's a sign you're producing more stomach acid and therefore need less supplemental HCl. At this point, reduce the dosage by one capsule for your next meal. Continue with this process until you plateau or don't need to use HCl anymore.

Will I Need to Take HCl Forever?

I hear this question from many of my clients. They experience remarkable results from optimizing their stomach acid but begin to wonder if they will become "addicted" to using the Betaine HCl for life. The answer is, maybe.

Some people who are already reasonably healthy can regain optimal HCl production and maintain that with the right diet. Older individuals or those who have suffered from chronic health problems may need continued stomach acid support. Fortunately, Betaine HCl supplements are some of the less expensive supplements on the market. A few dollars a month will enable you to keep plenty of HCl in stock.

Take the time and effort to do the testing. Optimizing stomach acid levels will make a significant difference in your health and quality of life and make your keto journey so much more enjoyable.

Thyroid Support

Throughout this book, I've discussed several issues involving thyroid problems. Chapter 13, in particular, contains some helpful ways to determine whether you may need thyroid support as well as a comprehensive list of ideas for improving the health of your thyroid. If you have a weak thyroid, your keto metabolic breakthrough will not be as successful as you want it to be, so give this critical endocrine organ the attention it deserves.

Essential nutrients for thyroid function include iodine, selenium, iron, B12, zinc, vitamin A, vitamin D, amino acids, and magnesium. If you're eating a nutrient-dense diet that includes the top keto foods I recommend in Chapter 9, you should already be getting these nutrients. However, if you suffer from low stomach acid, poor digestion, or certain autoimmune conditions, you may not be absorbing them properly. In such cases, I recommend getting tested to see what deficiencies you may have and then supplementing with a high-quality, professional grade multivitamin.

Glandular and Herbal Supplements

I often start clients with weak thyroid function on adaptogenic herbs such as ashwagandha, rhodiola, and lemon balm to help balance stress hormones and improve thyroid hormone expression.

I've also found that using a nonprescription bovine (cow) glandular supplement along with herbs and supportive nutrients can be a game-changer. A bovine glandular supplement contains thyroid hormones and valuable nutrients such as iodine, selenium, and zinc. Bovine supplements are typically low cost, and I have one available in my online store called Thyroid Strong. I recommend starting with two capsules first thing in the morning and slowly progressing to as many as eight capsules until you notice positive changes. However, if you begin to experience hyperthyroid symptoms such as feeling hot, irritable, or anxious, lower the dosage or discontinue the supplement altogether.

When Medication Is Necessary

In some cases, prescription thyroid medication may be warranted. As a functional clinician, I typically recommend stronger medication if a bovine supplement does not affect any significant change.

If you're already taking thyroid medication and getting positive results, don't stop taking it. Instead, talk to your prescribing physician about how to make dosage changes safely. As your new, healthier choices become habits, your need for medication may lessen over time. Keep an open mind and find a doctor who's willing to take the journey with you to help you find the right dosage.

In the meantime, focus on improving your lifestyle and addressing blood sugar, digestive, and chronic inflammatory issues, and you will undoubtedly continue to see marked improvements in your thyroid function and overall health.

Glutathione

Glutathione is the body's master antioxidant—and it has a truly profound impact on reducing inflammation in the body. It's also a critical component in the second phase of liver detox, where ingested toxins are excreted from the body, and it protects intracellular DNA and mitochondria from oxidative stress and damage.

Pure glutathione is broken down by the digestive system, but thankfully, you can boost your glutathione levels with a variety of supplements. N-acetyl L-cysteine (NAC) is a glutathione precursor that helps to replenish intracellular glutathione.

The most beneficial and bioavailable versions of glutathione are the S-acetyl and liposomal forms. These forms of glutathione can bypass the digestive tract and pass into the bloodstream and directly into the cells.

You can supplement with 200 to 400 milligrams of NAC or 100 to 200 milligrams of S-Acetyl or liposomal glutathione each day. Each can be taken with or without food, although many people believe it's best to take these supplements separately from eating so your body can readily absorb them with no competition from any food you've consumed. There isn't enough research to clarify this at this time, so my recommendation is that you take it at the time that's most convenient for you.

Mitochondrial Support

The mitochondria within every cell are where ketones are burned and where cellular energy is produced. Thanks to unhealthy diets, genetics, and chronic stress, many people experience a deficiency in the nutrients required for optimal mitochondrial health, including coenzyme Q10, acetyl-L-carnitine, alpha lipoic acid, B vitamins, and magnesium. Glutathione also plays a significant role in protecting the mitochondria, so boosting your glutathione levels with precursors such as NAC can be extremely helpful. Some individuals may have trouble producing enough glutathione from precursors alone and need S-Acetyl or liposomal glutathione supplementation to support overall glutathione levels. Here are some conditions that may require additional nutrients that support mitochondrial health:

- Autoimmune conditions

- Cancer

- Chronic fatigue and fibromyalgia

- Dementia, Alzheimer's, and poor memory

- Diabetes

THE BEST FOOD SOURCES OF COENZYME Q10 (CoQ10)

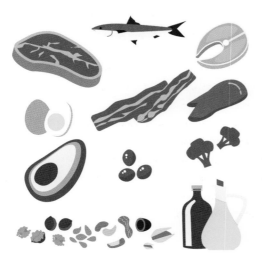

- **Pasture-raised meats**
- **Organ meats such as heart, liver, and kidney (which are the richest source)**
- **Wild-caught fish**
- **Pasture-raised egg yolk**
- **Grass-fed butter**

The following are the best vegan sources:
- **Avocados**
- **Olives and olive oil**
- **Broccoli, cauliflower, and sweet potato**
- **Nuts and seeds: pistachios, walnuts, sesame seeds, and hazelnuts**

- Heart disease

- Lyme disease

- Neurodegenerative diseases

If you've been on medications for lowering cholesterol (statins) or blood pressure, blood thinning agents, antidepressants, and certain diabetic medications, you have a higher risk of mitochondrial dysfunction and will benefit from additional support.

I recommend three supplements aside from glutathione for mitochondrial health. If you're interested in finding the precise dosage you need, you can have lab testing done. In my clinic, we conduct organic acid tests and micronutrient tests to help patients determine the correct dosage of these supplements:

- **CoQ10:** CoQ10 is a potent intracellular and intramitochondrial antioxidant that is necessary for the production of cellular energy. It's available in several forms, including ubiquinone, ubiquinol, and pyrroloquinoline quinone (PQQ). These supplements are fat-soluble, which means they work best when taken with meals. Starting dosages range from 50 to 100 milligrams daily, and you can increase your dosage to as much as 1,000 milligrams daily. Increase a little at a time until you find the dose that gives you sufficient energy.

- **Acetyl-L-carnitine:** Up to 70 percent of the energy produced by muscle cells (including the heart) comes from fat metabolism. Carnitine is the gatekeeper that allows fatty acids to pass into the mitochondrial furnace effectively. If you don't have enough carnitine, you can't adequately produce ketones from long-chain fats, which means you need to supplement daily with MCT or SCT oil to achieve ketosis. Starting dosages range from 200 to 400 milligrams, and you can slowly increase intake up to 2 to 3 grams per day if you have a significant deficiency.

- **Magnesium:** This plays a role in more than 300 different enzymatic functions and is one of the biggest nutritional deficiencies in our society. I recommend getting at least 200 to 400 milligrams of a good quality magnesium each day. If you take too much magnesium, you will end up with loose stools. If this happens, simply back down your dosage until your bowels become normalized again.

- **B vitamins:** B vitamins play a vital role in cellular energy production, neurotransmitter function, liver function, cellular reproduction, and much more. The table provides you with a recommended dosage range for the B vitamins.

B Vitamin	Starting Dose	Max Dose
B1: Thiamine HCl or benfotiamine	10 mg daily	600 mg daily
B2: Riboflavin 5'-phosphate (R5P)	10 mg daily	200 mg daily
B3: Niacinamide	10 mg daily	1,000 mg daily
B5: D-calcium pantothenate	10 mg daily	500 mg daily
B6: Pyridoxal 5'-phosphate (P5P)	10 mg daily	200 mg daily
B7: Biotin	500 mcg daily	10,000 mcg daily
B9: Methyltetrahydrofolate or methylfolate	200 mcg daily	10,000 mcg daily
B12: Methylcobalamin or Methyl B12	200 mcg daily	10,000 mcg daily

The most effective way to take in these essential vitamins is through a B-complex that contains all the varieties in one pill. You may also find a multivitamin with a B-complex included.

Most people don't need to take all of these supplements to see results on their keto journey, but one or more may be very beneficial and help you get faster and better overall results.

Be sure to get your supplements from a trusted place that does third-party testing for toxic contaminants. Do not get your supplements from a place that isn't known for promoting health—such as Walmart or Target! Find a functional health doctor or a great health food store that you trust to provide you with supplements. These professionals have done the research for you and found the top brands or, in some cases, they've worked with manufacturers to formulate specific products that really work.

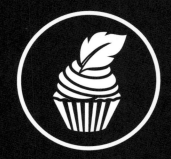

CHAPTER 16
THE BEST KETOGENIC SWEETENERS

Artificial sugars seemed like a real godsend when they first came on the market. All the sweetness of sugar with none of the calories? Sounds too good to be true!

It was. Researchers have since undeniably revealed that artificial sweeteners are toxic to the brain, disrupt the health of gut bacteria, and may lead to metabolic dysregulation and subsequent weight gain. (Ironic, right?)

Thanks to the widespread media coverage of the damaging effects of artificial sweeteners, some food manufacturers have jumped on the "natural" bandwagon and claim that their artificial sweeteners are now powered by healthier alternatives such as stevia. What they don't tell you is that their sweeteners are still primarily chemical sweeteners with just a *touch* of the natural stuff.

Fortunately, there are many exceptional natural sweeteners such as stevia, monk fruit (Lo Han), maple syrup, honey, coconut sugar, yacón syrup, and more. However, the most keto-friendly of them all are the ones with the lowest impact on blood sugar: stevia and monk fruit. Maple syrup, honey, coconut sugar, and yacón syrup are vastly better than sugar or artificial sweeteners, but they still spike your blood sugar and pull you out of ketosis.

Xylitol and erythritol are two sugar alcohols that are commonly used in keto desserts and recipes. However, some individuals find them disruptive to the gut, and these sugar alcohols can cause gas, bloating, and other digestive distress. Many people tolerate them well, but stevia and monk fruit are better options by far.

The World's Best Sweeteners

The stevia plant has been used for thousands of years. Its use was documented centuries ago in South America, where people believed the plant had healing properties and used its leaves and extracts to sweeten teas. This natural sweetener can be up to 300 times sweeter than sugar, so a little goes a long way.

Two primary components in the stevia plant are responsible for its sweet taste. First, stevioside compounds are sweet but also have a licorice-like aftertaste. Rebaudioside compounds are isolated in highly refined commercial stevia products because they provide sweetness without the licorice aftertaste. Although these isolated stevia components are still healthier than other chemical sweeteners, whole-plant extracts of stevia are a more wholesome option.

Monk fruit (also known as lo han or lo han guo) is a melon-like fruit that is native to southeast Asia, where it has been harvested and consumed for hundreds of years. This natural sweetener contains compounds called *mogrosides,* which are rated 300 times sweeter than sugar without any of sugar's drawbacks.

Monk fruit extracts have grown extremely popular in the United States and are sometimes combined with sugar alcohols such as erythritol and xylitol or a form of corn fiber that certain companies use as a nonglycemic sweetener.

Be aware that your favorite sweetener may include these ingredients. If you can tolerate sugar alcohols such as erythritol, then using those products is no problem. But people who don't tolerate sugar alcohols should be aware that most monk fruit–based sweeteners have sugar alcohols or corn fiber sweetener in them.

Read on to learn the four reasons why I love monk fruit and stevia more than the other natural sweetening agents.

BEST SWEETENERS CRITERIA

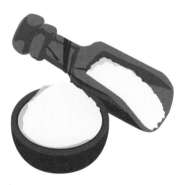

1. Whole food sourced
2. Minimal impact on blood sugar and insulin
3. Contain nutritional value
4. Provide health benefits
5. Good for the gut microbiome

No Effects on Blood Sugar

Although sweeteners such as coconut palm sugar are great alternatives to more processed and artificial products, stevia and monk fruit are the best for keto dieters because they have no impact on blood sugar levels!

In animal and human studies, researchers have found that stevia has beneficial effects on blood sugar balance.[1] Some emerging evidence even suggests that it may improve insulin signaling.[2]

Monk fruit also has a blood sugar–stabilizing effect. Although less research has been done on monk fruit and its components, preliminary studies indicate it may improve insulin signaling by protecting the pancreatic insulin-releasing cells from oxidative stress.[3, 4]

Added Nutritional Value

Stevia and monk fruit are also fantastic because, unlike sugar, they contain an array of nutrients. Not only do you get all the benefits that come from cutting sugar but you also get some added nutrition without any side effects!

Analysis of whole-leaf stevia extract uncovered a diverse array of nutrients. Stevia contains beneficial compounds, including polyphenols, carotenoids, chlorophyll compounds, and amino acids.[5] Although you should never use stevia as a primary source of nourishment, it adds a modest nutrient boost to your foods.

Analysis of monk fruit shows that it also contains a range of flavonoids, amino acids, polysaccharides, and triterpenes, which have cancer-fighting potential.[6] These components may be responsible for some of monk fruit's documented health benefits, including acting as an antioxidant, boosting immunity, and protecting the liver—all of which are the opposite of sugar's effects.

Anticancer Properties

Using stevia and monk fruit in place of sugar may provide anticancer benefits. So, as it turns out, you can have your cake and fight cancer, too!

Stevia contains compounds such as kaempferol, quercetin, and apigenin that have been shown to potentially reduce oxidative stress and help control the development of cancer.[7, 8] Another study found that whole-plant stevia extract had a higher anticancer effect than did stevioside alone, which further supports the importance of using stevia in whole-plant extract form.[9]

Mogrosides, the compounds in monk fruit that gives it its sweetness, have been isolated into five types. Researchers have found that mogroside V inhibits tumor growth in pancreatic cancer cells by interfering with cell division, preventing angiogenesis (blood flow to the tumor), and promoting cancer cell death.[10]

Immune and Gut Support

Replacing sugar with a natural sweetener that doesn't affect your blood sugar strengthens and balances your immune system. Also, steviosides and mogrosides have been shown to support a healthy immune response.[11]

Some evidence suggests that stevia has mild antimicrobial effects when taken internally, and it has promise in combating Lyme disease.[12, 13] Once again, monk fruit demonstrates nearly identical properties to stevia when it comes to immune support, with its immune-boosting and antimicrobial benefits.[14]

Another benefit of using stevia and monk fruit is that they don't provide fuel for harmful microbes in the gut. If you're trying to correct gut dysbiosis, using these sweeteners rather than sugar, artificial sweeteners, and sugar alcohols is a must!

Test and Then Enjoy!

It's essential that you test your blood sugar and ketones to see how your body responds to these sweeteners. Most people seem to tolerate them well, but they have also been known to knock a few people out of ketosis. So, test yourself to see how you respond.

Here are a few final things to consider:

- **Look for the purest forms.** Depending on availability, always buy the cleanest form or a whole-food extract. Stevia is much more readily available in stores than monk fruit. My favorite brand of stevia is the SweetLeaf brand, which is organic but not made from the whole leaf.

- **Stevia is linked to ragweed sensitivity.** Stevia is a member of the ragweed family. If you have had an adverse experience with stevia in the past, the reaction is most likely due to a ragweed allergy. In this case, avoid stevia and opt for monk fruit.

- **You can lessen the unmistakable stevia aftertaste.** Stevia is known to have a somewhat bitter, licorice aftertaste. Adding a pinch of pink salt to the stevia helps diminish this taste and give it a milder flavor.

- **Buy organic.** Plenty of organic stevia products exist, but finding organic monk fruit extract can be a challenge. However, the absence of an organic certification doesn't mean that a product is produced with the use of chemicals. A vast majority of monk fruit is harvested from its natural habitat and therefore would technically meet organic standards.

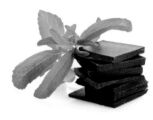

Just because you're on a ketogenic diet doesn't mean you have to forgo dessert or stop enjoying the sweeter things in life. As long as stevia and monk fruit agree with your digestive system and don't knock you out of ketosis, feel free to indulge from time to time in some stevia-sweetened chocolate bars, or use stevia and monk fruit as substitutes for sugar in your favorite dessert recipes. Just be sure to remember that they pack a potent sweet punch, so add them into foods slowly and sparingly.

But most importantly, enjoy life and all of its many flavors!

Afterword

I've reached the end of my explanation of the keto metabolic breakthrough, but the journey is just beginning. If you haven't already, I encourage you to start on the path to your unique keto metabolic breakthrough.

If you're not sure where to start, keep it simple. You know that to get your body into nutritional ketosis you have to stop giving it the old, less-effective fuel source (carbs and sugar) and start feeding it healthy fats. So, start there. Commit to eating fewer carbs and sugar today and develop a taste for clean, unprocessed fats. Opt for water instead of soda. Skip the toast with your eggs. Cook with avocado oil instead of processed, inflammatory canola or vegetable oils.

Every choice you make will get you one more step down the path toward your new ketogenic lifestyle. Will it be easy? No—but is there anything in life worth having that is?

If you want to be well, lose weight, and have more energy and vitality, now is your opportunity to choose to move in that direction. Select healthy, nutrient-dense foods over convenience. Opt to take the stairs. Decide to go to bed earlier. Small choices have exponential effects on your health and happiness.

Remember that you didn't get into this mess in only a few weeks, so you can't expect everything to be "all better" in such a short amount of time. With time and consistency, you will create a whole new lifestyle that will set you up to win!

To more fully support you and your keto metabolic breakthrough, I've provided some great-tasting recipes in the pages that follow. Review Chapter 12 to prepare your kitchen for your new lifestyle, and then start experimenting with some of the recipes I've shared.

I wish you only the best and happiest life. Please feel free to reach out to my team and me at DrJockers.com if you have any questions or if you think you would benefit from additional support.

If you received valuable insight from this book, it would also be a great honor if you shared it with your friends and family. Together we can make a big impact on the health of those closest to you!

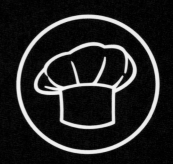

CHAPTER 17

RECIPES

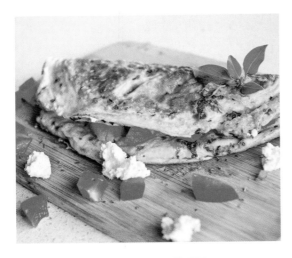

BREAKFAST

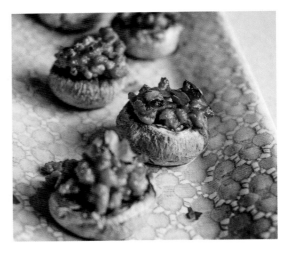

SNACKS, SIDES, AND CONDIMENTS

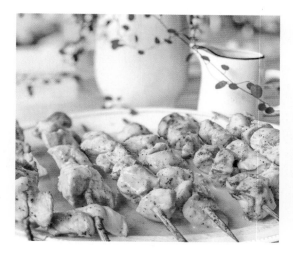

MAIN MEALS

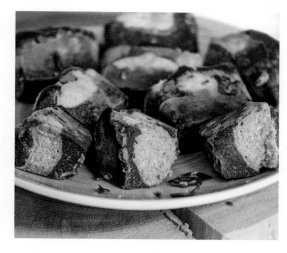

SWEET TREATS

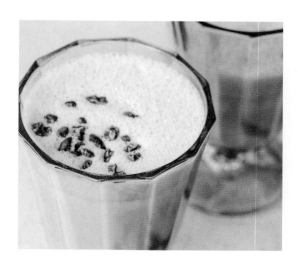

DRINKS

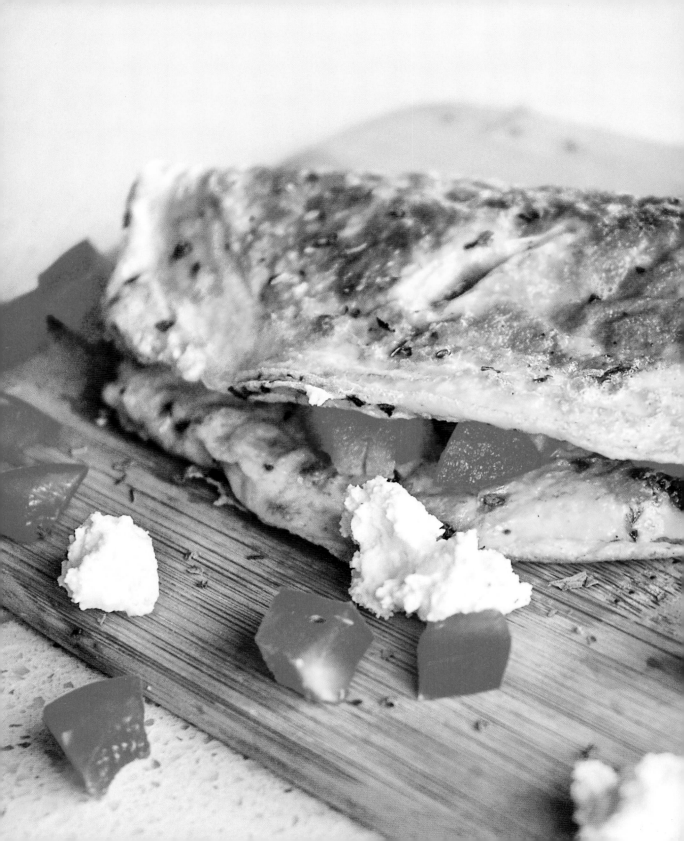

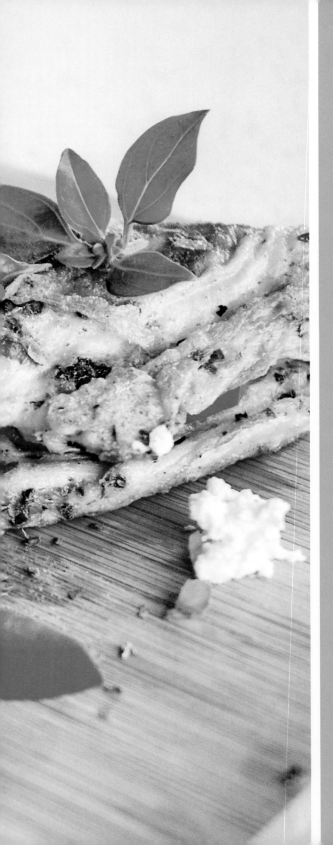

BREAKFAST

CHOCOLATE COLLAGEN GRANOLA

Yield: 3 cups, ¼ cup per serving   **Prep Time:** 15 minutes   **Cook Time:** 15 minutes

1 cup raw pumpkin seeds

1 cup raw hulled sunflower seeds

1 cup unsweetened coconut flakes

2 tablespoons chocolate-flavored collagen peptides

2 tablespoons unsalted butter, ghee, or coconut oil

2 tablespoons sugar-free maple syrup

1. Preheat the oven to 350°F and line a rimmed baking sheet with parchment paper.

2. Place the pumpkin seeds, sunflower seeds, coconut flakes, and protein powder in a high-powered blender or food processor and pulse until the seeds and coconut are broken into small pieces.

3. Melt the butter with the maple syrup, then pour it into the blender or food processor. Pulse until well combined. The texture will be like wet sand.

4. Use a tablespoon to scoop chunks of the mixture onto the prepared baking sheet.

5. Bake for 10 to 15 minutes, or until crunchy. (Check the granola each minute after 10 minutes have elapsed to ensure that it has the desired texture.) Remove from the oven. Let cool for 5 minutes.

6. Serve immediately or store in the refrigerator for up to a week.

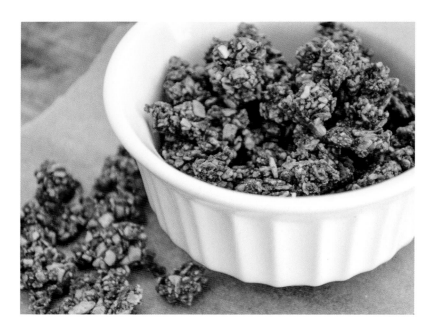

Calories: 269   **Fat:** 23g   **Protein:** 9g   **Carbs:** 8g   **Fiber:** 4g   **Sugar:** .5g

CINNAMON PANCAKES

Yield: 6 pancakes, 1 per serving   **Prep Time:** 10 minutes   **Cook Time:** 20 minutes

1 cup arrowroot flour

2 large eggs

⅓ cup full-fat coconut milk

⅓ cup chopped raw pecans

1 scoop vanilla-flavored protein powder (optional)

2 tablespoons filtered water

2 tablespoons powdered monk fruit sweetener

1 teaspoon vanilla extract

¾ teaspoon baking soda

¼ teaspoon fine sea salt

¼ teaspoon ground cinnamon

2 dropperfuls vanilla-flavored liquid stevia

2 dropperfuls cinnamon-flavored liquid stevia

Dash of ground nutmeg

1 tablespoon coconut oil, for the pan

1. Place all of the ingredients except the coconut oil in a medium bowl. Using an electric mixer, blend the ingredients thoroughly.

2. Warm the coconut oil in a skillet over medium heat. Pour ¼ cup of the batter into the pan. Cook two pancakes at a time.

3. Cook for 3½ to 4 minutes, then flip the pancakes and cook for 3 minutes on the other side.

4. Transfer the cooked pancakes to a plate. Repeat steps 2 and 3 until all of the batter has been used, making a total of 6 pancakes.

5. Serve immediately.

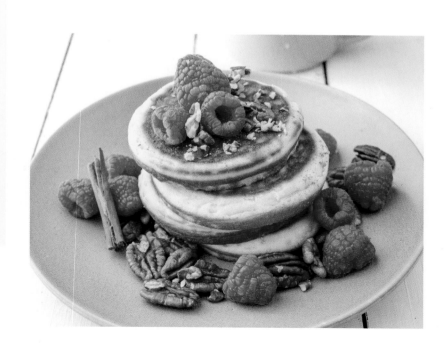

Calories: 190   **Fat:** 14g   **Protein:** 6g   **Carbs:** 10g   **Fiber:** 3g   **Sugar:** 1g

TOMATO BASIL OMELET

Yield: 1 serving   **Prep Time:** 5 minutes   **Cook Time:** 5 minutes

3 large eggs

1 teaspoon chopped fresh basil, or ¼ heaping teaspoon dried basil

1 teaspoon minced garlic

½ teaspoon fine sea salt

1 tablespoon coconut oil, ghee, or unsalted butter

1 small tomato, chopped

½ bell pepper (any color), sliced

Crumbled fresh (soft) goat cheese, for serving (optional)

1. In a small bowl, whisk together the eggs, basil, garlic, and salt.

2. In a skillet over medium heat, warm the coconut oil. Pour the egg mixture into the pan and cook without disturbing for 5 minutes, or until it is almost cooked. Add the tomato and bell pepper to the center of the eggs and then flip half of the cooked eggs over onto the other half to form an omelet.

3. Transfer the omelet to a plate and top with crumbled goat cheese, if desired.

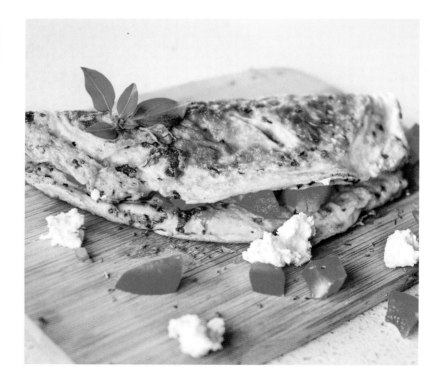

   Calories: 376   **Fat:** 29g   **Protein:** 20g   **Carbs:** 8g   **Fiber:** 2g   **Sugar:** 4g

TURKEY SAUSAGE BALLS

Yield: 12 to 15 meatballs, 1 per serving   **Prep Time:** 10 minutes   **Cook Time:** 20 minutes

1 pound ground turkey

½ cup blanched almond flour

1 large egg

3 tablespoons diced onions

1 teaspoon onion powder

1 teaspoon dried rosemary leaves

1 teaspoon paprika

1 teaspoon dried oregano leaves

1 teaspoon red pepper flakes

1 teaspoon fine sea salt

1 teaspoon freshly ground black pepper

1. Preheat the oven to 400°F. Line a baking sheet with parchment paper.

2. Place all of the ingredients in a medium bowl and use your hands to mix well.

3. Using a 1-tablespoon measuring spoon, scoop pieces of the mixture and roll them into balls. Place them on the prepared baking sheet.

4. Bake for 20 minutes, or until golden brown and no longer pink in the center. Remove from the oven and set aside to cool slightly.

5. Serve immediately.

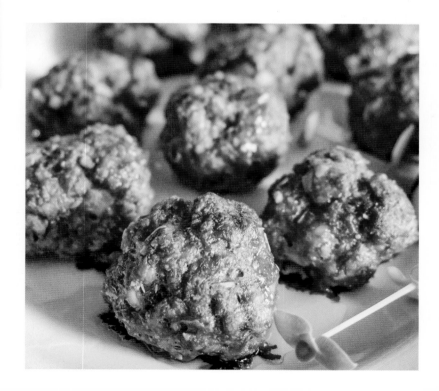

KETO HASH BROWNS

Yield: 12 hash browns, 1 per serving   **Prep Time:** 20 minutes   **Cook Time:** 20 minutes

1 head cauliflower, cored and roughly chopped

Boiling water, as needed

1 large egg

½ cup shredded cheddar cheese

1 tablespoon chopped fresh chives

1 teaspoon garlic powder

1 teaspoon fine sea salt

1 teaspoon freshly ground black pepper

½ teaspoon cayenne pepper

1. Preheat the oven to 400°F. Line a rimmed baking sheet with parchment paper or grease it with coconut oil.

2. Place the cauliflower in a high-powered blender or food processor and pulse it until it's finely chopped.

3. Transfer the cauliflower to a bowl and cover with boiling water. Set aside for 3 minutes.

4. Drain the cauliflower and place in the center of a kitchen towel for a minute to cool slightly. Wrap the cauliflower in the towel and squeeze out any remaining liquid.

5. Return the cauliflower to the blender or food processor and add the remaining ingredients. Blend until a dough forms.

6. Using a 1-tablespoon measuring spoon, scoop pieces of the dough and roll them into balls, making a total of 12 balls. Place them on the prepared baking sheet. Using a fork, flatten the balls into small rounds.

7. Bake for 20 minutes, or until golden brown. Remove from the oven and set aside to cool slightly.

8. Serve immediately or store in an airtight container in the refrigerator for up to 5 days.

Calories: 38   **Fat:** 2g   **Protein:** 3g   **Carbs:** 3g   **Fiber:** 1g   **Sugar:** 1g

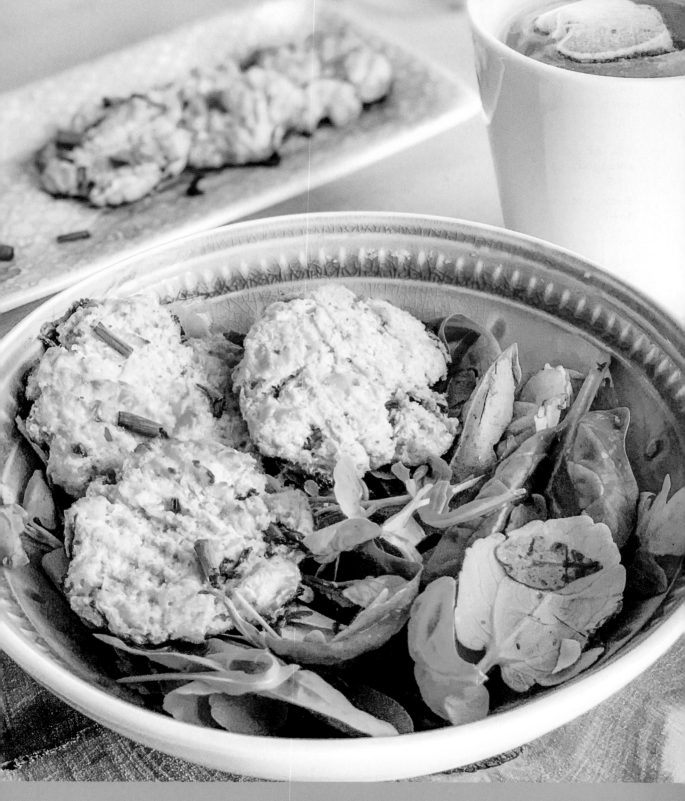

SAVORY SALMON PANCAKES

Yield: 8 pancakes, 1 per serving   **Prep Time:** 10 minutes   **Cook Time:** 16 minutes

FOR THE PANCAKES:

4 ounces (½ cup) cream cheese, softened

4 large eggs

1 teaspoon ground cinnamon

1 tablespoon coconut oil, unsalted butter, or ghee, for cooking

FOR THE CREAM CHEESE SPREAD:

4 ounces (½ cup) cream cheese, softened

2 teaspoons chopped fresh fennel fronds

2 ounces cold-smoked wild-caught salmon, diced

1 teaspoon freshly squeezed lemon juice

1. Make the pancakes: Place the cream cheese, eggs, and cinnamon in a high-powered blender and blend until well combined. (You also can use an electric mixer.)

2. Make the cream cheese spread: In a medium bowl, mix together the cream cheese and fennel. Add the salmon to the cream cheese and mix until well combined. Add the lemon juice to the mixture and mix one more time.

3. Warm the coconut oil in a medium-sized skillet over medium heat. Pour about 2 tablespoons of the pancake batter into the skillet and cook for 1 minute. Turn the pancake over and cook on the other side for 1 minute more. Remove the pancake to a plate. Repeat until you've used all of the batter, adding more coconut oil to the pan as needed.

4. To assemble, place a dollop of the cream cheese spread on top of each pancake and spread it to the edges.

5. Serve immediately.

Calories: 120   **Fat:** 11g   **Protein:** 5g   **Carbs:** 2g   **Fiber:** 0g   **Sugar:** 0g

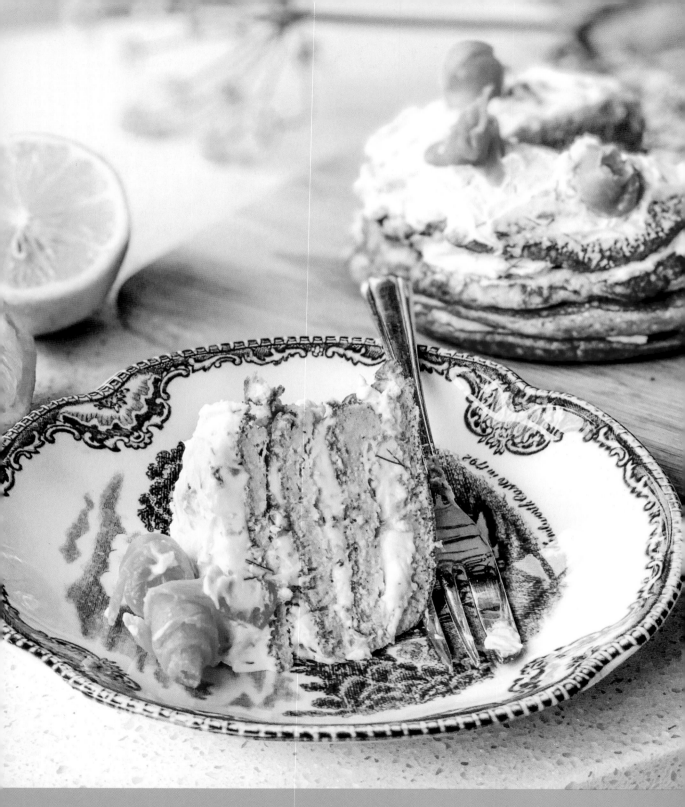

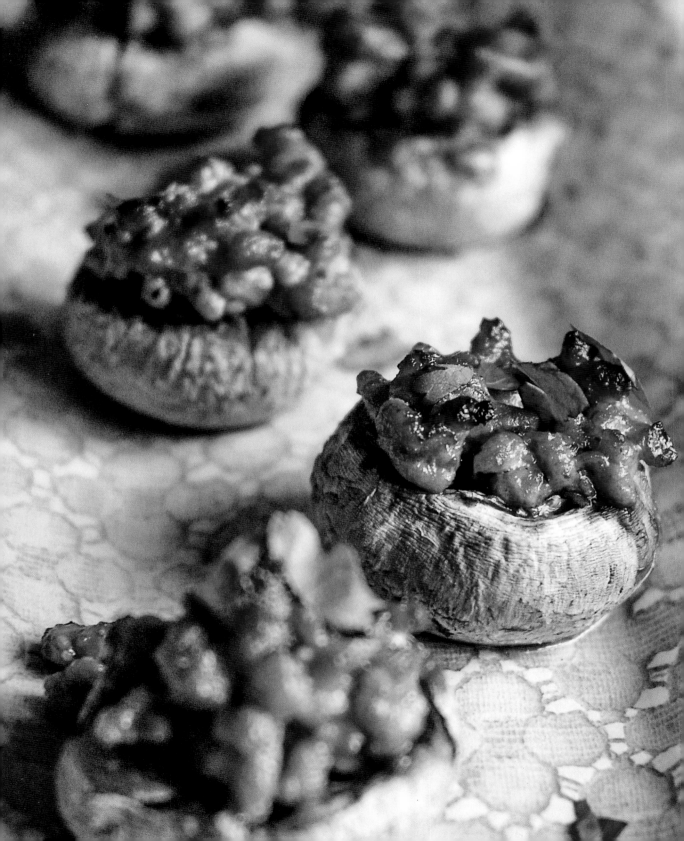

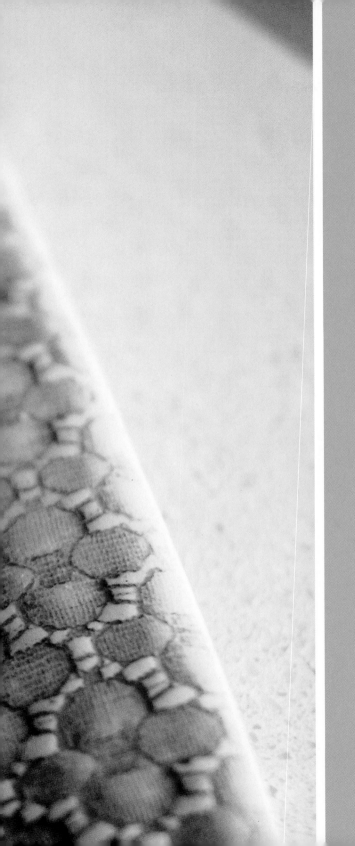

SNACKS, SIDES, AND CONDIMENTS

SMOKED SALMON SUSHI ROLLS

Yield: 2 servings   **Prep Time:** 15 minutes   **Cook Time:** —

1 cucumber, peeled

1 avocado, pitted and skinned

2 tablespoons avocado oil mayonnaise (optional)

2 pinches fine sea salt

2 nori seaweed sheets

6 ounces cold-smoked wild-caught salmon, such as Nova lox, cut into strips

1. Slice the cucumber into strips. Set aside.

2. Place the avocado in a small bowl with the mayonnaise (if using) and salt and mash together until well combined.

3. Spread an equal amount of the avocado mixture on each sheet of the nori. Add equal amounts of the cucumber and smoked salmon to each.

4. Roll the nori sheets into sushi rolls. Slice into individual pieces.

5. Serve immediately.

Tip: This recipe is easily doubled. If you make a bunch of rolls at a time, you can store them in the refrigerator for up to 2 days.

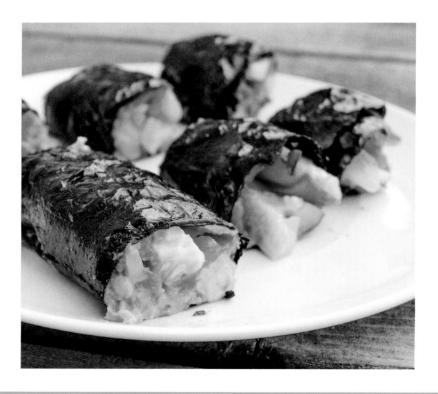

Calories: 96   **Fat:** 6g   **Protein:** 6g   **Carbs:** 4g   **Fiber:** 2g   **Sugar:** 1g

PALEO STUFFED MUSHROOMS

Yield: 10 mushrooms, 2 per serving   **Prep Time:** 15 minutes   **Cook Time:** 30 minutes

10 white mushrooms (about 1½ inches in diameter), stemmed

1 teaspoon coconut oil, for cooking

8 ounces bulk buffalo sausage, beef sausage, or ground beef

½ cup chopped red onions

½ cup chipotle lime avocado oil mayonnaise

1 teaspoon parsley or chives, chopped (optional)

1. Preheat the oven to 375°F. Arrange the mushroom caps on a baking sheet.

2. In a medium sauté pan over high heat, warm the coconut oil, then cook the sausage and onions for 5 minutes, or until the meat is cooked through. Remove from the heat and stir in the mayonnaise.

3. Use a spoon to evenly divide the filling among the mushroom caps.

4. Bake for 20 to 25 minutes, or until the stuffing is beginning to brown nicely along with the mushroom caps. Remove from the oven.

5. Garnish with parsley, if desired. Serve immediately.

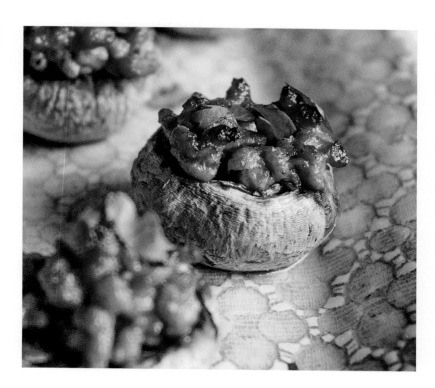

Calories: 195   **Fat:** 16g   **Protein:** 10g   **Carbs:** 3g   **Fiber:** 1g   **Sugar:** 2g

SEED CRACKERS

Yield: 12 crackers, 2 per serving   **Prep Time:** 15 minutes   **Cook Time:** 20 minutes

½ cup sesame seeds

½ cup hulled raw sunflower seeds

½ teaspoon garlic powder

½ teaspoon onion powder

½ teaspoon fine sea salt

2 tablespoons filtered water

1. Preheat the oven to 350°F.

2. Place the sesame seeds, sunflower seeds, garlic powder, onion powder, and salt in a high-powered blender or food processor and blend until the mixture takes on the consistency of meal.

3. With the blender or food processor still running, drizzle in the water until the mixture takes on the consistency of dough and clumps together into a ball.

4. Transfer the dough to a 14-inch-square piece of parchment paper and place another sheet of the same size on top of it. Using a rolling pin, roll out the dough as thin as you like. If it's on the thicker side, about ¼ inch, the crackers will be much sturdier.

5. Remove the top sheet of parchment paper and transfer the rolled dough, still on the bottom sheet of parchment, to a baking sheet. Using a pizza cutter or sharp knife, cut the dough into 12 rectangles, but do not separate the pieces.

6. Bake for 15 to 20 minutes, or until golden brown. Remove from the oven and set aside to cool completely on the baking sheet.

7. Break the crackers along the cut lines. Serve or store in an airtight container in the refrigerator for up to a week.

Calories: 115   **Fat:** 9g   **Protein:** 4g   **Carbs:** 5g   **Fiber:** 3g   **Sugar:** 0g

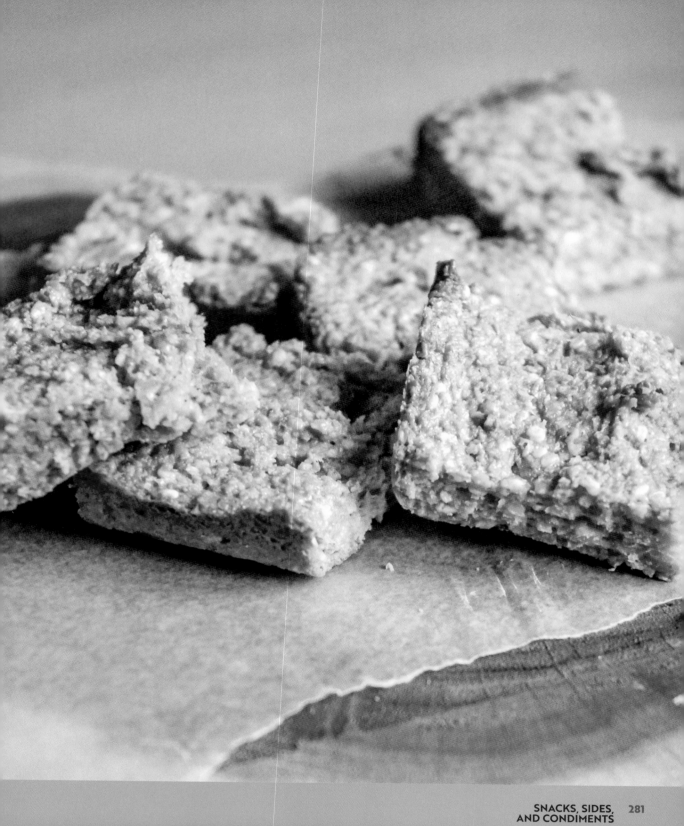

CRUNCHY GARLIC CHIPS

Yield: 6 servings, about ½ cup per serving   **Prep Time:** 25 minutes, plus 20 minutes to rest   **Cook Time:** 15 minutes

1¼ cups chia and/or flax seed powder

1 tablespoon nutritional yeast

2 teaspoons garlic powder

1 teaspoon onion powder

½ cup filtered water

1. Preheat the oven to 400°F.

2. In a large bowl, whisk together all of the ingredients except the water. Add the water and, using a rubber spatula, mix until a smooth dough forms. Set aside to rest for 10 minutes.

3. Transfer the dough to a 14-inch-square piece of parchment paper and place an equal-size sheet on top of it. Using a rolling pin, roll out the dough as thin as you like. (If it's on the thicker side, the result will be more like crackers than chips.)

4. Remove the top sheet of parchment paper and transfer the rolled dough, still on the bottom sheet of parchment, to a baking sheet.

5. Bake until golden brown, 10 to 15 minutes, depending on the thickness. After 10 minutes, check each minute to ensure the dough is baking to the right level of crispness.

6. Remove from the oven, turn off the oven, and break into chips. Return to the oven, with the door left slightly ajar, for 10 minutes to make the chips crispy.

7. Serve or store in the refrigerator in an airtight container for up to a week.

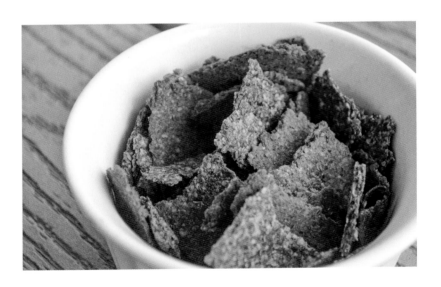

Calories: 272   **Fat:** 17g   **Protein:** 11g   **Carbs:** 17g   **Fiber:** 14g   **Sugar:** 0g

PROTEIN POPPING POWER BALLS

Yield: 16 balls, 1 per serving   **Prep Time:** 15 minutes   **Cook Time:** —

Warm filtered water, as needed

1 cup coconut butter

½ cup unsweetened coconut flakes

½ cup chia seeds

1 scoop vanilla-flavored protein powder

1 teaspoon vanilla extract

1 teaspoon fine sea salt

1. Pour the warm water into a medium-sized pan. Place the coconut butter in a glass bowl and set the bowl on top of the pan of water. Set aside until the coconut butter is slightly softened.

2. Add the remaining ingredients to the bowl with the coconut butter and mix well. Roll the mixture into 16 equal-size balls, about 1 to 2 inches in diameter.

3. Serve immediately or store in an airtight container in the refrigerator for up to a week or in the freezer for up to 3 months.

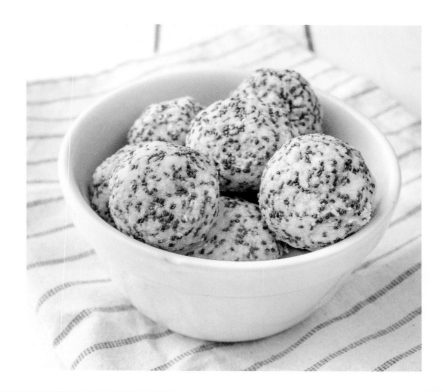

GRAIN-FREE KALE FLATBREAD

Yield: 12 slices, 1 per serving   **Prep Time:** 15 minutes   **Cook Time:** 50 to 65 minutes

2 cups tightly packed destemmed kale

½ large onion, roughly chopped

1 cup hulled raw sunflower seeds

1 cup chopped raw walnuts

2 large eggs

2 tablespoons unsalted butter, ghee, or coconut oil

1 teaspoon fine sea salt

½ teaspoon freshly squeezed lemon juice

1. Preheat the oven to 300°F. Grease a baking sheet or baking stone with coconut oil cooking spray.

2. Place all of the ingredients in a high-powered blender or food processor and blend, pausing periodically to scrape down the sides of the container, until the mixture has a smooth, doughlike consistency and all of the chunks have been eliminated. This could take several minutes.

3. Using a rubber spatula, spread the mixture evenly onto the prepared baking sheet; make it as thin and even as you can get it.

4. Bake for 50 to 65 minutes, depending on thickness. To check for doneness, gently insert a fork or toothpick into the flatbread; if it comes out clean, it's ready. Remove from the oven.

5. Cut into 12 slices and serve. Store leftovers in an airtight container in the refrigerator for up to 3 days.

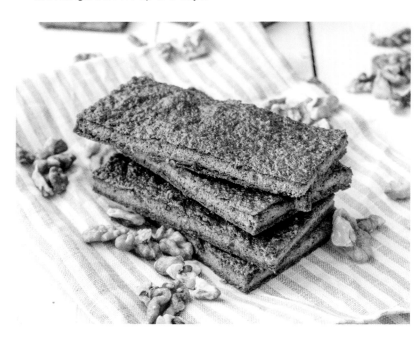

Calories: 243   **Fat:** 22g   **Protein:** 8g   **Carbs:** 7g   **Fiber:** 4g   **Sugar:** 1g

CREAMY LEMONY SUPERFOOD GUACAMOLE

Yield: 6 servings   **Prep Time:** 15 minutes   **Cook Time:** —

3 ripe avocados, pitted, skinned, and mashed

½ cup full-fat coconut milk

Juice of 1 lemon

2 tablespoons apple cider vinegar

1 tablespoon dried oregano leaves, dill weed, or cilantro leaves

1 teaspoon fine sea salt

FOR SERVING:

Sliced cucumbers, red cabbage leaves, celery stalks, or sliced red bell peppers

Besides serving this creamy guacamole with veggie dippers, you could also serve it as a spread for coconut flour wraps, with Fast and Easy Fajitas (page 316), or as a dip for Seed Crackers (page 280).

1. In a large bowl, mix together the avocados, coconut milk, lemon juice, and vinegar until well combined. Stir in the herbs and salt until the mixture is fully combined.

2. Serve with the dippers of your choice.

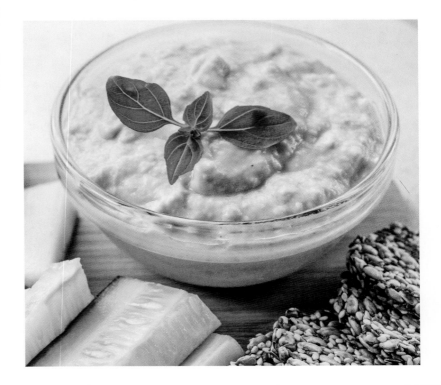

Calories: 198   **Fat:** 19g   **Protein:** 2g   **Carbs:** 10g   **Fiber:** 7g   **Sugar:** 1g

AVOCADO PESTO

Yield: 2 cups, ¼ cup per serving   **Prep Time:** 15 minutes   **Cook Time:** —

2 cups fresh kale, destemmed

1 avocado, pitted and skinned

½ cup filtered water

¼ cup freshly squeezed lemon juice

¼ cup extra-virgin olive oil

¼ cup fresh basil leaves, or 2 teaspoons dried basil leaves

¼ cup fresh thyme leaves, or 2 teaspoons dried thyme leaves

4 cloves garlic, peeled

1 teaspoon fine sea salt

½ teaspoon freshly ground black pepper

This is a fantastic recipe to serve with zucchini noodles or another low-carb noodle option. You also can use it as a dip for veggies or one of the bread recipes in this book.

1. Place all of the ingredients in a high-powered blender or food processor and blend until smooth and creamy.

2. Transfer to a serving dish and serve immediately or store in an airtight container in the refrigerator for up to 2 days.

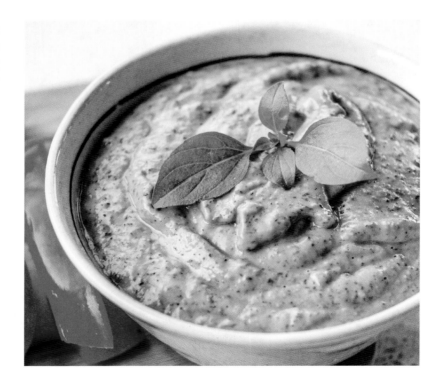

Calories: 115   **Fat:** 11g   **Protein:** 1g   **Carbs:** 5g   **Fiber:** 2.5g   **Sugar:** .5g

RANCH DRESSING

Yield: 1 cup, 2 tablespoons per serving   **Prep Time:** 10 minutes   **Cook Time:** —

½ cup avocado oil mayonnaise, plus more as desired

½ cup full-fat coconut milk, plus more as desired

1 tablespoon dried parsley

1 teaspoon garlic powder

½ teaspoon onion powder

½ teaspoon fine sea salt

¼ teaspoon freshly ground black pepper

This recipe makes a thick and creamy dressing. If you'd like a thinner dressing, simply thin with a little more coconut milk; if you like it to be the consistency of a dip for veggies or homemade Seed Crackers (page 280), thicken it with additional mayonnaise.

1. In a small bowl, whisk together the mayonnaise and coconut milk until well combined. Stir in the parsley, garlic powder, onion powder, salt, and pepper until thoroughly combined.

2. Add more coconut milk if a thinner consistency is desired or more mayonnaise if a thicker consistency is desired.

3. Serve or transfer to an airtight container and store in the refrigerator for up to a week. The dressing will thicken as it chills.

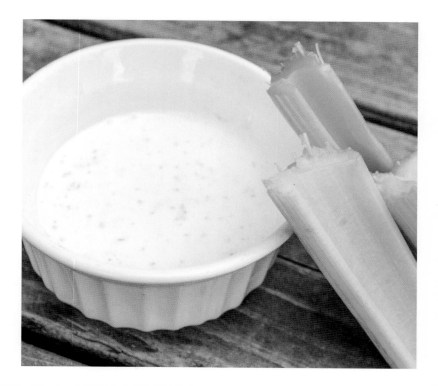

Calories: 126   **Fat:** 15g   **Protein:** 0g   **Carbs:** 0g   **Fiber:** 0g   **Sugar:** 0g

CASHEW ARTICHOKE DIP

Yield: 6 servings, ¼ cup per serving   **Prep Time:** 20 minutes, plus 2 hours to soak cashews   **Cook Time:** 10 minutes

2 cups raw cashews

Filtered water, as needed

1 (20-ounce) package frozen spinach, thawed and drained

1 tablespoon coconut oil

½ cup chopped onions

2 cloves garlic, crushed to a paste

2 (14-ounce) cans artichoke hearts, rinsed, drained, and finely chopped

1 teaspoon fine sea salt

1 teaspoon onion powder

½ teaspoon garlic powder

Pinch of freshly ground black pepper

1 tablespoon freshly squeezed lemon juice

1. Place the cashews in a medium bowl, cover with filtered water, and refrigerate for at least 2 hours or overnight.

2. Drain the cashews and put them in a food processor or high-powered blender with enough fresh filtered water to barely cover them. Blend until smooth and set aside.

3. Wrap the spinach in paper towels and squeeze out the excess liquid. Set aside in a colander to drain further.

4. In a medium saucepan over medium heat, warm the coconut oil. Add the onions and sauté for 10 minutes, or until soft. Add the garlic and sauté for 1 minute.

5. Add the artichoke hearts, salt, onion powder, garlic powder, and pepper and stir to combine. Cook until heated through.

6. Add the spinach and lemon juice. Stir to combine and cook until heated through.

7. Stir in the cashew cream. Cook, stirring often, until heated through and well blended.

8. Serve warm.

Tip: I like to throw the cooked mixture into the food processor or blender and pulse it for a minute or two; it makes the dip creamier.

Calories: 188   Fat: 13g   Protein: 9g   Carbs: 15g   Fiber: 6g   Sugar: 3g

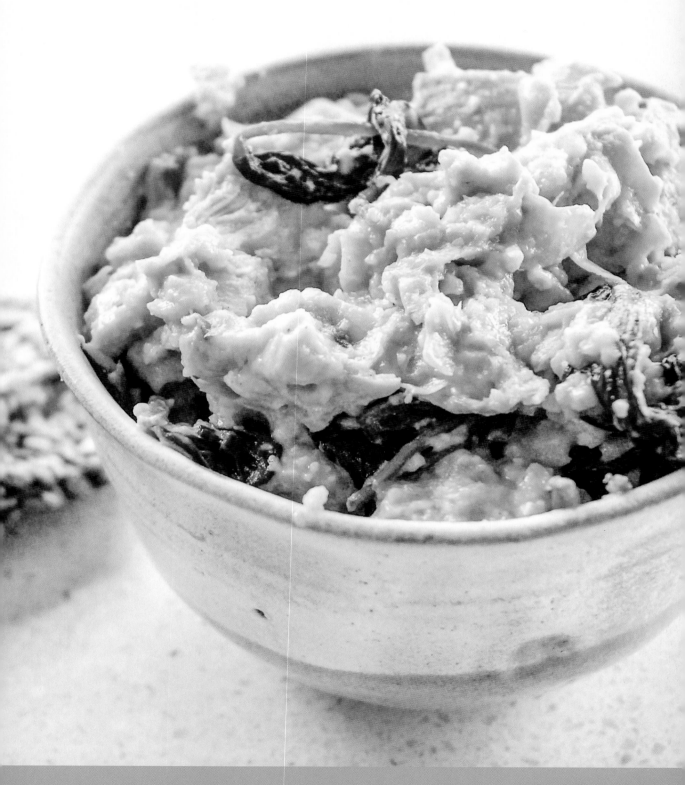

PROTEIN BARS

Yield: 12 bars, 1 per serving   **Prep Time:** 10 minutes, plus 1 hour to chill   **Cook Time:** —

1 cup creamy nut butter of choice (almond and cashew are good choices)

¼ cup coconut oil, melted

¼ cup sugar-free chocolate chips or cacao nibs (optional)

2 scoops vanilla-flavored protein powder

1 teaspoon ground cinnamon (optional)

½ teaspoon fine sea salt

10 to 15 drops vanilla-flavored liquid stevia, or 1 teaspoon powdered stevia or monk fruit sweetener

1. In a large bowl, stir together all of the ingredients.

2. Transfer the contents of the bowl to a loaf pan or baking dish and smooth the top. Freeze for 1 hour, or until firm.

3. Slice into bars. Serve or store in an airtight container in the refrigerator for up to a week or in the freezer for up to 3 months and enjoy when you want a delicious boost!

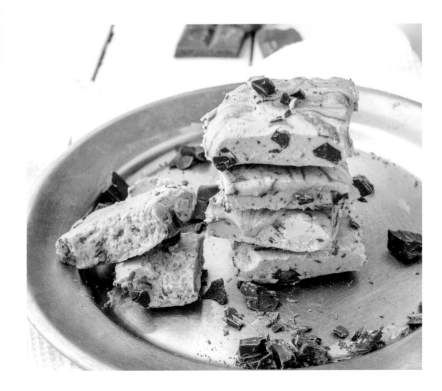

Calories: 180   Fat: 15g   Protein: 6g   Carbs: 5g   Fiber: 2g   Sugar: 2g

COCONUT FLOUR BREAD

Yield: 1 (8½ by 4½-inch) loaf, 12 servings   **Prep Time:** 20 minutes   **Cook Time:** 30 minutes

5 large eggs

1 cup creamy cashew or almond butter

¼ cup coconut flour

2 teaspoons apple cider vinegar

½ teaspoon baking powder

½ teaspoon baking soda

1. Preheat the oven to 350°F. Grease an 8½ by 4½-inch loaf pan with coconut oil cooking spray.

2. Allow all of the ingredients to sit out at room temperature for 5 minutes.

3. Place all of the ingredients in a food processor or high-powered blender and process until well combined and smooth. Transfer the batter to the prepared loaf pan.

4. Bake for 25 to 30 minutes, or until a toothpick inserted in the center of the loaf comes out clean.

5. Let the bread cool for 5 minutes, then remove it from the baking pan.

6. Serve or store in an airtight container in the refrigerator for up to a week.

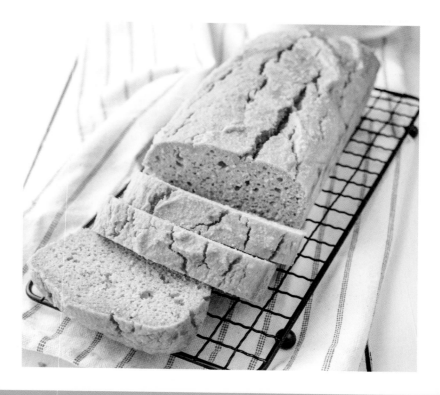

Calories: 166   **Fat:** 14g   **Protein:** 8g   **Carbs:** 6g   **Fiber:** 3g   **Sugar:** 1g

GARLIC AND ROSEMARY BREAD

Yield: 1 (9 by 5-inch) loaf, 18 servings   **Prep Time:** 20 minutes   **Cook Time:** 50 minutes

1 medium head cauliflower (about 1½ pounds), cored and cut into florets

10 large eggs

¼ teaspoon cream of tartar

1¼ cups coconut flour

6 tablespoons (¾ stick) unsalted butter, melted

6 cloves garlic, crushed

1½ tablespoons baking powder

1 teaspoon fine sea salt

1 tablespoon dried rosemary leaves

1 tablespoon dried parsley

1. Preheat the oven to 350°F. Line a 9 by 5-inch loaf pan with parchment paper.

2. Place the cauliflower in a food steamer over medium-low heat and steam the cauliflower until it's tender, about 6 minutes.

3. Remove the pot from the heat, uncover, and allow the cauliflower to cool slightly. Move the cauliflower to a food processor and pulse until the cauliflower has the texture of rice.

4. Place the riced cauliflower in a piece of muslin or a clean towel and press to extract any remaining liquid. Set aside.

5. Separate the egg whites from the yolks; place the whites in a medium bowl and the yolks in the food processor.

6. Add the cream of tartar to the bowl with the egg whites. Use an electric mixer to beat the whites and cream of tartar until stiff peaks form. Set aside.

7. Add the coconut flour, melted butter, garlic, baking powder, salt, and one-quarter of the whipped egg whites to the food processor and blend until combined.

8. Add the cauliflower to the coconut flour mixture in the food processor and process until well combined.

9. Add the remaining whipped egg whites to the food processor. Use a rubber spatula to gently fold them into the flour mixture, then pulse the food processor a few times to combine. Add the rosemary and parsley and stir gently to combine.

10. Transfer the batter to the prepared loaf pan and bake for 40 to 45 minutes, until the top of the loaf is golden brown. Remove the pan from the oven, allow the loaf to cool in the pan for 10 to 15 minutes, and then turn the bread onto a wire rack to cool completely before slicing and serving.

Calories: 116   Fat: 8g   Protein: 6g   Carbs: 7g   Fiber: 3g   Sugar: 2g

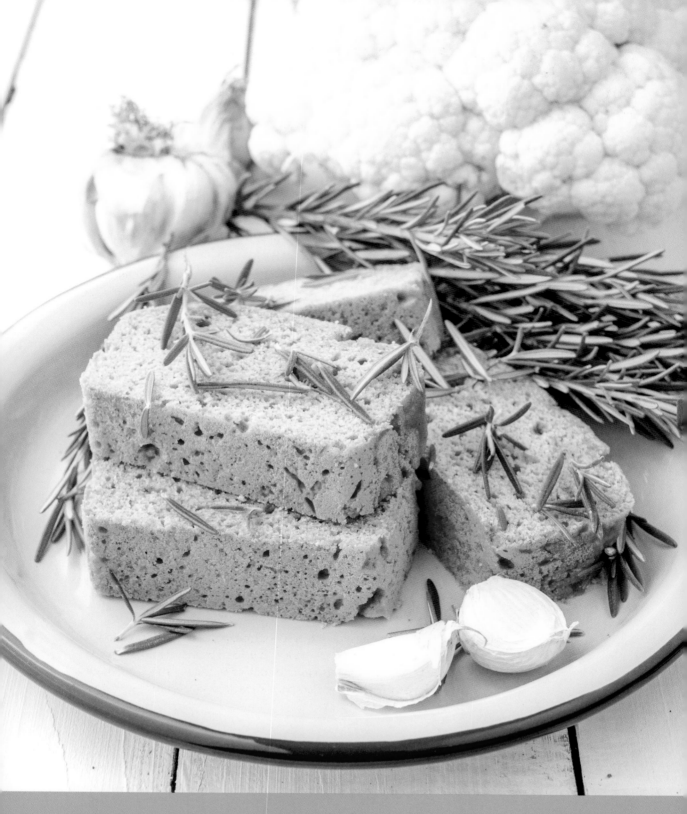

SNACKS, SIDES,
AND CONDIMENTS   293

ALMOND BUTTER BREAD

Yield: 2 (3 by 5-inch) mini loaves, 6 servings per loaf   **Prep Time:** 5 minutes   **Cook Time:** 30 minutes

1 cup creamy almond butter

3 large eggs

½ teaspoon baking soda

1 tablespoon apple cider vinegar

10 to 20 drops vanilla-flavored liquid stevia (optional)

1. Preheat the oven to 350°F. Grease two 3 by 5-inch mini loaf pans with coconut oil cooking spray.

2. Place all of the ingredients in a food processor or high-powered blender and process until smooth. Divide the batter equally between the loaf pans.

3. Bake for 25 minutes, then remove from the oven. Insert a toothpick in the center of each loaf to check for doneness; if it comes out clean, the bread is fully baked. If the toothpick is not clean, return the loaves to the oven and continue checking them every 5 minutes until done. Remove the pans from the oven, allow the loaves to cool in the pans for 10 minutes, and then turn the bread onto a wire rack to cool completely before slicing and serving.

4. Serve or store in an airtight container in the refrigerator for up to a week.

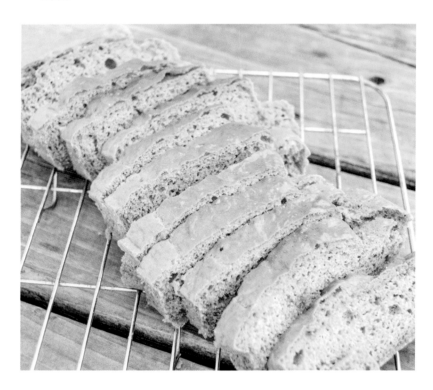

Calories: 144   **Fat:** 13g   **Protein:** 6g   **Carbs:** 5g   **Fiber:** 3g   **Sugar:** 2g

ZUCCHINI NOODLES

Yield: 2 servings   **Prep Time:** 20 minutes   **Cook Time:** 5 minutes

4 medium zucchini or yellow squash, peeled

2 tablespoons unsalted butter or coconut oil

1 teaspoon fine sea salt

¼ teaspoon freshly ground black pepper

Grated fresh ginger, for topping (optional)

Grated fresh turmeric, for topping (optional)

2 tablespoons extra-virgin olive oil

Chopped fresh herbs (such as basil, flat-leaf parsley, oregano, and thyme), for garnish (optional)

1. Using a spiral slicer or a knife, slice the squash into noodles.

2. In a skillet over high heat, warm the butter. Add the noodles to the pan, season with the salt and pepper, and sauté for 1 to 2 minutes. Remove from the heat.

3. Top the noodles with fresh ginger and turmeric, if using. Drizzle on the olive oil and garnish with herbs, if desired.

4. Serve immediately.

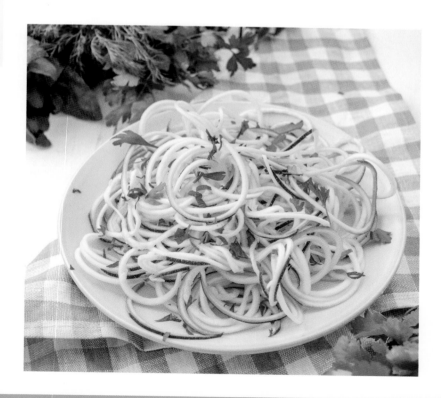

GARLIC HERB GREEN BEANS

Yield: 6 servings   **Prep Time:** 20 minutes   **Cook Time:** 10 minutes

3 tablespoons coconut oil

3 tablespoons unsalted butter or ghee

1 pound green beans, trimmed

2 cups chicken broth, plus more if needed

1 medium onion, diced

3 cloves garlic, crushed

1 tablespoon Italian seasoning or seasoning salt

1½ teaspoons fine sea salt

1. In a large saucepan over high heat, warm the coconut oil and butter. Add the remaining ingredients and cook for 10 minutes, or until tender. Add more chicken broth if needed to keep the beans moist as they cook.

2. Transfer to a serving bowl and serve.

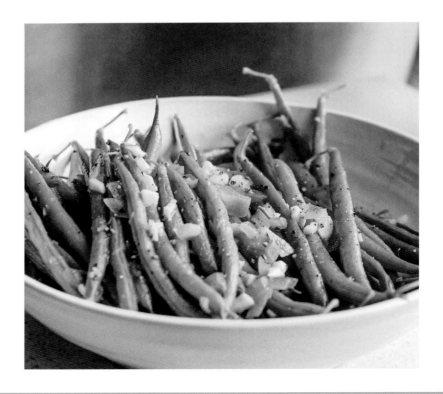

Calories: 155   **Fat:** 13g   **Protein:** 2g   **Carbs:** 8g   **Fiber:** 3g   **Sugar:** 2g

CAULIFLOWER MASH

Yield: 3 servings   **Prep Time:** 15 minutes   **Cook Time:** 15 minutes

1 head cauliflower, cored and roughly chopped

2 tablespoons unsalted butter, ghee, or coconut oil

Fine sea salt and freshly ground black pepper

1 to 2 cloves garlic (optional)

Chopped fresh dill (optional)

Turmeric powder (optional)

Chopped fresh herbs (such as flat-leaf parsley, basil, oregano, and thyme), for garnish

1. Place the cauliflower in a food steamer over medium-low heat and steam it until tender, about 5 minutes.

2. Place the cauliflower in a food processor or high-powered blender. Add the butter and season with salt and pepper. If desired, add the garlic, dill, and/or turmeric. Blend to the desired consistency.

3. Transfer to a serving dish, garnish with herbs, and enjoy!

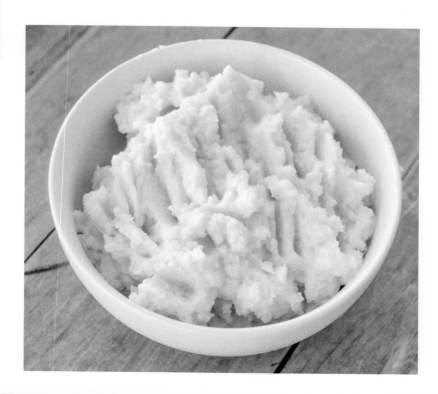

Calories: 115   **Fat:** 9g   **Protein:** 4g   **Carbs:** 10g   **Fiber:** 4g   **Sugar:** 3.5g

CAULIFLOWER "POTATO" SALAD

Yield: 6 servings   **Prep Time:** 10 minutes   **Cook Time:** 15 minutes

FOR THE DRESSING:

1½ cups avocado oil mayonnaise

¾ tablespoon Dijon mustard

¾ tablespoon apple cider vinegar

Fine sea salt and freshly ground black pepper

FOR THE SALAD:

1 head cauliflower, cored and roughly chopped

5 ounces turkey or grass-fed beef bacon, cooked until crisp and crumbled

3 stalks celery, chopped

½ medium red onion, finely chopped

2 tablespoons chopped fresh chives

Fine sea salt and freshly ground black pepper

1. Make the dressing: In a small bowl, whisk together the mayonnaise, mustard, and vinegar until well combined. Add the salt and pepper to taste.

2. Place the cauliflower in a food steamer over medium-low heat and steam until it's tender, about 3 to 5 minutes.

3. Make the salad: Place the steamed cauliflower in a large bowl and add the bacon, celery, red onion, and chives. Mix well.

4. Pour the dressing over the salad and toss lightly until well combined. Add more salt and pepper to taste. Serve warm or chilled.

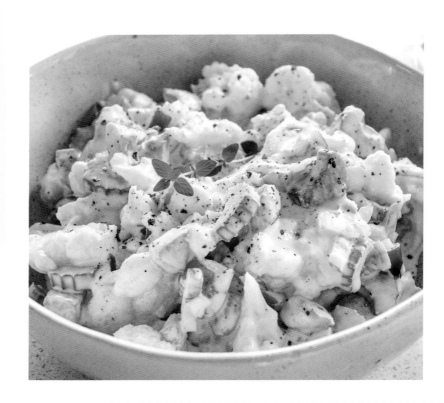

Calories: 126   **Fat:** 11g   **Protein:** 4g   **Carbs:** 3.5g   **Fiber:** 1.5g   **Sugar:** 1.5g

CAULIFLOWER FRIED RICE

Yield: 3 servings   **Prep Time:** 15 minutes   **Cook Time:** 5 minutes

1 medium head cauliflower (about 1½ pounds), cored

1½ tablespoons unsalted butter, ghee, or coconut oil, plus more if desired

2 tablespoons coconut aminos

½ teaspoon fine sea salt

Freshly ground black pepper, to taste

2 teaspoons turmeric powder (optional)

½ teaspoon ginger powder (optional)

1. Chop the cauliflower into large chunks and place them in a high-powered blender or food processor. Pulse the cauliflower into small pieces that resemble grains of rice.

2. In a large sauté pan over medium heat, melt the butter. Add the riced cauliflower, coconut aminos, salt, and pepper and sauté for 5 minutes, or until tender.

3. Transfer the contents of the pan to a serving bowl and stir in the turmeric and/or ginger, if desired. Optionally, melt up to 2 tablespoons more butter and mix in as well.

4. Serve immediately.

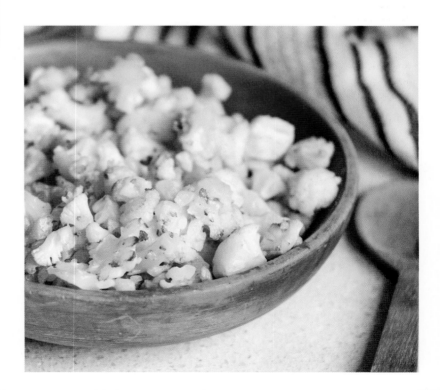

Calories: 54   **Fat:** 3g   **Protein:** 2g   **Carbs:** 6g   **Fiber:** 2g   **Sugar:** 3g

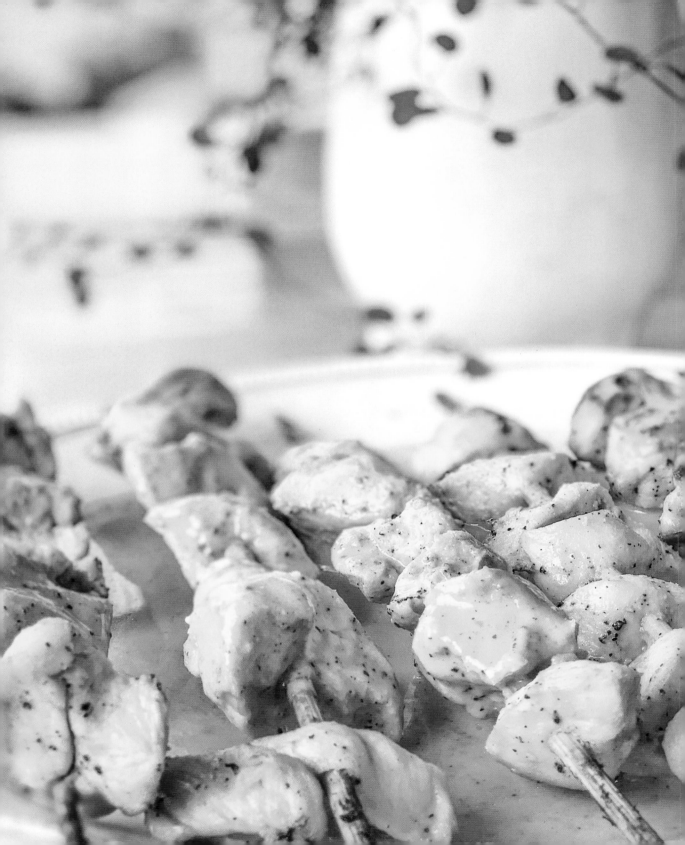

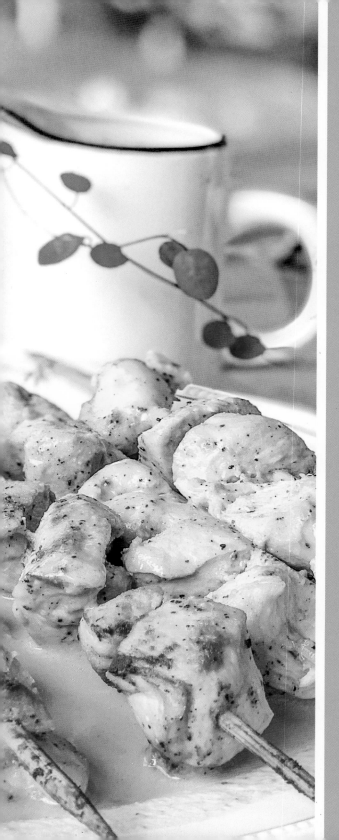

MAIN MEALS

CHICKEN AVOCADO CHILI

Yield: 4 servings   **Prep Time:** 10 minutes   **Cook Time:** 20 minutes

1 tablespoon coconut oil or unsalted butter

¼ cup chopped onions

½ cup chopped green bell peppers

3 cups chicken broth

2 cups shredded cooked chicken or turkey

1 cup fresh spinach

¼ cup chopped green onions

Pinch of fine sea salt

2 avocados, pitted, skinned, and diced, for garnish

Chopped fresh cilantro leaves, for garnish

1. In a medium saucepan over medium heat, warm the coconut oil. Add the onions and bell peppers and sauté for 10 minutes, or until soft.

2. Raise the heat to medium-high, then add the chicken broth, chicken, spinach, green onions, and salt. Stir until well combined and bring to a boil.

3. Reduce the heat to medium-low, cover, and simmer for at least 5 minutes to allow the flavors to develop. Remove from the heat.

4. Serve warm garnished with the avocados and cilantro.

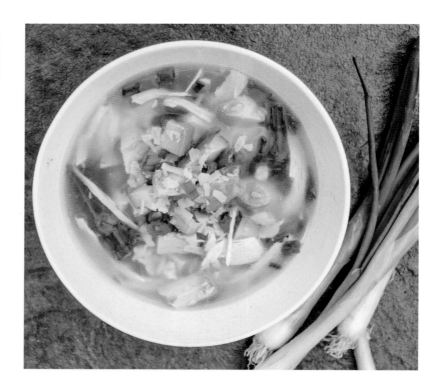

Calories: 287   **Fat:** 20g   **Protein:** 16g   **Carbs:** 13g   **Fiber:** 7g   **Sugar:** 2g

CHICKEN LO MEIN

Yield: 3 servings   **Prep Time:** 20 minutes   **Cook Time:** 8 minutes

1 tablespoon coconut oil

2 cups coarsely chopped fresh broccoli or cauliflower florets

½ cup chopped shiitake mushrooms

¼ cup chopped celery

2 cups shredded cabbage

½ cup sliced green onions

¼ cup chopped raw almonds

1 tablespoon grated fresh ginger

2 cloves garlic, minced

¾ tablespoon coconut aminos

¼ teaspoon fine sea salt

1½ cups cooked chicken, cut into bite-sized pieces

½ cup extra-virgin olive oil or MCT oil

Cauliflower Fried Rice (page 299), for serving (optional)

1. In a skillet over high heat, warm the coconut oil. Add the broccoli, mushrooms, and celery and sauté for 2 minutes. Add the cabbage, green onions, almonds, ginger, garlic, and coconut aminos and cook for 2 to 3 minutes, or until the cabbage softens. Season with the salt. Remove from the heat, add the cooked chicken, and toss until well combined and heated through.

2. Pour the oil over the mixture and toss until well coated.

3. Serve hot over cauliflower rice, if using.

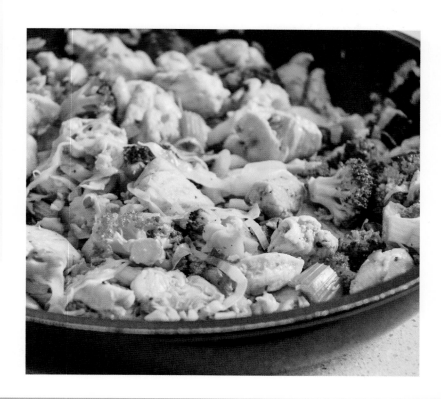

GOLDEN LIME CHICKEN KEBABS

Yield: 8 servings   **Prep Time:** 10 minutes, plus 20 minutes to marinate   **Cook Time:** 20 minutes

FOR THE SAUCE:

½ cup freshly squeezed lime juice

⅓ cup avocado oil

⅓ cup apple cider vinegar

2 cloves garlic, minced

2 teaspoons turmeric powder

2 teaspoons onion powder

1 teaspoon pink salt or fine sea salt

1 teaspoon freshly ground black pepper

2¼ pounds boneless, skinless chicken breasts

Special equipment:

8 (8-inch) bamboo or wood skewers

1. Preheat the oven to 400°F and grease a rimmed baking sheet with coconut oil cooking spray.

2. Make the sauce: Place all of the sauce ingredients in a blender and blend until well combined. Set aside.

3. Cut the chicken into 2-inch cubes and place on the prepared baking sheet. Pour the sauce over the chicken and set aside to marinate for 20 minutes.

4. Slide the marinated chicken onto the bamboo or wood skewers, placing 4 to 5 ounces of chicken on each skewer.

5. Place the kebabs on the baking sheet and bake for 20 minutes, or until cooked through in the center and golden brown.

6. Serve immediately.

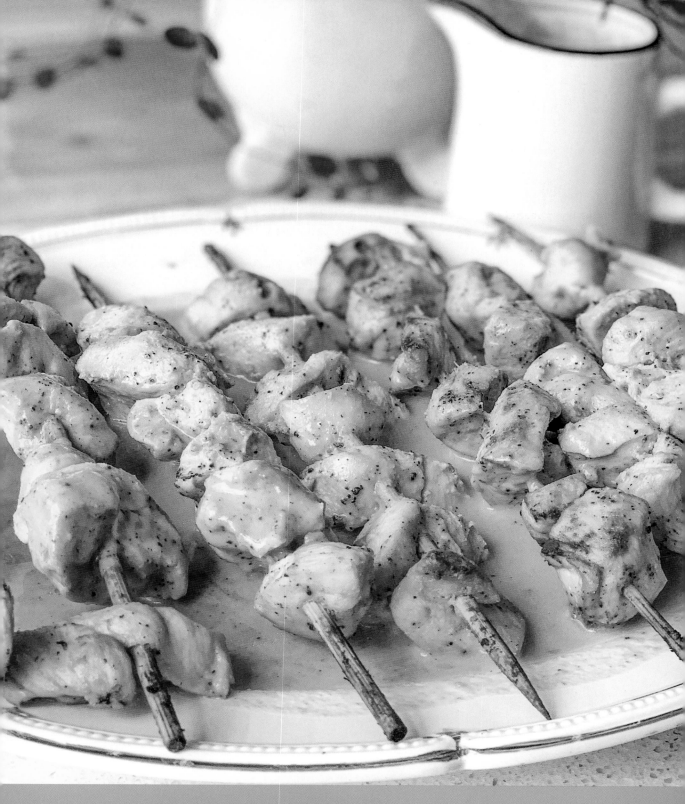

CHICKEN FAJITA SALAD

Yield: 2 servings   **Prep Time:** 15 minutes   **Cook Time:** 20 to 25 minutes

FOR THE MEXICAN SPICE BLEND:
(Makes 1 tablespoon plus 2 teaspoons)

2 teaspoons chili powder

1½ teaspoons ground cumin

½ teaspoon ground coriander

½ teaspoon fine sea salt

½ teaspoon freshly ground black pepper

¼ red bell pepper, thinly sliced

¼ yellow bell pepper, thinly sliced

¼ green bell pepper, thinly sliced

¼ medium yellow or red onion, finely chopped

2 boneless, skinless chicken breasts (about 6 ounces each), cut into strips

2 teaspoons Mexican Spice Blend (from above)

1 clove garlic, minced

2 tablespoons extra-virgin olive oil, avocado oil, or MCT oil

Mixed greens, as needed

2 tablespoons ranch dressing, homemade (page 287) or store-bought (see Tip), for serving

Sliced avocado or guacamole, for topping (optional)

1. Preheat the oven to 400°F.

2. In a small bowl, whisk together all of the ingredients for the Mexican Spice Blend. Set aside 2 teaspoons for use in this recipe. Store the rest in an airtight container for up to 6 months.

3. Arrange the bell peppers and onion on a rimmed baking sheet. Top with the strips of chicken and evenly sprinkle the Mexican spice blend and garlic over everything. Drizzle the oil over the vegetables and chicken and toss until all of the ingredients are well coated with the spices and oil. Spread the ingredients out on the baking sheet, making sure that none of the chicken is overlapping.

4. Roast, tossing once halfway through the cooking time, for 20 to 25 minutes, or until the vegetables and chicken are tender and cooked through. Remove from the oven.

5. Arrange a handful of mixed greens on each of two plates and top each with equal portions of the roasted vegetables and chicken. Drizzle the salads with the ranch dressing and top with the avocado.

6. Serve immediately.

Tip: When buying a premade ranch dressing, I recommend Primal Kitchen's ranch dressing.

Calories: 609   **Fat:** 40g   **Protein:** 46g   **Carbs:** 21g   **Fiber:** 12g   **Sugar:** 3g

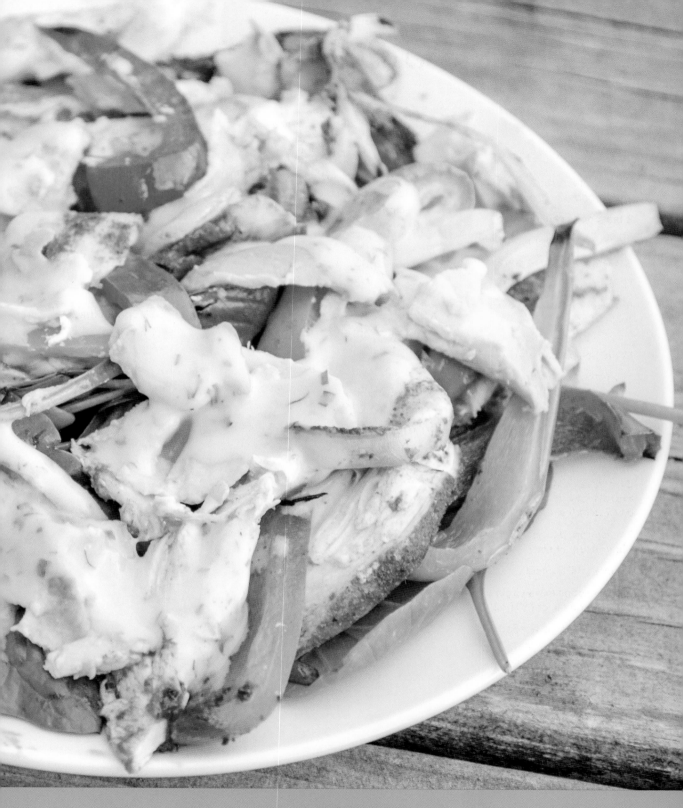

LIME HERB LAMB CHOPS

Yield: 6 servings   **Prep Time:** 8 minutes   **Cook Time:** 16 minutes

6 (6-ounce) lamb chops

Grated zest of 2 limes

Juice of 2 limes

1 tablespoon dried
rosemary leaves

1 tablespoon dried basil

Fine sea salt

1. Set the broil setting in your oven to 350°F.

2. Place the lamb chops in a glass baking dish and pour the lime juice over them. Gently massage the juice into the chops.

3. In a small bowl, mix together the lime zest, rosemary, and basil and rub the mixture on both sides of the lamb chops. Season the chops on both sides with salt.

4. Broil the chops for 5 minutes on each side for medium-rare chops (the thickest part of the chop should be 145°F). Broil them longer if more well-done chops are desired, checking every couple of minutes. Remove from the oven and allow to rest for 2 minutes before serving.

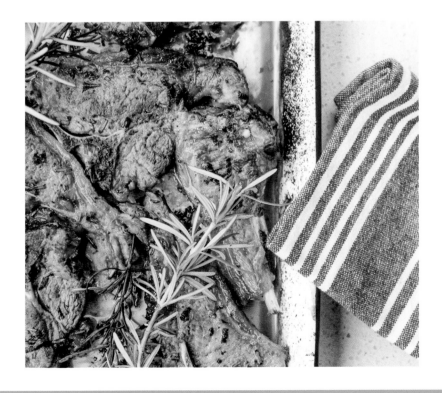

Calories: 139   **Fat:** 15g   **Protein:** 13g   **Carbs:** 2g   **Fiber:** 0g   **Sugar:** 0g

BEEF AND BUTTERED BROCCOLI

Yield: 4 servings   **Prep Time:** 15 minutes   **Cook Time:** 20 minutes

2 tablespoons coconut oil

1 pound sirloin steak, cut into 1-inch pieces

3 cloves garlic, finely chopped

2 heads fresh broccoli, chopped into bite-sized florets, or 1 (1-pound) bag frozen chopped broccoli

3 tablespoons unsalted butter or ghee

1 teaspoon seasoning salt

¼ cup coconut aminos

Black sesame seeds, for garnish

1. In a large skillet over high heat, warm the coconut oil, then add the beef and garlic and cook for 20 minutes, or until fully cooked through.

2. Place the broccoli in a food steamer over medium-low heat and steam the broccoli for 20 minutes, or until soft.

3. Combine the cooked beef and broccoli in a large serving bowl, then add the butter. Season with the seasoning salt and coconut aminos and stir gently to combine.

Tip: The Cauliflower Fried Rice (page 299) makes a good accompaniment for this dish.

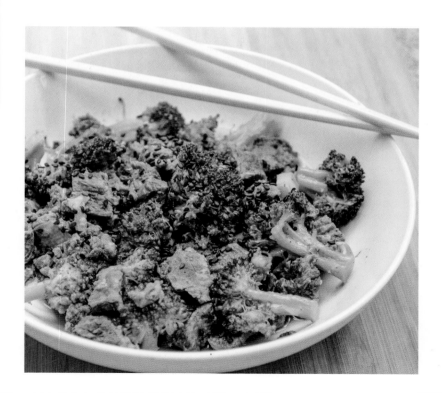

NAKED KALE BURGER SAUTÉ

Yield: 4 servings   **Prep Time:** 15 minutes   **Cook Time:** 15 minutes

1 pound grass-fed ground beef

4 tablespoons coconut oil, divided

2 curly kale leaves, stems removed and discarded

1 medium carrot (about 2½ ounces), peeled and grated (see Tip)

1 cup diced bell peppers (any color)

1 to 2 cloves garlic, crushed

Grated fresh ginger, to taste

2 avocados, pitted, skinned, and sliced

2 ounces grass-fed raw semi-hard or hard cheese of choice, sliced (optional)

2 lemons, halved

2 tablespoons extra-virgin olive oil

Fine sea salt and freshly ground black pepper

Leaves from ½ stem fresh flat-leaf parsley, finely chopped, for garnish

1. Form the beef into four burgers.

2. In a stainless-steel skillet over high heat, warm 2 tablespoons of the coconut oil. Place the burgers in the hot pan and cook for 5 minutes on each side. Remove the pan from the heat.

3. In a separate skillet over high heat, warm the remaining 2 tablespoons of coconut oil. Add the kale and carrot and sauté for 5 minutes, or until the kale is wilted, then stir in the bell peppers, garlic, and ginger until combined.

4. Arrange equal portions of the kale mixture on four serving plates and top each with a burger. Arrange equal portions of the avocado slices and cheese, if using, on each burger. Once the meat and vegetables are plated, squeeze ½ lemon over each plate and then drizzle each burger with an equal portion of the olive oil.

5. Season each serving with salt and pepper. Garnish with the parsley and serve.

Tip: Use the carrot only if you are fully keto-adapted, practicing intermittent fasting, and engaging in high-intensity exercise.

Calories: 616   **Fat:** 53g   **Protein:** 25g   **Carbs:** 15g   **Fiber:** 8g   **Sugar:** 3g

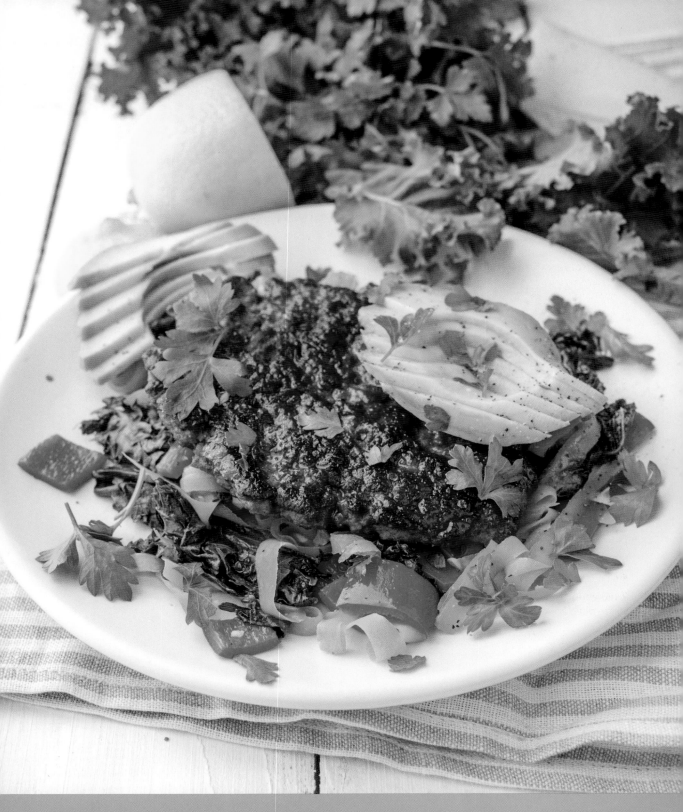

TACO LETTUCE WRAPS

Yield: 8 servings   **Prep Time:** 20 minutes   **Cook Time:** 20 minutes

2 tablespoons coconut oil

2 pounds grass-fed ground beef

¼ cup coconut aminos

½ teaspoon ground cumin

¼ teaspoon ground coriander

FOR SERVING:

8 large butter lettuce leaves, tender collard green leaves, or coconut flour wraps

1 cup chopped red onions

1 small avocado, sliced or 1 cup guacamole

1 cup shredded cheddar cheese

1 cup sour cream or coconut milk kefir (optional)

Black sesame seeds, for garnish

1. In a large skillet over high heat, warm the coconut oil, then add the beef and cook for 10 minutes, stirring occasionally to break up the chunks of meat.

2. Season the beef with the coconut aminos, cumin, and coriander and mix well. Cook for another 10 minutes, until the beef is cooked through. Transfer the beef to a serving bowl.

3. Serve the beef with the lettuce leaves, onion, guacamole, cheese, and sour cream.

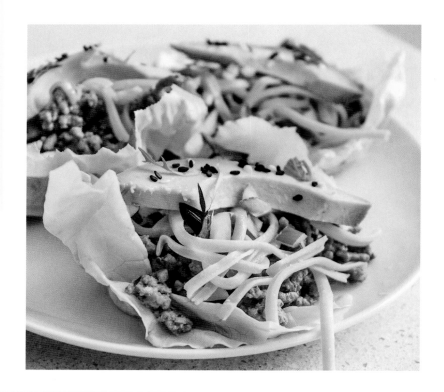

Calories (with lettuce leaves): 451 **Fat:** 34g **Protein:** 27g **Carbs:** 10g **Fiber:** 2g **Sugar:** 4g

COCONUT LIME SEARED SALMON

Yield: 2 servings   **Prep Time:** 10 minutes, plus 30 minutes to marinate   **Cook Time:** 6 minutes

FOR THE COCONUT LIME MARINADE/SAUCE:

½ (13½-ounce) can full-fat coconut milk

Handful of unsweetened shredded coconut

Grated zest of 1 lime

¼ cup freshly squeezed lime juice

FOR THE SALMON:

2 (6-ounce) fresh or frozen and thawed wild-caught salmon fillets, with skin

2 tablespoons coconut oil, for frying

1 teaspoon dried dill weed

1 teaspoon grated fresh ginger

1 teaspoon grated lemon zest

Fine sea salt and freshly ground black pepper

1 lime, sliced into wedges, for garnish

Unsweetened shredded coconut, for garnish

1. Stir together all of the sauce ingredients in a large bowl. Set aside.

2. Place the salmon in a gallon-size zip-top bag and pour in roughly two-thirds of the marinade. Seal the bag and refrigerate the salmon for at least 30 minutes to allow the flavors to meld. Reserve the remaining sauce for serving.

3. In a medium-sized skillet over high heat, warm the coconut oil. Add the salmon fillets to the pan and cook for 2 to 3 minutes on each side, until the fish flakes easily with a fork. Transfer the fillets to a platter.

4. Drizzle the reserved coconut lime sauce over the salmon fillets. Sprinkle the dill, ginger, lemon zest, salt, and pepper over the fillets and then garnish with the lime wedges and coconut. Serve while hot.

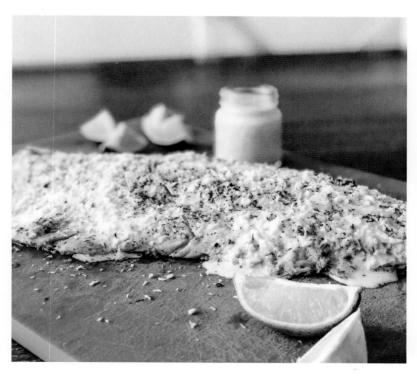

| Calories: 710 | Fat: 58g | Protein: 39g | Carbs: 7g | Fiber: 1g | Sugar: 1g | MAIN MEALS 313 |

SUPER SPROUT CHICKEN SALAD

Yield: 2 servings   **Prep Time:** 5 minutes   **Cook Time:** —

4 handfuls organic spring mix

1 medium carrot (about 2½ ounces), diced or grated

4 radishes, peeled and diced or grated

2 handfuls fresh sprouts (broccoli, kale, arugula, etc.)

1 cucumber, peeled and diced

1 cup pitted black olives

1 avocado, pitted, skinned, and diced (optional)

8 ounces cooked chicken breast strips

1 (1-inch) piece fresh turmeric, grated

1 (1-inch) piece fresh ginger, grated

¼ cup extra-virgin olive oil

Juice of 1 lemon

2 tablespoons dried oregano leaves

1 teaspoon fine sea salt

Pinch of freshly ground black pepper

1. Place the spring mix in a large serving bowl. Add the carrot, radishes, sprouts, cucumber, olives, and avocado, if using, and toss lightly to combine.

2. Add the chicken, turmeric, and ginger. Drizzle with the olive oil and lemon juice and season with the oregano, salt, and pepper. Toss all of the ingredients until thoroughly blended.

3. Serve immediately.

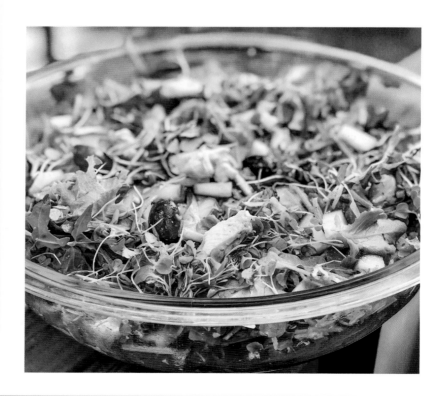

Calories: 595   **Fat:** 46g   **Protein:** 31g   **Carbs:** 21g   **Fiber:** 10g   **Sugar:** 5g

SUPER SALMON SALAD

Yield: 4 servings   **Prep Time:** 10 minutes   **Cook Time:** 15 minutes

2 tablespoons coconut oil

4 (6-ounce) fresh or frozen and thawed wild-caught salmon fillets

1 cup fresh or frozen and thawed shelled English peas

2 red or yellow bell peppers, diced

1 avocado, pitted, skinned, and diced

2 stalks celery, diced

¼ cup extra-virgin olive oil

Juice of 1 lemon or lime

1 teaspoon dried oregano leaves

Fine sea salt and freshly ground black pepper

½ cup chopped fresh parsley or cilantro, for garnish

1. In a large skillet over medium-low heat, warm the coconut oil. Add the salmon and cook for 10 minutes, or until just cooked through and the fish flakes easily with a fork. Remove the salmon from the pan and set aside.

2. Place the peas in a food steamer over medium-low heat and steam them until just softened, about 5 minutes. Remove the peas from the steamer and set aside.

3. Arrange equal portions of the peas, bell peppers, avocado, and celery on four serving plates. Top the arranged vegetables with the warm salmon.

4. Drizzle the plates with the olive oil and lemon juice and sprinkle with the oregano. Season to taste with salt and pepper, then garnish with the parsley and serve.

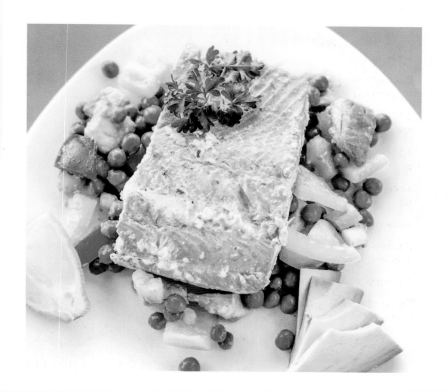

Calories: 660   **Fat:** 49g   **Protein:** 41g   **Carbs:** 15g   **Fiber:** 6g   **Sugar:** 4g

FAST AND EASY FAJITAS

Yield: 6 servings   **Prep Time:** 10 minutes   **Cook Time:** 15 minutes

3 tablespoons coconut oil

4 cups sliced mixed vegetables, such as yellow, orange, or red bell peppers and red onions

Juice of ½ lime

1 pound cooked chicken, cut into strips

1 teaspoon fine sea salt

1 teaspoon sesame seeds

¼ teaspoon dried basil

1 teaspoon ground cumin

⅛ teaspoon cayenne pepper

⅛ teaspoon chili powder

⅛ teaspoon garlic salt

⅛ teaspoon onion powder

1 teaspoon turmeric powder

Dash of freshly ground black pepper

6 turmeric-flavored Nuco Organic Coconut Wraps

FOR SERVING (OPTIONAL):

½ cup shredded grass-fed cheddar cheese and/or 1 cup guacamole

1. In a large skillet over medium heat, warm the coconut oil. Add the vegetables and lime juice and cook for 5 minutes.

2. Add the cooked chicken and all of the seasonings and herbs except the turmeric and black pepper. Cover and cook, stirring occasionally, for 10 minutes. Remove from the heat and stir in the turmeric and pepper.

3. Arrange the vegetables and chicken in the coconut wraps and serve with the cheese and/or guacamole, if desired.

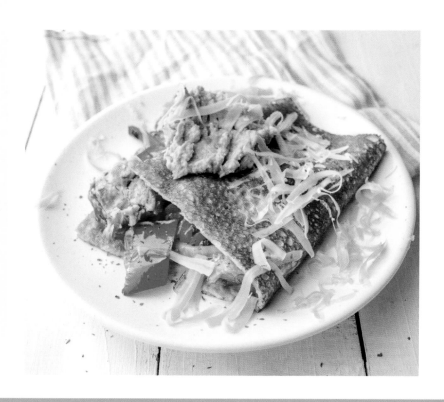

Calories: 324   **Fat:** 24g   **Protein:** 20g   **Carbs:** 8g   **Fiber:** 3g   **Sugar:** 2g

EGG DROP SOUP

Yield: 4 servings   **Prep Time:** 10 minutes   **Cook Time:** 17 minutes

1 tablespoon unsalted butter, ghee, or coconut oil

½ onion, diced

1 stalk celery, diced

1 quart chicken broth

1 handful fresh spinach

1 teaspoon coconut aminos

1 teaspoon extra-virgin olive oil

1 teaspoon fine sea salt

½ teaspoon freshly ground black pepper

8 large eggs, lightly beaten

2 tablespoons chopped green onions, for garnish

1. In a large saucepan over medium-low heat, melt the butter. Add the onion and celery and cook until softened.

2. Add the chicken broth, spinach, coconut aminos, olive oil, salt, and pepper to the pan and bring to a boil over high heat.

3. Very slowly, in a steady stream, pour the beaten eggs into the broth. As you pour, gently stir the broth in a clockwise direction until thin streams or ribbons of egg form.

4. Ladle the soup into bowls, garnish with the green onions, and serve.

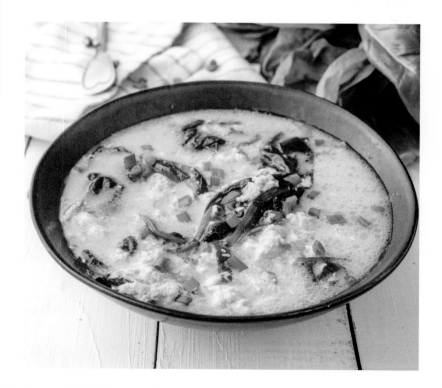

Calories: 214   **Fat:** 15g   **Protein:** 15g   **Carbs:** 6g   **Fiber:** 1g   **Sugar:** 2g

COCONUT CURRY SOUP

Yield: 6 servings   **Prep Time:** 10 minutes   **Cook Time:** 30 minutes

2 tablespoons coconut oil

½ cup chopped red onions

1 tablespoon grated fresh ginger

1 clove garlic, minced

2 (13½-ounce) cans full-fat coconut milk

1 cup chicken or vegetable broth

1 cup chopped broccoli

1 cup destemmed and chopped kale

1 tablespoon curry powder

1 teaspoon turmeric powder

½ teaspoon fine sea salt

6 ounces chopped cooked meat of choice (optional)

2 tablespoons chopped fresh cilantro, for garnish

This is an easy, versatile soup. You can add or substitute other vegetables, such as cauliflower and mushrooms, as desired.

1. In a medium saucepan over low heat, warm the coconut oil. Add the onions, ginger, and garlic and cook until tender.

2. Add the coconut milk, broth, cauliflower, kale, curry powder, turmeric, and salt and stir until well combined. Raise the heat to medium and cook, stirring often, for 10 minutes.

3. Reduce the heat to low and simmer, stirring often, for 15 minutes. Remove from the heat and stir in the meat, if using.

4. Ladle the soup into bowls and garnish with the cilantro. Serve immediately.

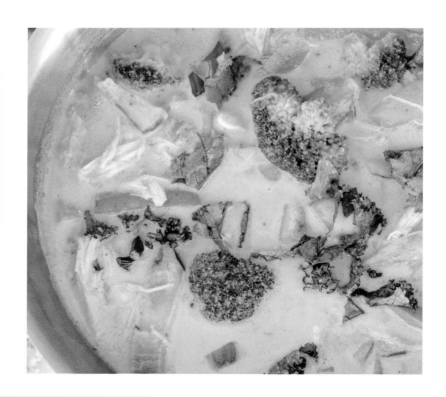

   Calories: 297   **Fat:** 30g   **Protein:** 3g   **Carbs:** 8g   **Fiber:** 1g   **Sugar:** 1.5g

SUPER AVOCADO SALAD

Yield: 2 servings   **Prep Time:** 10 minutes   **Cook Time:** —

½ small bunch kale, destemmed

2 large handfuls baby spinach

3 stalks celery, diced

1 avocado, pitted, skinned, and cut into chunks

½ red bell pepper, diced

½ yellow or orange bell pepper, diced

¼ red onion, diced

4 ounces grass-fed cheese of choice, cut into chunks

½ lemon

¼ cup extra-virgin olive oil

½ teaspoon dried oregano leaves

½ teaspoon dried thyme leaves

½ teaspoon dried basil leaves

Grated fresh ginger, for topping

If you're sensitive to cow's milk cheese, you can substitute goat cheese for this recipe, or replace the cheese altogether with chopped hard-boiled eggs or chopped cooked chicken.

1. Place the kale, spinach, celery, avocado, bell peppers, onion, and cheese in a large salad bowl. Toss lightly to mix.

2. Squeeze the lemon half over the salad and drizzle on the olive oil. Sprinkle on the herbs and ginger.

3. Serve immediately and enjoy!

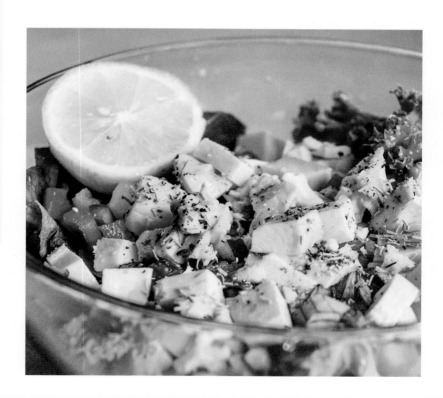

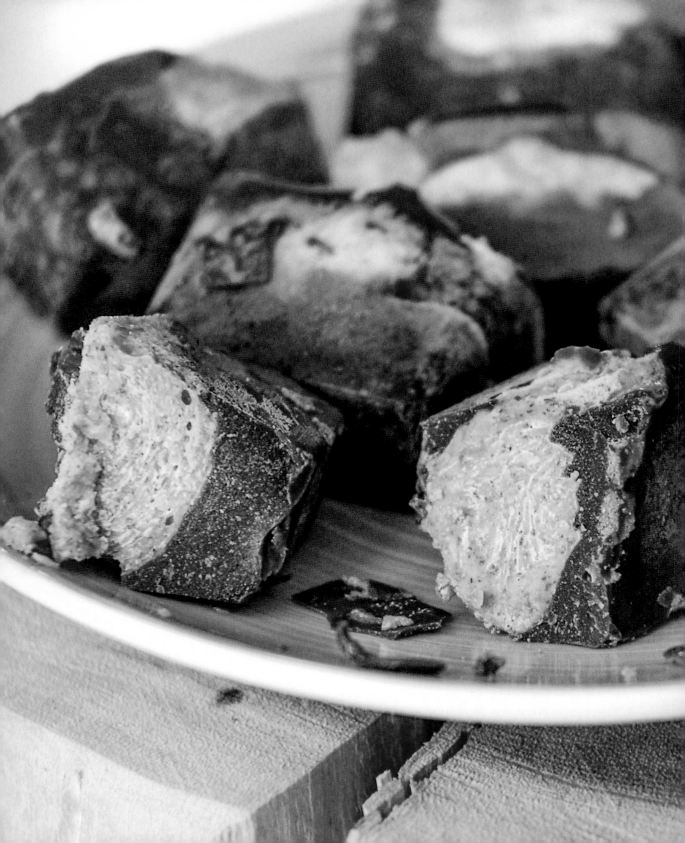

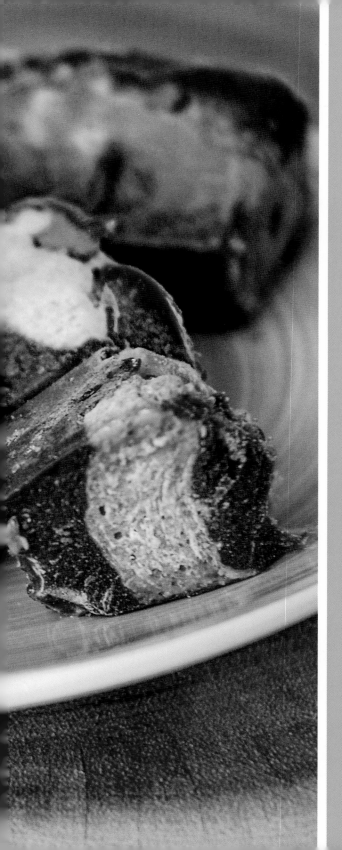

SWEET TREATS

CHOCOLATE RASPBERRY CREAM

Yield: 2 servings   **Prep Time:** 10 minutes, plus 12 hours to chill coconut milk   **Cook Time:** —

1 (13½-ounce) can full-fat coconut milk

¼ cup frozen raspberries

2 scoops chocolate-flavored protein powder

3 tablespoons raw cacao powder

1 tablespoon turmeric powder

Pinch of freshly ground black pepper

10 drops unflavored liquid stevia, or more to taste

Pinch of fine sea salt, or more to taste

1. Turn the can of coconut milk upside down and place it in the refrigerator for 12 hours to separate the cream from the water. When you turn the can right side up and open it, you will see water on top. Pour the water into an airtight container and store it in the refrigerator for later use (such as smoothies and shakes). Remove the cream from the can.

2. Place the cream, raspberries, protein powder, cacao powder, turmeric, and pepper in a high-powered blender and blend until smooth and creamy.

3. Mix in the stevia and salt and taste. Add more stevia or salt as desired.

4. Serve immediately.

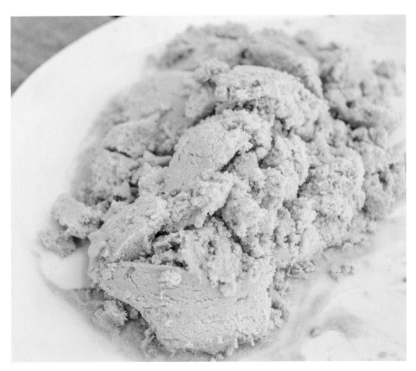

Calories: 516   **Fat:** 45g   **Protein:** 18g   **Carbs:** 15g   **Fiber:** 5g   **Sugar:** 2g

COCONUT SNOWBALLS

Yield: 10 snowballs, 1 per serving   **Prep Time:** 20 minutes, plus 1 hour to chill   **Cook Time:** —

2 cups unsweetened shredded coconut

¼ cup full-fat coconut milk, plus more as needed

2 tablespoons powdered stevia or monk fruit sweetener, plus more for sprinkling if desired

20 drops peppermint essential oil (optional)

⅛ teaspoon vanilla extract

Pinch of fine sea salt

Ground cinnamon, for sprinkling (optional)

1. In a food processor or high-powered blender, blend the coconut on high until it takes on a powdery texture. Add the coconut milk, stevia, peppermint oil (if using), vanilla extract, and salt and blend on high until a thick batter forms. Add a little more coconut milk if the batter is too crumbly.

2. Line a plate with parchment paper. Slightly wet your hands and form the batter into small balls, about 2 inches in diameter. Place the balls on the prepared plate.

3. Sprinkle with extra sweetener or cinnamon, if desired, and refrigerate for 1 hour, or until the snowballs are firm.

4. Serve or store in an airtight container in the refrigerator for up to a week.

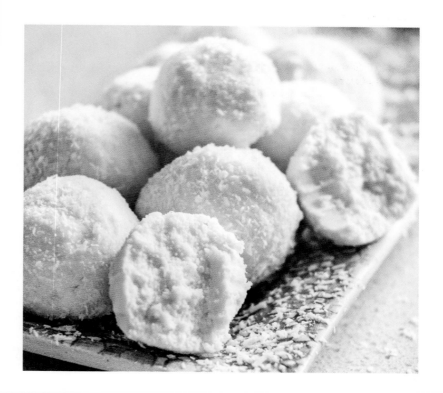

Calories: 128   Fat: 12g   Protein: 1g   Carbs: 4g   Fiber: 2g   Sugar: 1g

CHOCOLATE COLLAGEN SQUARES

Yield: 12 (2-inch) squares, 1 per serving   **Prep Time:** 20 minutes, plus 1 hour to chill   **Cook Time:** 2 minutes

½ cup coconut oil

5 tablespoons raw cacao powder

2 tablespoons creamy nut butter of choice

½ teaspoon vanilla extract

2 tablespoons chocolate-flavored collagen peptides (see Tip)

1 tablespoon MCT oil (optional)

Pinch of fine sea salt

1. Line a 9 by 5-inch loaf pan with parchment paper.

2. In a small saucepan over low heat, melt the coconut oil. Add the cacao powder, nut butter, and vanilla extract; then add the collagen, MCT oil (if using), and salt. Cook, whisking constantly, until well blended and there are no lumps remaining.

3. Transfer the mixture to the prepared loaf pan and refrigerate for 1 hour, or until firm.

4. Cut into 12 squares or bars. Enjoy immediately or store in an airtight container in the refrigerator for up to a week.

Tip: Chocolate-flavored collagen peptides is sweetened with stevia and tastes amazing, so if you use it, you won't need to use any additional sweetener. If you instead use plain collagen peptides, also add 1 to 2 teaspoons of chocolate-flavored liquid stevia.

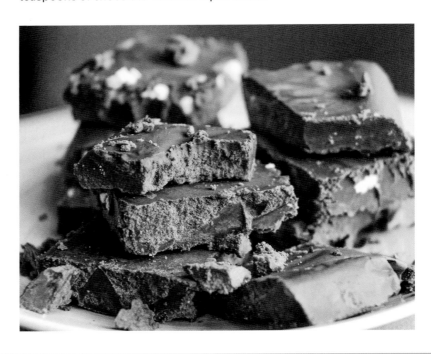

Calories: 124   **Fat:** 12g   **Protein:** 2g   **Carbs:** 3g   **Fiber:** 1g   **Sugar:** 0g

CHOCOLATE AVOCADO TRUFFLES

Yield: 12 truffles, 1 per serving   **Prep Time:** 15 minutes, plus 30 minutes to chill   **Cook Time:** 5 minutes

¾ cup unsweetened chocolate chips

1 avocado, pitted and skinned

1 teaspoon chocolate-flavored liquid stevia

½ teaspoon vanilla extract

Pinch of ground cinnamon

Pinch of fine sea salt

1 to 2 teaspoons raw cacao powder, for coating

1. Place a medium saucepan with 1 inch of water over low heat. Set a heat-safe glass bowl on top of the saucepan. Place the chocolate in the bowl and allow it to melt slowly, stirring occasionally.

2. In a separate bowl, mash the avocado. When the chocolate has fully melted, pour it into the bowl containing the mashed avocado. Stir them together, then add the stevia, vanilla extract, cinnamon, and salt. Stir until fully combined and free of lumps. Refrigerate for 30 minutes, or until cooled and hardened.

3. Using a spoon, scoop the mixture into 12 equal-size balls and roll the balls between your palms until they are smooth.

4. Place the cacao powder in a shallow bowl. Roll each ball in the cacao powder and serve immediately. Store leftovers in an airtight container in the refrigerator for up to a week.

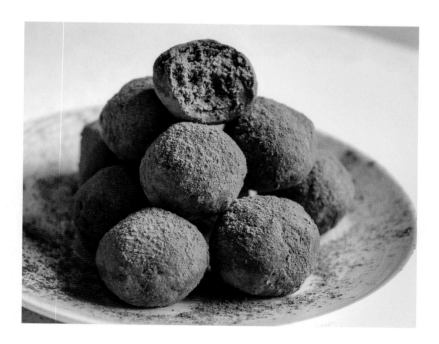

Calories: 129   **Fat:** 11g   **Protein:** 2g   **Carbs:** 6g   **Fiber:** 3g   **Sugar:** 0g

PEPPERMINT PATTIES

Yield: 6 patties, 1 per serving   **Prep Time:** 15 minutes, plus 30 minutes to chill   **Cook Time:** 5 minutes

½ cup plus 1 tablespoon coconut oil, divided

1 teaspoon unflavored liquid stevia or monk fruit sweetener

½ teaspoon vanilla extract

3 drops peppermint essential oil or peppermint extract

1 cup sugar-free chocolate chips

Pinch of fine sea salt

1. If your coconut oil is rock-hard, warm ½ cup of it in a small saucepan over low heat until softened. Line a plate with parchment paper.

2. In a bowl, combine the softened coconut oil, stevia, vanilla extract, and peppermint oil, mashing any clumps of coconut oil against the side of the bowl until the mixture is smooth. Refrigerate for 10 minutes to allow it to harden somewhat.

3. Using a 1-tablespoon scoop, form the mixture into 6 balls and place them on the prepared plate. Freeze for 5 to 10 minutes to allow them to firm up.

4. Lay a second sheet of parchment paper on top of the balls and, using your hands, press down to flatten the patties to the desired thickness. (I like them on the thicker side.)

5. Place a medium saucepan with 1 inch of water over low heat. Set a heat-safe glass bowl on top of the saucepan. Place the chocolate chips and the remaining 1 tablespoon of coconut oil in the bowl and allow to slowly melt, stirring occasionally to break up any solid pieces. Remove the bowl from the heat and set aside to cool slightly.

6. Line another plate with parchment paper.

7. Dip the chilled patties into the melted chocolate. You can gently drop the patties into the chocolate for maximum coverage and use a fork to remove them from the bowl, allowing excess chocolate to drip back into the bowl.

8. Place the patties on the prepared plate and place in the freezer for 10 to 15 minutes, or until hardened.

9. Serve immediately or store in an airtight container in the freezer for up to a week.

    Calories: 315   **Fat:** 32g   **Protein:** 3g   **Carbs:** 16g   **Fiber:** 11g   **Sugar:** 0g

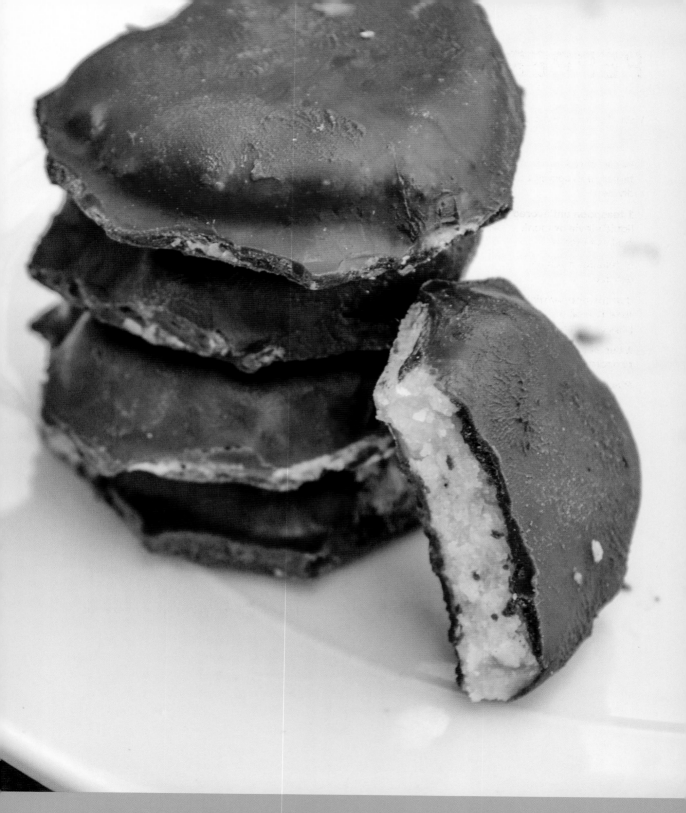

KETO BROWNIES

Yield: 8 brownies, 1 per serving   **Prep Time:** 15 minutes   **Cook Time:** 20 minutes

½ cup coconut almond butter or creamy almond butter

½ cup mashed avocado

3 tablespoons raw cacao powder

2 tablespoons monk fruit maple-flavored syrup or maple-flavored liquid stevia

1 tablespoon coconut oil, plus more for greasing

½ cup sugar-free chocolate chips

1. Preheat the oven to 325°F. Grease a 9 by 5-inch loaf pan with coconut oil or line it with parchment paper.

2. Place the coconut almond butter, avocado, cacao powder, sweetener, and 1 tablespoon of the coconut oil in a food processor or high-powered blender and blend on high until smooth. The batter will be very thick. Using a spoon, stir in the chocolate chips.

3. Transfer the batter to the prepared loaf pan. Using the back of a spoon, do your best to spread the batter evenly across the pan.

4. Bake for 20 minutes. To test for doneness, insert a toothpick in the middle of the brownies. It should come out fairly clean. If it has a lot of chocolate on it, bake for another 5 minutes, then test with the toothpick again. Remove the pan from the oven and set aside to cool.

5. Cut into 8 squares and serve or store in an airtight container at room temperature for up to a week or in the freezer for up to 3 months.

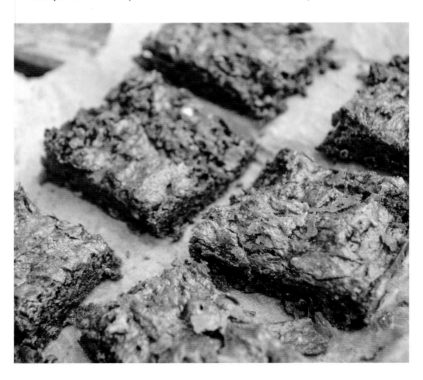

    Calories: 208   **Fat:** 18g   **Protein:** 5g   **Carbs:** 13g   **Fiber:** 8g   **Sugar:** 2g

COCONUT CUSTARD LEMON PIE

Yield: 1 (9-inch) pie, 12 servings   **Prep Time:** 8 minutes   **Cook Time:** 25 minutes

2 large eggs

1 cup full-fat coconut milk

¾ cup powdered monk fruit sweetener

¼ cup coconut flour

2 tablespoons unsalted butter, melted

1 teaspoon vanilla extract

1 teaspoon grated lemon zest

¾ teaspoon baking powder

1 cup unsweetened shredded coconut, plus more for garnish

1. Preheat the oven to 350°F. Spray a 9-inch pie pan with coconut oil cooking spray and set aside.

2. In a medium bowl, whisk together all of the ingredients except the shredded coconut until well combined and the mixture has a custardlike texture.

3. Fold the shredded coconut into the custard. Pour the mixture into the prepared pie pan and bake for 20 to 25 minutes, until the custard is set and the top is golden brown.

4. Remove the pie from the oven and let cool down completely before serving.

5. Cover any leftover pie and store it at room temperature for up to 5 days.

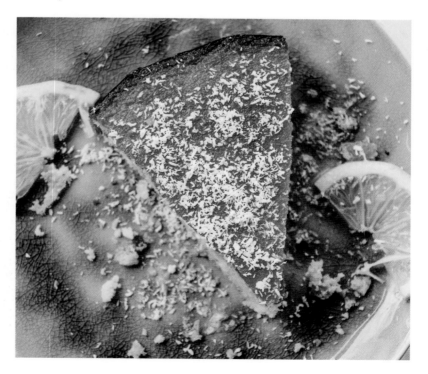

TURMERIC COCONUT CREAM CUPS

Yield: 12 candy cups, 1 per serving   **Prep Time:** 30 minutes, plus 20 minutes to chill   **Cook Time:** 5 minutes

½ cup (1 stick) unsalted butter or ghee

½ teaspoon turmeric powder

Pinch of freshly ground black pepper

1½ cups unsweetened shredded coconut

½ cup coconut butter

½ cup coconut oil

1 teaspoon freshly squeezed lemon juice

1 teaspoon unflavored liquid stevia or monk fruit sweetener (optional)

These cream cups are super satisfying—one goes a long way!

1. Have on hand a silicone or metal mini muffin pan.

2. In a small saucepan over low heat, melt the butter. Add the turmeric and pepper and stir until well combined. Remove the pan from the heat and set aside.

3. Place the shredded coconut, coconut butter, coconut oil, lemon juice, and stevia in a food processor and process until well blended.

4. Place about 2 tablespoons of the coconut mixture in each of 12 wells in the mini muffin pan. Gently press down on the mixture to even it out.

5. Pour equal portions of the turmeric butter over the coconut mixture in each well until the coconut is completely covered.

6. Freeze for about 20 minutes, or until the coconut mixture is frozen.

7. Serve immediately or store in a tightly sealed container in the refrigerator for up to a week or in the freezer for up to 3 months.

Calories: 291   **Fat:** 30g   **Protein:** 1g   **Carbs:** 5g   **Fiber:** 3g   **Sugar:** 1g

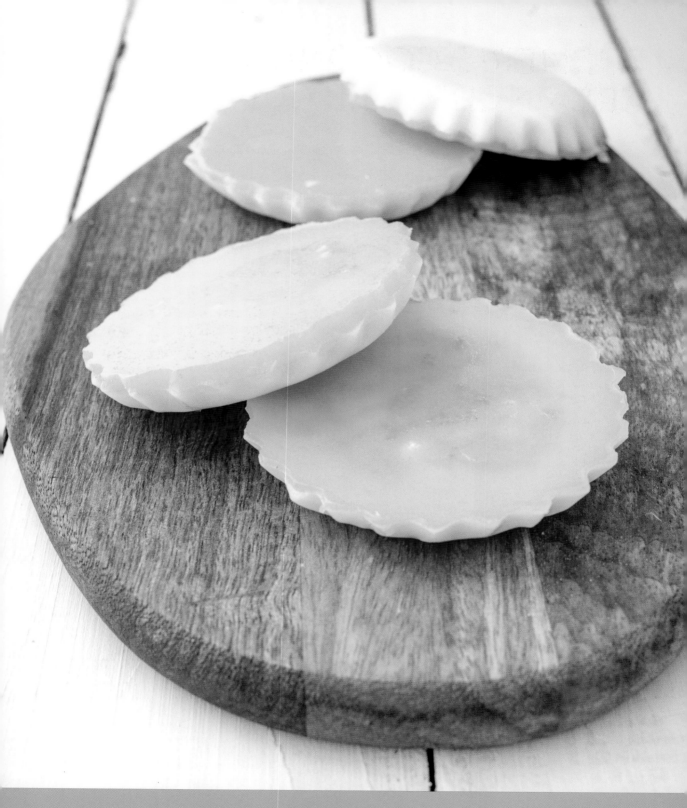

FROZEN COCONUT ALMOND BUTTER CUPS

Yield: 12 candy cups, 1 per serving   **Prep Time:** 25 minutes, plus 10 to 20 minutes to chill   **Cook Time:** 5 minutes

½ cup sugar-free chocolate chips

1 tablespoon coconut oil

¼ cup coconut almond butter or creamy almond butter

1 teaspoon chocolate-flavored liquid stevia, or to taste

Pinch of fine sea salt

1. Grease 12 wells of a standard-size silicone ice cube tray with coconut oil cooking spray.

2. Melt the chocolate chips and coconut oil in a small saucepan over low heat. Stir until well combined.

3. Pour half of the chocolate mixture into the prepared ice cube tray, dividing it evenly among the greased wells. This will form the bottom layer of the cups.

4. In a small bowl, mix together the coconut almond butter and stevia.

5. Top the chocolate mixture in the ice cube tray with the coconut almond butter mixture, putting about 1 teaspoon in each well. This will form the middle layer of the cups.

6. Evenly cover the coconut almond butter in each well with the remaining chocolate mixture. This will form the top layer of the cups.

7. Place the ice cube tray in the freezer for 10 to 20 minutes, or until the candy cups become firm.

8. Remove from the freezer and enjoy immediately or store in a zip-top bag in the freezer for up to 3 months. If storing, remove from the freezer about 30 minutes before enjoying to allow them to thaw slightly and make them easier to remove from the ice cube tray.

Calories: 76   **Fat:** 7g   **Protein:** 2g   **Carbs:** 5g   **Fiber:** 3g   **Sugar:** 1g

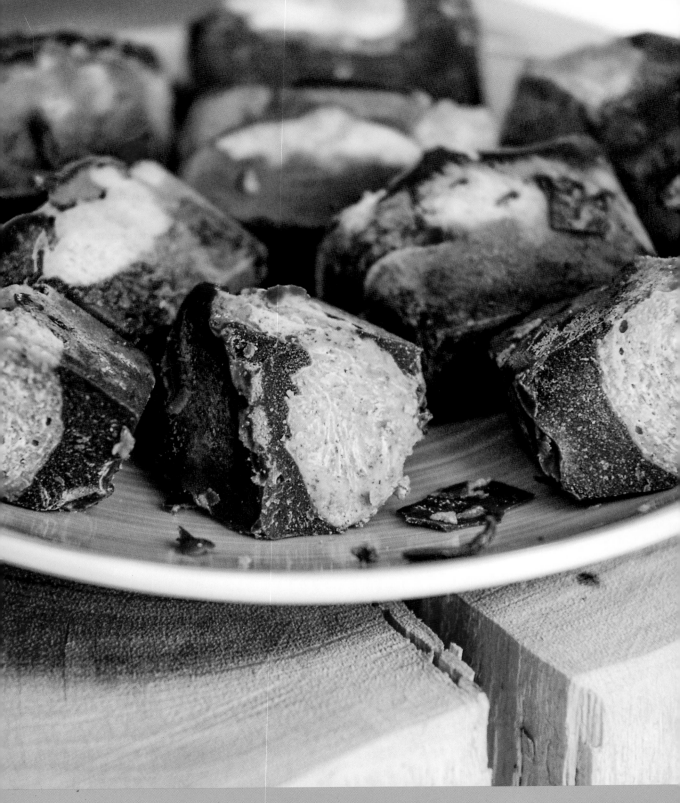

NO-CHURN COCONUT MILK ICE CREAM

Yield: 2 cups, ½ cup per serving   **Prep Time:** 10 minutes, plus time to freeze   **Cook Time:** —

2 (13½-ounce) cans full-fat coconut milk

1 teaspoon vanilla extract

1 teaspoon unflavored liquid stevia or monk fruit sweetener

Pinch of fine sea salt

The fat in the coconut milk makes this ice cream super satisfying. Better yet, you don't need an ice cream maker for this recipe.

1. Line a deep baking dish with parchment paper. Pour the coconut milk into the dish and freeze for several hours, or until hard.

2. Once frozen, pull the coconut milk off the parchment paper and break it into chunks.

3. In a food processor or high-powered blender, combine the coconut milk chunks with the remaining ingredients and process on high until smooth, scraping down the sides as necessary. Continue processing until the mixture reaches the desired ice cream texture.

4. Serve immediately or store in the freezer for up to a week. To serve stored ice cream, allow it to thaw for 20 minutes and then blend it before scooping it into serving dishes.

VARIATION: CHOCOLATE COCONUT MILK ICE CREAM

Follow the recipe as written, but in step 3, use 5 to 15 drops chocolate-flavored liquid stevia in place of the unflavored liquid stevia and add ¼ cup raw cacao powder.

Calories: 350   **Fat:** 38g   **Protein:** 3g   **Carbs:** 5g   **Fiber:** 0g   **Sugar:** 0g

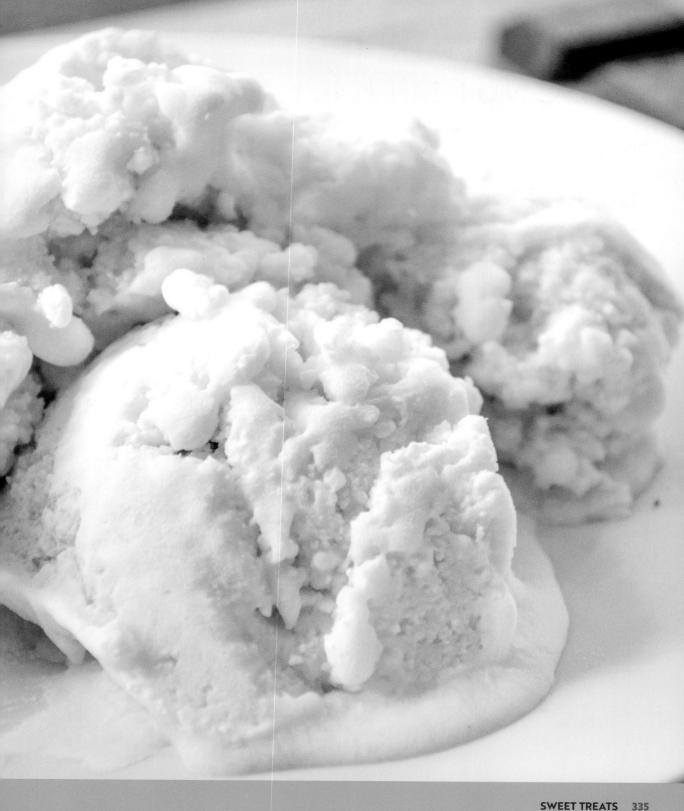

NO-BAKE TURMERIC COOKIES

Yield: 6 cookies, 1 per serving   **Prep Time:** 15 minutes, plus 45 minutes to chill   **Cook Time:** —

1 cup unsweetened shredded coconut

2 teaspoons coconut oil

3 tablespoons tahini, almond butter, cashew butter, or slightly melted coconut butter

1 scoop unflavored protein powder

1 tablespoon turmeric powder

1 teaspoon unflavored liquid stevia or monk fruit sweetener

1. In a food processor or high-powered blender, combine the coconut flakes and coconut oil and blend on high until the mixture takes on the consistency of coconut butter—creamy and smooth.

2. Add the tahini and continue blending until well combined.

3. Transfer the mixture to a bowl and add the protein powder, turmeric, and stevia. Using a fork, mix it into a crumbly dough.

4. Line a baking sheet with parchment paper.

5. Measure 2 tablespoons of the dough and form it into a ball. Place on the prepared baking sheet. Using your hands, flatten each cookie into a round shape. Repeat with the remaining dough, making a total of 6 cookies.

6. Transfer the baking sheet to the refrigerator and chill for 45 minutes. As the cookies chill, they will solidify and take on a great texture.

7. Serve immediately or place in an airtight container and store in the refrigerator for up to a week.

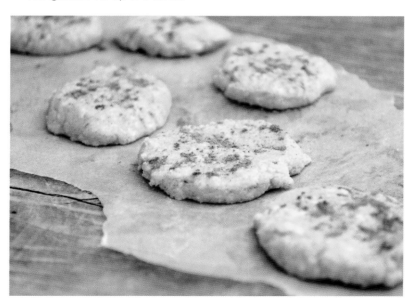

   Calories: 171   **Fat:** 15g   **Protein:** 6g   **Carbs:** 5g   **Fiber:** 3g   **Sugar:** 1g

COCONUT SHORTBREAD COOKIES

Yield: 6 cookies, 1 per serving   **Prep Time:** 25 minutes   **Cook Time:** 8 to 10 minutes

¼ cup plus 2 tablespoons coconut flour

5 tablespoons unsalted butter, melted but not hot

2 large eggs

2 dropperfuls vanilla-flavored liquid stevia

¼ teaspoon vanilla extract

1. Preheat the oven to 350°F. Line a baking sheet with parchment paper.

2. Place all of the ingredients in a bowl and mix until the dough has the consistency of a thick paste.

3. Shape the dough into 6 equal-size balls and place them on the prepared baking sheet, spacing them about 2 inches apart. Press down gently on the tops of the cookies with a fork, making a crosshatch pattern.

4. Bake the cookies for 8 to 10 minutes, or until they're lightly browned on the bottom. Remove from the oven and let cool completely on the baking sheet; otherwise, they will crumble.

5. Serve immediately or store in the refrigerator for up to a week or in the freezer for up to 3 months.

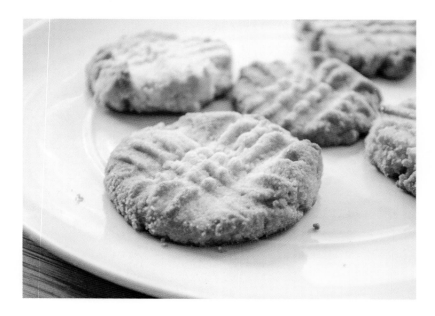

CHOCOLATE CHIP COOKIES

Yield: 21 cookies, 1 per serving   **Prep Time:** 20 minutes   **Cook Time:** 10 minutes

1 cup creamy almond butter

¼ cup powdered monk fruit sweetener

1 large egg

1 teaspoon vanilla extract

½ teaspoon baking soda

½ teaspoon fine sea salt

3 dropperfuls unflavored liquid stevia

2 dropperfuls vanilla-flavored liquid stevia

¼ cup sugar-free chocolate chips

¼ cup chopped raw walnuts

1. Preheat the oven to 350°F. Line a baking sheet with parchment paper.

2. Place all of the ingredients except the chocolate chips and walnuts in a medium bowl. Using an electric mixer, mix into a smooth dough.

3. Add the chocolate chips and walnuts to the dough and mix with a spoon.

4. Place 1 heaping tablespoon of dough on the prepared baking sheet. Repeat, spacing the cookies about 2 inches apart, until you've used all of the dough. You should get about 21 cookies. Using your hands, flatten each cookie into a round shape.

5. Bake for 10 minutes. To check for doneness, gently insert a fork or toothpick into a cookie; if it comes out clean, they're ready. If not, return to the oven for 1 to 2 minutes. Remove from the oven and set aside to cool on the baking sheet for 20 minutes.

6. Using a spatula, transfer the cookies to a cooling rack to finish cooling. They will harden and become less crumbly as they cool.

7. Serve immediately or store in the refrigerator for up to a week or in the freezer for up to 3 months.

Calories: 95   **Fat:** 8g   **Protein:** 3g   **Carbs:** 4g   **Fiber:** 2g   **Sugar:** 0g

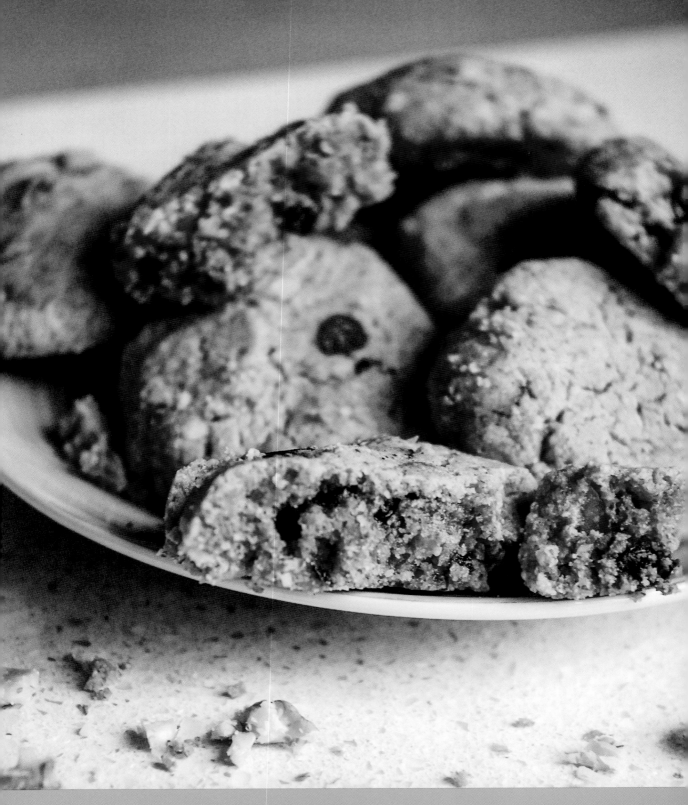

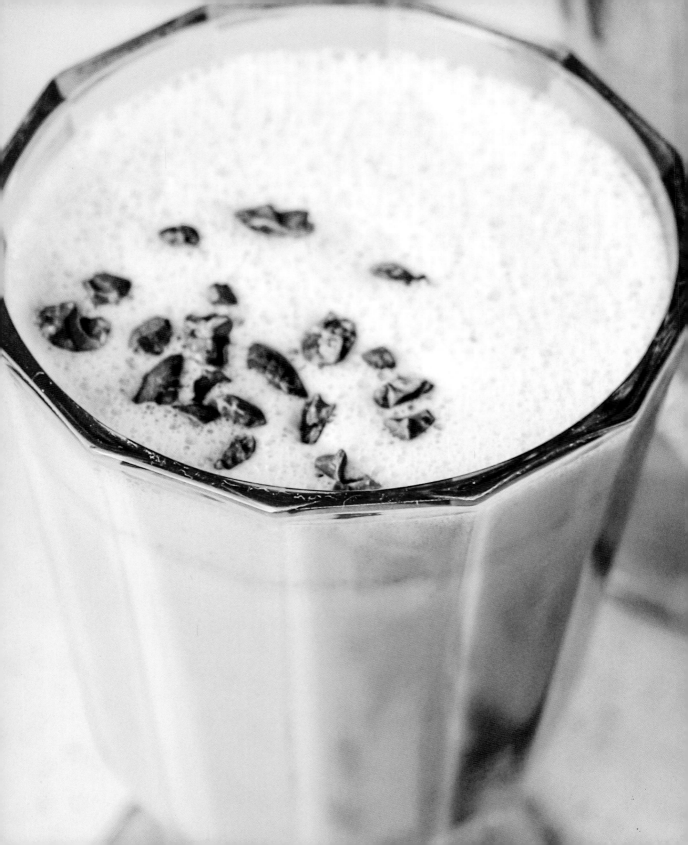

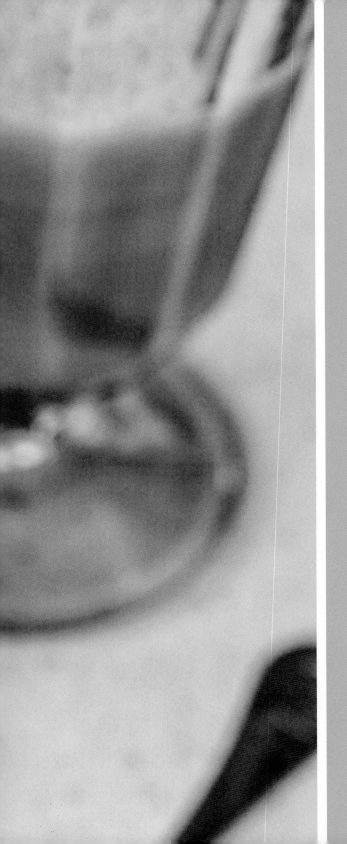

DRINKS

CHOCOLATE CHIA SUPER SMOOTHIE

Yield: 2 servings   **Prep Time:** 5 minutes   **Cook Time:** –

2 cups unsweetened almond or light coconut milk (from a carton)

1 tablespoon raw cacao powder

1 tablespoon coconut butter

1 teaspoon chia seeds

1 teaspoon flax seeds

1 scoop unflavored protein powder

½ avocado, pitted and skinned (optional)

½ teaspoon vanilla extract (optional)

Ice, as needed

1. Place all of the ingredients in a blender, using more or less almond milk and ice depending on the desired thickness of the smoothie. Blend until smooth and creamy.

2. Transfer to two 10-ounce serving glasses and enjoy!

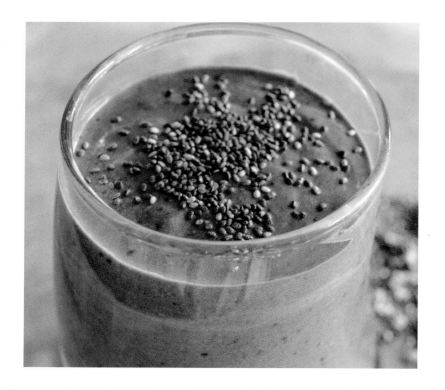

Calories: 163   **Fat:** 10g   **Protein:** 13g   **Carbs:** 7g   **Fiber:** 4g   **Sugar:** 1g

KEY LIME PIE SMOOTHIE

Yield: 2 servings   **Prep Time:** 5 minutes, plus time to soak cashews overnight   **Cook Time:** —

1 cup full-fat coconut milk

1 cup filtered water

½ cup raw cashews, soaked overnight and drained

1 avocado, pitted and skinned

1 large handful spinach

Juice of 1 lime

¼ teaspoon vanilla extract

5 to 10 drops vanilla-flavored liquid stevia (optional)

1. Place all of the ingredients in a high-powered blender and blend until smooth and creamy.

2. Transfer to two 10-ounce serving glasses and enjoy!

Tip: If you prefer, you can use light coconut milk that comes in a carton instead of a can; in that case, use 2 cups of milk and omit the water.

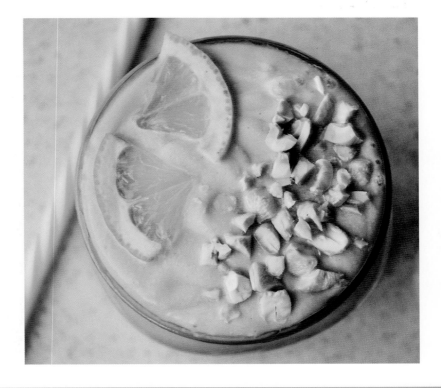

CINNAMON COCONUT SMOOTHIE

Yield: 2 servings   **Prep Time:** 5 minutes   **Cook Time:** —

½ cup full-fat coconut milk

½ cup filtered water

2 tablespoons creamy almond butter, or 1 handful raw walnuts and/or almonds

1 scoop vanilla-flavored protein powder (optional)

¼ teaspoon vanilla extract

20 drops vanilla-flavored liquid stevia, or to taste

Pinch of fine sea salt

½ teaspoon ground cinnamon, for sprinkling

1. Place all of the ingredients except the cinnamon in a blender and blend until smooth and creamy.

2. Transfer to two 6-ounce serving glasses. Top with the cinnamon and enjoy!

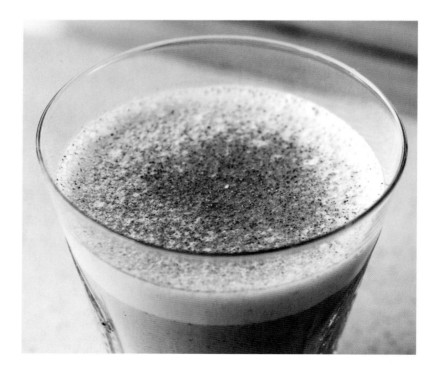

Calories: 243   **Fat:** 20g   **Protein:** 14g   **Carbs:** 5g   **Fiber:** 2g   **Sugar:** 1g

CHOCOLATE COCONUT MILKSHAKE

Yield: 2 servings   **Prep Time:** 5 minutes, plus 2 hours to freeze coconut milk   **Cook Time:** —

2 cups full-fat coconut milk, divided

2 tablespoons coconut almond butter or other nut butter of choice

2 scoops unflavored protein powder

1 dropperful vanilla-flavored liquid stevia

¼ cup raw cacao nibs or sugar-free chocolate chips

1. Pour 1 cup of the coconut milk into an ice cube tray and freeze for at least 2 hours, or until completely frozen.

2. Place the remaining 1 cup of coconut milk, the coconut almond butter, protein powder, and stevia in a high-powered blender and blend until smooth.

3. Add the coconut milk ice cubes to the blender and blend just until the mixture is smooth and no ice chunks remain. (Don't blend it too much, or the ice will begin to melt and you'll lose that thick milkshake-like consistency.)

4. Add the cacao nibs and pulse just until they are evenly distributed and flecked throughout the milkshake.

5. Transfer to two 10-ounce serving glasses and serve immediately.

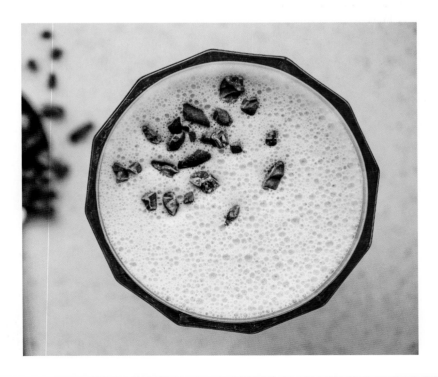

SWEET RASPBERRY SHAKE

Yield: 2 servings   **Prep Time:** 5 minutes   **Cook Time:** —

½ (13½-ounce) can full-fat coconut milk

1 scoop vanilla-flavored protein powder

¼ cup frozen raspberries or strawberries

1 teaspoon ground cinnamon

Unflavored liquid stevia, to taste

1. Place all of the ingredients in a blender and blend until smooth and creamy.

2. Transfer to two 6-ounce serving glasses and enjoy!

Tip: If you prefer, you can use light coconut milk that comes in a carton instead of canned; in that case, I suggest adding 1 tablespoon of coconut oil or coconut butter to boost the fat content.

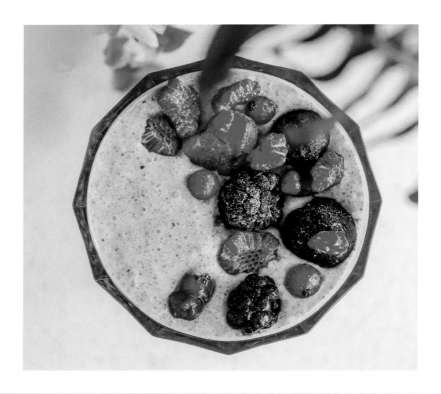

Calories: 226   **Fat:** 17g   **Protein:** 11g   **Carbs:** 4g   **Fiber:** 1g   **Sugar:** 1g

DE-INFLAMING LEMONADE

Yield: 4 to 6 servings   **Prep Time:** 5 minutes   **Cook Time:** —

1 cup freshly squeezed lemon juice (from 4 to 6 lemons)

4 to 6 cups filtered water

1 tablespoon coconut oil or MCT oil (optional)

1 teaspoon ground cinnamon

1 teaspoon grated fresh ginger (optional)

1 teaspoon turmeric powder

½ teaspoon unflavored liquid stevia, or to taste

Pinch of fine sea salt

Pinch of freshly ground black pepper (optional)

The pepper in this recipe is optional, but using it will dramatically improve the absorption of the curcuminoids in the turmeric, which absorb best when ingested along with good fats and piperine, the main ingredient in black pepper.

1. Place all of the ingredients in a blender and blend until fully combined.

2. Serve immediately in four 12-ounce or six 8-ounce glasses, or store in an airtight container in the refrigerator for up to a week. You will need to mix well each time you want to drink it if you let it sit for a while.

Tip: Drink this lemonade regularly. People who suffer from crippling pain have reported that their symptoms improved significantly after they made this an everyday drink.

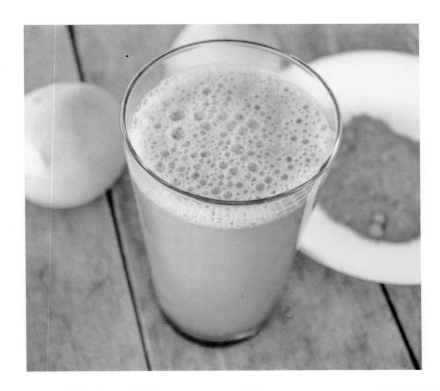

Calories: 11   **Fat:** 0g   **Protein:** 0g   **Carbs:** 4g   **Fiber:** 1g   **Sugar:** 1g

MATCHA TEA

Yield: 1 serving   **Prep Time:** 5 minutes   **Cook Time:** 5 minutes

1 cup filtered water

2 tablespoons full-fat coconut milk

½ teaspoon matcha tea leaves, or 1 or 2 matcha tea bags

Unflavored liquid stevia, to taste

1 teaspoon coconut oil or MCT oil

½ teaspoon unsalted butter or ghee (optional)

Option 1

1. In a small saucepan, bring the water and coconut milk to a light boil. Add the tea and stevia and stir until fully combined. Remove the pan from the heat and remove and discard the tea leaves or bags.

2. Add the contents of the saucepan, coconut oil, and butter, if using, to a glass blender (the heat from the tea can cause chemicals in plastic to leach into the beverage) and blend for 30 seconds to 1 minute, or until creamy.

3. Transfer to a 10-ounce serving cup and serve immediately.

Option 2

1. In a small saucepan, bring the water to a light boil. Add the tea and stir until fully combined. Set aside for 5 minutes.

2. Remove and discard the tea leaves or bags. Return the saucepan to the heat, add the coconut milk and stevia, and return to a light boil.

3. Place the contents of the saucepan, coconut oil, and butter, if using, in a glass blender and blend for 30 seconds to 1 minute, or until creamy.

4. Transfer to a serving cup and serve immediately.

Tip: If you like your matcha creamier, change the proportions to ½ cup coconut milk and ½ cup water and follow the steps of Option 1.

Calories: 101   **Fat:** 10g   **Protein:** 1g   **Carbs:** 2g   **Fiber:** 1g   **Sugar:** 0g

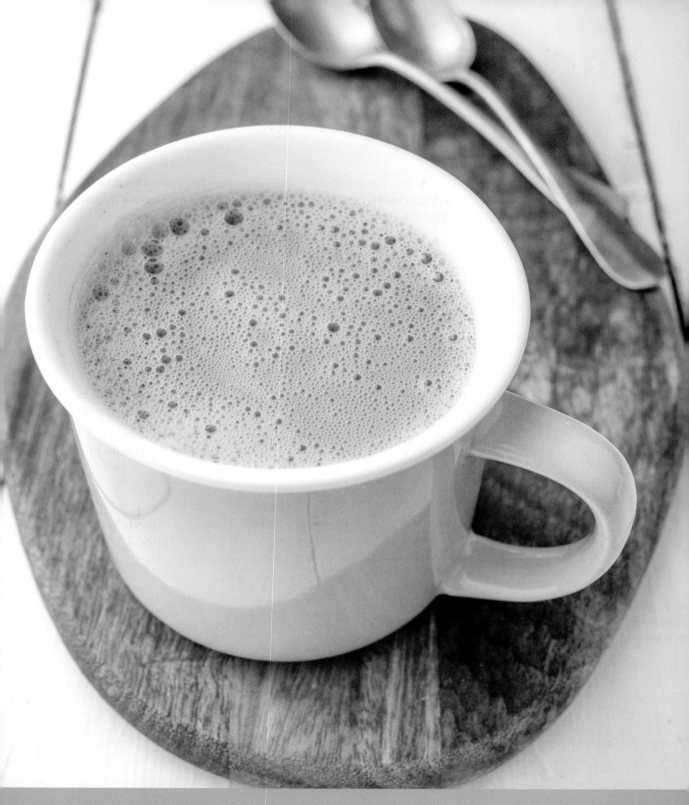

FAT-BURNING TURMERIC COFFEE

Yield: 2 servings   **Prep Time:** 5 minutes   **Cook Time:** —

2 cups freshly brewed coffee, very hot

1 teaspoon MCT oil or coconut oil

1 teaspoon unsalted butter

¼ teaspoon ground cinnamon

¼ teaspoon turmeric powder

1 dropperful vanilla-flavored liquid stevia

1 dropperful English toffee–flavored liquid stevia

Dash of fine sea salt

1. Place all of the ingredients in a blender and blend until thoroughly combined.

2. Transfer to two 10-ounce serving cups and serve immediately.

Tips: This recipe is easily doubled or tripled.

Be sure to use a glass blender for this recipe; the heat from the coffee can cause chemicals in plastic to leach into the beverage.

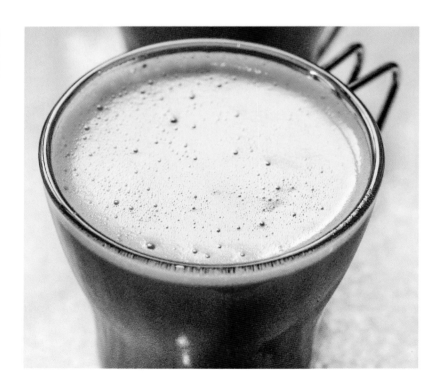

Calories: 43   **Fat:** 5g   **Protein:** 1g   **Carbs:** .5g   **Fiber:** 0g   **Sugar:** 0g

GOLDEN MILK

Yield: 2 servings   **Prep Time:** 5 minutes   **Cook Time:** 10 minutes

1 cup full-fat coconut milk

½ teaspoon ginger powder

½ teaspoon turmeric powder

Pinch of freshly ground black pepper

Unflavored liquid stevia, to taste

Ground cinnamon, for sprinkling

Coconut cream, for topping (optional; see Tip)

1. In a saucepan over medium heat, whisk together the coconut milk, ginger, turmeric, and pepper until the mixture starts to bubble.

2. Reduce the heat to low and simmer for about 5 minutes, allowing the flavors to meld.

3. Transfer to two 8-ounce serving glasses and stir in the stevia. Top with cinnamon and coconut cream, if desired. Enjoy!

Tip: To get coconut cream, refrigerate a can of coconut milk overnight. When you open the can, you can scrape the cream off the top.

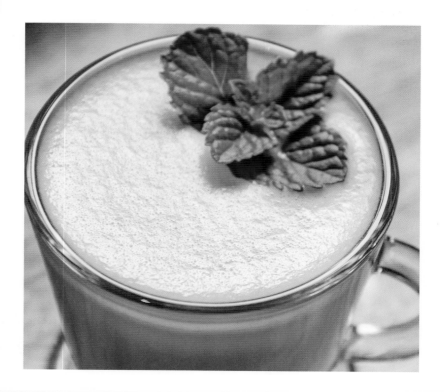

Calories: 423   **Fat:** 45g   **Protein:** 3g   **Carbs:** 7g   **Fiber:** 0g   **Sugar:** 0g

ACKNOWLEDGMENTS

There are so many people I would like to thank for this book, especially my amazing wife, Angel, and my children, David, Joshua, and Joyful. You guys are my inspiration and bring me so much life and energy with your smiles!

Thank you to my mother, Barbara Jockers, who first got me interested in natural health and nutrition and taught me a lot in the kitchen back when I was a teenager. Mom, you were the first to encourage me in health and nutrition, and I am forever grateful!

This project would not have been accomplished without the help of my writing assistant, Jen Brown, and my DrJockers.com team: my assistant, Alyse Martinez; my brother and web administrator, James Jockers; my graphic designer, Stephen Johnson; my customer service specialist, Deb Larrabee; my health coaches, Melissa Nohr and Danielle Dellaquila; and my social media manager, Chene Sonnekus.

I also want to thank my business partner, Brett Farrell, and his assistants, Tracy and Corina. I want to thank my team at Exodus Health Center, including Dr. Audrey Bedford, and customer service specialists, Jayne Goss and Courtney McTaggart.

Much love to all of my health clients and fans who have trusted me and my recommendations. It is through you that I have had the opportunity to learn much in regard to leadership, healing, faith, and life. It's still one of my greatest joys to see people achieve new breakthroughs in their life and health. I've been blessed by so many of you who have had the discipline and focus to change your lives and reach a new level of health!

RESOURCES

Testing for Ketones

Blood Testing

Testing your blood ketones is the gold standard for measuring your state of ketosis. The following units offer one meter that can test both blood glucose and ketones through two different strips.

- Keto-Mojo (keto-mojo.com): This company offers a blood glucose and ketone meter and testing strips for the best value on the market.
- Precision Xtra (abbottstore.com/diabetes-management/precision-brand.html): Abbott sells both the blood glucose and ketone meter and testing strips. The ketone strips for this device cost more than the strips for the Keto-Mojo device.

Breath Testing

If you want to track your ketones and fat-burning state through breath, you can try one of the following devices, which are the main units on the market. At the time of writing, I don't trust the measurements of other devices. Both devices are great and offer apps that you can use to track your numbers over time on your cell phone.

- Ketonix (ketonix.com): This device is the less expensive of the two and is much easier to use than the LEVL.
- LEVL (levlnow.com): This device continually recalibrates and is thought to be more accurate.

Calorie-Tracking Apps

You can find some great apps for tracking your macros and monitoring how your body is adapting to the keto lifestyle. Search the app store for your device to find these apps, or visit the listed website:

- Carb Manager (carbmanager.com)
- Cronometer (cronometer.com)
- KetoDiet (ketodietapp.com)
- MyFitnessPal (myfitnesspal.com)
- Total Keto Diet App (totalketodiet.com)

Biomarker Tracking App

The Heads Up Health app enables you to sync your calorie-tracking app, your blood and breath ketone levels, and your lab tests so you can see them and follow them in real time. If you enjoy observing your biological data, then you'll love this app. Visit headsuphealth.com or find it in your app store.

Phone Apps for Specific Eating Plans

If you're looking for specific meal plans and shopping instructions that follow the ketogenic diet principles, here are some helpful apps you can use on your phone:

- Keto Diet app (ketodietapp.com)
- Low Carb app (lazyketo.app)
- Senza (www.senza.us)
- Suggestic (suggestic.com)
- Total Keto Diet (totalketodiet.com)

Check out the Dr. Jockers Keto Challenge in the Suggestic app. Get started at ketochallenge. premium.suggestic. com.

Premade Keto Meals

If you're looking for delicious premade keto meals that can be delivered to your home each week, then check out these companies:

- Factor 75 (factor75.com)
- Green Chef (greenchef.com)
- Keto Fridge (ketofridge.com)

Great Keto Websites

Here are some of my favorite websites for keto-related information.

- Diet Doctor (dietdoctor.com)
- Dr. Axe (draxe.com)
- Dr. Perlmutter (drperlmutter.com)
- Keto Connect (ketoconnect.net)
- Mike Mutzel (highintensityhealth.com)
- Perfect Keto (perfectketo.com)
- Ruled Me (ruled.me)

My website is full of helpful information, including in-depth articles on ketosis, the keto diet, intermittent fasting, keto recipes, and so much more. You can find it at drjockers.com.

RECOMMENDED PRODUCTS

You may have some questions about the products I use in my recipes, so I've compiled some information about my favorite choices for some items. Many of these products are available at your local grocery store, but if you have difficulty finding something locally, try an online grocery retailer such as Amazon.com

Baking Ingredients

Almond flour: Almond flour works great for baking. It's rich in healthy fats and high-quality fiber, it's gluten-free, and it's very low in net carbs.

Bob's Red Mill Paleo Baking Flour: This paleo baking flour is a combination of coconut flour, almond flour, arrowroot starch, and tapioca root flour. This product is a bit higher in net carbs because it includes arrowroot and tapioca, but when you mix it well with full-fat coconut milk, butter, and eggs, it bakes well, and the overall fats reduce the net carbs per serving.

Coconut flakes: Unsweetened coconut flakes are in the baking section of most grocery stores. I always recommend that you use an organic brand, if possible.

Coconut flour: This is the fiber of the coconut, and you can use it for baking! It's rich in good coconut fats and high-quality fiber. It's also gluten-free and very low in net carbs.

Dairy and Dairy Alternatives

Almond milk: You can substitute unsweetened almond milk in some recipes. However, remember that almond milk is lower in fat than coconut milk, so making this ingredient substitution will change the texture and macronutrient content of the recipe.

Coconut milk: You can buy coconut in cans or cartons. When you purchase the canned variety, make sure to pick a brand that comes in a BPA-free can. The brand I prefer is Natural Value. You're likely to use a lot of canned coconut milk when you have a keto lifestyle, so I recommend buying cans by the case. The brand of carton-packaged coconut milk that I prefer is So Delicious unsweetened coconut milk because it doesn't include any sweetener or carrageenan (a common food additive).

Cow's dairy products: I always recommend organic dairy products; ideally, you'd use dairy from pasture-raised animals. *Organic* means that the animals weren't consuming pesticide-sprayed grains. *Pasture-raised* means the animals were able to roam on pasture and eat what grows wild.

Pasture-raised dairy products have the most nutrient density and least amount of toxins. You can find products from pasture-raised animals at grocery stores like Whole Foods and health food stores. You also can order it online from places like US Wellness Meats (grasslandbeef.com).

Meat and Seafood

I always recommend organic meat. You can find organic poultry at your local health food store, in many grocery stores, and via online stores such as US Wellness Meats. When shopping for red meat, look for grass-fed or pasture-raised products because they have the highest nutrient density.

I recommend wild-caught as opposed to farm-raised seafood. Wild-caught seafood has more nutrients and fewer environmental toxins, so it's much better for your health. You can find wild-caught seafood at your local health food store, at many grocery stores, and through online vendors.

Pantry Items

Avocado oil mayo: This awesome mayonnaise alternative is made with avocado oil and has great health benefits. I prefer the Primal Kitchen Mayo brand, which is free of sweeteners. Primal Kitchen offers several flavors; I use the Chipotle Lime variety in the Paleo Stuffed Mushrooms (page 279).

Chicken broth: I always recommend the highest quality organic, pasture-raised bone broth. Although you can make your own bone broth (you can find many recipes online), it does take quite a bit of time, and it's a messy process. Using store-bought broth in place of homemade is just fine. My favorite brand of store-bought broth is Kettle & Fire.

Coconut almond butter: This product is relatively new on the nut butter scene. It's a combination of coconut butter and almond butter. It has smooth and creamy texture and tastes great. You can use it as a spread or in any recipe that calls for nut butter.

Coconut aminos: This soy sauce alternative is made from coconut. It is soy-free and hypoallergenic, and it's well-tolerated by most individuals. It works well in stir-fries, meat dishes, and any other recipe that calls for soy sauce.

Coconut butter: Coconut butter (also known as coconut manna for some brands) is a combination of coconut oil and coconut flour, which makes it a smooth and fibrous mixture. It's great to use in keto recipes that call for nut butter, or you can sometimes use it as a dairy alternative.

Coconut flour wraps: These wraps are similar to flour tortillas except they're grain-free and made from coconut meat. They're thinner than your typical wheat-based wraps, they have a great flavor and texture, and they're keto-friendly. Nuco is my favorite brand, and I love the turmeric coconut wrap, which includes the healing spice turmeric for an added health benefit without affecting the great flavor.

Protein Powders

When you shop for protein powder, look for high-quality, organic products that are low in carbs. They should be less than 5 grams of net carbs per serving and ideally have 2 grams or less of net carbs per serving.

I'm a huge fan of collagen and bone broth proteins, which provide key amino acids that support your gut lining, joints, skin, and immune system. Our ancestors got a lot of their protein from tendons and joints in the animals they consumed. In our society, we mostly eat muscle meat because the regions of the meat that contain collagen are harder to chew and less tasty, so we typically discard them. Consuming bone broth and using a good-quality collagen or bone broth protein is a way to ingest those key amino acids.

Other good protein powder sources include egg protein, nondenatured grass-fed whey protein, and beef protein. For vegan sources, I suggest pea protein, hemp protein, chia, and flax protein. Soy protein is a poor source, so I suggest you avoid it. Also, look for protein powders that are either unsweetened or sweetened with stevia or monk fruit.

My website store (store.DrJockers.com) includes the protein powders I recommend and use personally.

Sweeteners and Sweets

Chocolate: I use organic unsweetened dark chocolate or cacao powder in recipes that require chocolate. Cacao powder is the most minimally processed version of chocolate. In recipes that call for *unsweetened chocolate chips,* I use Lily's brand baking chips, which are flavored with stevia and erythritol. They are low-carb and keto-friendly.

ChocZero products: ChocZero offers several syrups of different flavors (such as maple and caramel) and keto bark flavored with monk fruit and non-GMO corn fiber. These products are sugar-free, low in net carbs, and free of sugar alcohols. The fiber content of ChocZero increases the total carbohydrates of a recipe but not the net carbs. Read Chapter 4 for more information on calculating net carbs, which are the carbs that elevate blood sugar levels.

In recipes where I specify *sugar-free maple syrup,* I used either ChocZero or Lakanto brand.

Lakanto Monk Fruit Sweetener: This brand has powdered monk fruit and erythritol sweeteners that are easy to bake with. These products are sugar-free and low in net carbs. In the recipe section, I used the Lakanto brand dried sweetener wherever you see *dried monk fruit sweetener* in the ingredients list.

Stevia: This natural sweetener is 100 times stronger than sugar and has no ill effect on blood sugar, and it's my preferred sweetener. I recommend the SweetLeaf brand of liquid stevia droplets.

In my experience, people like the flavor of liquid stevia better than the white powder. The drops also come in a variety of flavors, some of which are ingredients in some of the recipes in this book. Regardless of the type of stevia you use, if you notice an unpleasant aftertaste, try adding a bit more salt to your dish. The salt blunts the aftertaste of the stevia.

ENDNOTES

Introduction

1. J. Weaver. "More People Search for Health Online." *Telemedicine on NBCNEWS. com* website, July 16, 2013. Accessed at http://www.nbcnews.com/id/3077086/t/more-people-search-health-online/#.W8irZ5NKiqA.

Chapter 1

1. C. M. Hales, M. D. Carroll, C. D. Fryar, and C. L. Ogden. "Prevalence of Obesity Among Adults and Youth: United States, 2015–2016." *NCHS Data Brief* no. 288 (2017). Accessed at https://www.cdc.gov/nchs/data/databriefs/db288.pdf.

2. G. Levy. "Sharp Increase in Obesity Rates, Over Last Decade, Federal Data Show." *U.S. News & World Report* website. March 26, 2018. Accessed at https://www.usnews.com/news/data-mine/articles/2018-03-26/sharp-increase-in-obesity-rates-over-last-decade-federal-data-show.

3. H. Cai, W. N. Cong, S. Ji, S. Rothman, S. Maudsley, and B. Martin. "Metabolic Dysfunction in Alzheimer's Disease and Related Neurodegenerative Disorders." *Current Alzheimer Research* 9, no. 1 (2012):5–17.

4. Partnership to Fight Chronic Disease. "The Growing Crisis of Chronic Disease in the United States." Accessed Jun 24, 2019 at https://www.fightchronicdisease.org/sites/default/files/docs/GrowingCrisisofChronicDiseaseintheUSfactsheet_81009.pdf.

5. B. Shilhavy. "Time Magazine: We Were Wrong About Saturated Fats." *Health Impact News* website. Accessed June 24, 2019 at https://healthimpactnews.com/2014/time-magazine-we-were-wrong-about-saturated-fats/.

Chapter 2

1. J. D. Bremner. "Traumatic Stress: Effects on the Brain." *Dialogues in Clinical Neuroscience* 8, no. 4 (2006): 445–61.

2. L. Stojanovich and D. Marisavljevich. "Stress as a Trigger of Autoimmune Disease." *Autoimmunity Reviews* 7, no. 3 (2008): 209–13.

3. U. Meier and A. M. Gressner. "Endocrine Regulation of Energy Metabolism: Review of Pathobiochemical and Clinical Chemical Aspects of Leptin, Ghrelin, Adiponectin, and Resistin." *Clinical Chemistry* 50, no. 9 (2004): 1511–25.

4. Ibid.

5. M. Scacchi, A. I. Pincelli, and F. Cavagnini. "Growth Hormone in Obesity." *International Journal of Obesity and Related Metabolic Disorders* 23, no. 3 (1999): 260–71.

6. See note 3 above.

7. G. Wilcox. "Insulin and Insulin Resistance." *Clinical Biochemist Reviews* 26, no. 2 (2005): 19–39.

8. L. Manuel-Apolinar et al. "Role of Prenatal Undernutrition in the Expression of Serotonin, Dopamine and Leptin Receptors in Adult Mice: Implications of Food Intake." *Molecular Medicine Reports* 9, no. 2 (2014): 407–12.

9. See note 3 above.

10. P. Koutkia et al. "Characterization of Leptin Pulse Dynamics and Relationship to Fat Mass, Growth Hormone, Cortisol, and Insulin." *American Journal of Physiology* 285, no. 2 (2003): E372–9.

11. See note 3 above.

12. S. D. Hewagalamulage et al. "High Cortisol Response to Adrenocorticotrophic Hormone Identifies Ewes with Reduced Melanocortin Signaling and Increased Propensity to Obesity." *Journal of Neuroendocrinology* 27, no. 1 (2015): 44–56.

13. E. Y. Joo, C. W. Yoon, D. L. Koo, D. Kim, and S. B. Hong. "Adverse Effects of 24 Hours of Sleep Deprivation on Cognition and Stress Hormones." *Journal of Clinical Neurology (Seoul, Korea)* 8, no. 2 (2012):146–50.

14. F. Raygan et al. (2016). "Comparative Effects of Carbohydrate Versus Fat Restriction on Metabolic Profiles, Biomarkers of Inflammation and Oxidative Stress in Overweight Patients with Type 2 Diabetic and Coronary Heart Disease: A Randomized Clinical Trial." *ARYA Atherosclerosis* 12, no. 6 (2016): 266–73.

15. N. Steckhan et al. (2016). "Effects of Different Dietary Approaches on Inflammatory Markers in Patients with Metabolic Syndrome: A Systematic Review and Meta-Analysis." *Nutrition* 32, no. 3 (2016): 338–48.

16. W. Mertz. "The Essential Trace Elements." *Science* 213, no. 4514 (1981): 1332–8.

17. See note 12 above.

18. R. Nagel. "Living with Phytic Acid." *Weston A. Price Foundation* website. March 26, 2010. Accessed at https://www.westonaprice.org/health-topics/vegetarianism-and-plant-foods/living-with-phytic-acid/.

Chapter 3

1. C. Kearns, L. Schmidt, and S. Glantz. "Sugar Industry and Coronary Heart Disease Research: A Historical Analysis of Internal Industry Documents." *JAMA Internal Medicine* 176, no. 11 (2016): 1680–5.

2. G. D. Lawrence. "Dietary Fats and Health: Dietary Recommendations in the Context of Scientific Evidence." *Advances in Nutrition* 4, no. 3 (2013): 294–302.

3. M. Dehghan et al. "Associations of Fats and Carbohydrate Intake with Cardiovascular Disease and Mortality in 18 Countries from Five Continents (PURE): A Prospective Cohort Study." *The Lancet* 390, no. 10107 (2017): P2050–62.

4. M. N. Roberts et al. "A Ketogenic Diet Extends Longevity and Healthspan in Adult Mice." *Cell Metabolism* 26, no. 3 (2017): P539–46.

5. B. Burgess, H. A. Raynor, and B. J. Tepper. "PROP Nontaster Women Lose More Weight Following a Low-Carbohydrate Versus a Low-Fat Diet in a Randomized Controlled Trial." *Obesity (Silver Spring)* 25, no. 10 (2017): 1682–90.

6. Y. Gao et al. "Dietary Sugars, Not Lipids, Drive Hypothalamic Inflammation." *Molecular Metabolism* 6, no. 8 (2017): 897–908.

7. Y. Meng et al. "Efficacy of Low Carbohydrate Diet for Type 2 Diabetes Mellitus Management: A Systematic Review and Meta-Analysis of Randomized Controlled Trials." *Diabetes Research and Clinical Practice* no. 131 (2017): 124–31.

8. J. C. Bradberry and D. E. Hilleman. "Overview of Omega-3 Fatty Acid Therapies." *Pharmacy & Therapeutics* 38, no. 11 (2013): 681–91.

9. S. C. Dyall and A. T. Michael-Titus. "Neurological Benefits of Omega-3 Fatty Acids." *NeuroMolecular Medicine* 10, no. 4 (2008): 219–35.

10. See note 8 above.

11. S. Egert, M. Kratz, F. Kannenberg, M. Fobker, and U. Wahrburg. "Effects of High-Fat and Low-Fat Diets Rich in Monounsaturated Fatty Acids on Serum Lipids, LDL Size and Indices of Lipid Peroxidation in Healthy Non-Obese Men and Women When Consumed Under Controlled Conditions." *European Journal of Nutrition* 50, no. 1 (2011): 71–9.

12. L. G. Gillingham, S. Harris-Janz, and P. J. H. Jones. "Dietary Monounsaturated Fatty Acids Are Protective Against Metabolic Syndrome and Cardiovascular Disease Risk Factors." *Lipids* 46, no. 3 (2011): 209–28.

13. J. Zhao et al. "Dietary Fat Intake and Endometrial Cancer Risk: A Dose Response Meta-Analysis." *Medicine (Baltimore)* 95, no. 27 (2016): e4121.

14. D. Sparks. "Trans Fat Is Double Trouble for Your Heart Health." *Mayo Clinic News Network* website. May 24, 2018. Accessed at https://newsnetwork.mayoclinic.org/discussion/transfat-is-double-trouble-for-your-heart-health/.

15. A. Sanchez-Villegas et al. "Dietary Fat Intake and the Risk of Depression: The SUN Project." *PLoS ONE* 6, no. 1 (2011): e16268.

Chapter 4

1. S. F. Sleiman et al. "Exercise Promotes the Expression of Brain Derived Neurotrophic Factor (BDNF) Through the Action of the Ketone Body β-hydroxybutyrate." *eLife* 5 (2016): e15092.

2. C. Vandenberghe et al. "Caffeine Intake Increases Plasma Ketones: An Acute Metabolic Study in Humans." *Canadian Journal of Physiology and Pharmacology* 95, no. 4 (2016): 455–8.

3. G. A. Mitchell et al. "Medical Aspects of Ketone Body Metabolism." *Clinical and Investigative Medicine* 18, no. 3 (1995): 193–216.

4. W. A. Wolpert. "Use of Continuous Glucose Monitoring in the Detection and Prevention of Hypoglycemia." *Journal of Diabetes Science and Technology* (Online) 1, no. 1 (2007): 146–50.

Chapter 5

1. N. Steckhan et al. "Effects of Different Dietary Approaches on Inflammatory Markers in Patients with Metabolic Syndrome: A Systematic Review and Meta-Analysis." *Nutrition* 32, no. 3 (2016): 338–48.

2. F. Raygan et al. (2016). "Comparative Effects of Carbohydrate Versus Fat Restriction on Metabolic Profiles, Biomarkers of Inflammation and Oxidative Stress in Overweight Patients with Type 2 Diabetic and Coronary Heart Disease: A Randomized Clinical Trial." *ARYA Atherosclerosis* 12, no. 6 (2016): 266–73.

3. T. Greco, T. C. Glenn, D. A. Hovda, and M. L. Prins. (2015). "Ketogenic Diet Decreases Oxidative Stress and Improves Mitochondrial Respiratory Complex Activity." *Journal of Cerebral Blood Flow & Metabolism* 36, no. 9 (2015): 1603–13.

4. A. Maiorana et al. "Ketogenic Diet in a Patient with Congenital Hyperinsulinism: A Novel Approach to Prevent Brain Damage." *Orphanet Journal of Rare Diseases* 10, no.1 (2015): 120.

5. M. Lucas et al. (2014). "Inflammatory Dietary Pattern and Risk of Depression Among Women." *Brain, Behavior, and Immunity* 36 (2014): 46–53.

6. R. D. Pitceathly and C. Viscomi. "Effects of Ketosis in Mitochondrial Myopathy: Potential Benefits of a Mitotoxic Diet." *EMBO Molecular Medicine* 8, no. 11 (2016): 1231–3.

7. M. Maalouf, J. M. Rho, and M. P. Mattson. "The Neuroprotective Properties of Calorie Restriction, the Ketogenic Diet, and Ketone Bodies." *Brain Research Reviews* 59, no. 2 (2009): 293–315.

8. P. D'Aquila, D. Bellizzi, and G. Passarino. "Mitochondria in Health, Aging and Diseases: The Epigenetic Perspective." *Biogerontology* 16, no. 5 (2015): 569–85.

Chapter 6

1. F. Raygan, et al. (2016). "Comparative Effects of Carbohydrate Versus Fat Restriction on Metabolic Profiles, Biomarkers of Inflammation and Oxidative Stress in Overweight Patients with Type 2 Diabetic and Coronary Heart Disease: A Randomized Clinical Trial." *ARYA Atherosclerosis* 12, no. 6 (2016): 266–73.

2. N. Steckhan et al. "Effects of Different Dietary Approaches on Inflammatory Markers in Patients with Metabolic Syndrome: A Systematic Review and Meta-Analysis." *Nutrition* 32, no. 3 (2016): 338–48.

3. M. Lucas et al. (2014). "Inflammatory Dietary Pattern and Risk of Depression Among Women." *Brain, Behavior, and Immunity* 36 (2014): 46–53.

4. R. D. Pitceathly and C. Viscomi. "Effects of Ketosis in Mitochondrial Myopathy: Potential Benefits of a Mitotoxic Diet." *EMBO Molecular Medicine* 8, no. 11 (2016): 1231–3.

5. R. D. Feinman, M. C. Vernon, and E. C. Westman. (2006). "Low Carbohydrate Diets in Family Practice: What Can We Learn from an Internet-Based Support Group." *Nutrition Journal* 5 (2006): 26.

6. V. Iebba et al. "Eubiosis and Dysbiosis: The Two Sides of the Microbiota." *New Microbiologica* 39, no. 1 (2016): 1–12.

7. J. C. Clemente, L. K. Ursell, L. W. Parfrey, and R. Knight. "The Impact of the Gut Microbiota on Human Health: An Integrative View." *Cell* 148, no. 6 (2012): 1258–70.

8. C. Newell et al. "Ketogenic Diet Modifies the Gut Microbiota in a Murine Model of Autism Spectrum Disorder." *Molecular Autism* 7, no. 1 (2016): 37.

9. A. Swidsinski et al. "Reduced Mass and Diversity of the Colonic Microbiome in Patients with Multiple Sclerosis and Their Improvement with Ketogenic Diet." *Frontiers in Microbiology* 8 (2017): 1141.

10. G. T. Macfarlane and S. Macfarlane. "Bacteria, Colonic Fermentation, and Gastrointestinal Health." *Journal of AOAC International* 95, no. 1 (2012): 50–60.

11. G. Xie et al. "Ketogenic Diet Poses a Significant Effect on Imbalanced Gut Microbiota in Infants with Refractory Epilepsy." *World Journal of Gastroenterology* 23, no. 33 (2017): 6164–71.

12. Y. Wang, D. Wang, and D. Guo. "Interictal Cytokine Levels Were Correlated to Seizure Severity of Epileptic Patients: A Retrospective Study on 1218 Epileptic Patients." *Journal of Translational Medicine* 13, no. 1 (2015): 378.

13. D. Tendler et al. "The Effects of a Low-Carbohydrate, Ketogenic Diet on a Nonalcoholic Fatty Liver Disease: A Pilot Study." *Digestive Diseases and Sciences* 52, no. 2 (2007): 589–93.

14. F. Haghighatdoost, A. Salehi-Abargouei, P. J. Surkan, and L. Azadbakht. "The Effects of Low Carbohydrate Diets on Liver Function Tests in Nonalcoholic Fatty Liver Disease: A Systematic Review and Meta-Analysis of Clinical Trials." *Journal of Research in Medical Sciences* 21, no. 1 (2016): 53.

15. M. R. Swain, M. Anandharaj, R. C. Ray, and R. P. Rani. "Fermented Fruits and Vegetables of Asia: A Potential Source of Probiotics." *Biotechnology Research International* 2014 (2014).

16. Y. M. C. Liu and H. S. Wang. "Medium-Chain Triglyceride Ketogenic Diet, an Effective Treatment for Drug-Resistant Epilepsy and a Comparison with Other Ketogenic Diets." *Biomedical Journal* 36, no. 1 (2013): 9–15.

17. K. A. Page et al. "Medium-Chain Fatty Acids Improve Cognitive Function in Intensively Treated Type 1 Diabetic Patients and Support in vitro Synaptic Transmission During Acute Hypoglycemia." *Diabetes* 58, no. 5 (2009): 1237–44.

18. See note 17 above.

19. R. West et al. "Better Memory Functioning Associated with Higher Total and Low-Density Lipoprotein Cholesterol Levels in Very Elderly Subjects Without the Apolipoprotein e4 Allele." *The American Journal of Geriatric Psychiatry* 16, no. 9 (2008): 781–5.

20. H. Iso, D. R. Jacobs, D. Wentworth, J. D. Neaton, and J. D. Cohen. (1989). "Serum High Cholesterol Levels and Six-Year Mortality from Stroke in 350,977 Men Screened for the Multiple Risk Factor Intervention Trial." *The New England Journal of Medicine* 320, no. 14 (1989): 904–10.

21. P. K. Elias, M. F. Elias, R. B. D'Agostino, L. M. Sullivan, and P. A. Wolf. "Serum Cholesterol and Cognitive Performance in the Framingham Heart Study." *Psychosomatic Medicine* 67, no. 1 (2005): 24–30.

22. D. M. Dreon, H. A. Fernstrom, B. Miller, and R. M. Krauss. "Low-Density Lipoprotein Subclass Patterns and Lipoprotein Response to a Reduced-Fat Diet in Men." *The FASEB Journal* 8, no. 1 (1994): 121–6.

23. R. M. Krauss and D. M. Dreon. "Low-Density-Lipoprotein Subclasses and Response to a Low-Fat Diet in Healthy Men." *The American Journal of Clinical Nutrition* 62, no. 2 (1995): 478S–87S.

24. T. D. Noakes and J. Windt. "Evidence that Supports the Prescription of Low-Carbohydrate High-Fat Diets: A Narrative Review." *British Journal of Sports Medicine* 51, no. 2 (2017): 133–9.

25. See note 1 above.

26. B. J. Van Lenten et al. "Anti-Inflammatory HDL Becomes Pro-Inflammatory During the Acute Phase Response. Loss of Protective Effect of HDL Against LDL Oxidation in Aortic Wall Cell Cocultures." *Journal of Clinical Investigation* 96, no. 6 (1996): 2758–67.

27. D. S. Grimes, E. Hindle, and T. Dyer. "Sunlight, Cholesterol and Coronary Heart Disease." *QJM* 89, no. 8 (1996): 579–89.

Chapter 7

1. F. Raygan et al. (2016). "Comparative Effects of Carbohydrate Versus Fat Restriction on Metabolic Profiles, Biomarkers of Inflammation and Oxidative Stress in Overweight Patients with Type 2 Diabetic and Coronary Heart Disease: A Randomized Clinical Trial." *ARYA Atherosclerosis* 12, no. 6 (2016): 266–73.

2. N. Steckhan et al. "Effects of Different Dietary Approaches on Inflammatory Markers in Patients with Metabolic Syndrome: A Systematic Review and Meta-Analysis." *Nutrition* 32, no. 3 (2016): 338–48.

3. C. E. Friedberg, M. van Buren, J. A. Bijlsma, and H. A. Koomans. "Insulin Increases Sodium Reabsorption in Diluting Segment in Humans: Evidence for Indirect Mediation Through Hypokalemia." *Kidney International* 40, no. 2 (1991): 251–6.

4. R. A. DeFronzo, C. R. Cooke, R. Andres, G. R. Faloona, and P. J. Davis. "The Effect of Insulin on Renal Handling of Sodium, Potassium, Calcium, and Phosphate in Man." *Journal of Clinical Investigation* 55, no. 4 (1975): 845–55.

5. A. H. Manninen. "Very-Low-Carbohydrate Diets and Preservation of Muscle Mass." *Nutrition & Metabolism* 3, no. 1 (2006): 9.

6. K. Brooks and J. Carter. "Overtraining, Exercise, and Adrenal Insufficiency." *Journal of Novel Physiotherapies* 3, no. 125 (2013): 11717.

7. J. M. Ren, C. F. Semenkovich, E. A. Gulve, J. Gao, and J. O. Holloszy. "Exercise Induces Rapid Increases in GLUT4 Expression, Glucose Transport Capacity, and Insulin-Stimulated Glycogen Storage in Muscle." *The Journal of Biological Chemistry* 269, no. 20 (1994): 14396–401.

Chapter 9

1. Y. J. Zhang et al. "Impacts of Gut Bacteria on Human Health and Diseases." *International Journal of Molecular Sciences* 16, no. 4 (2015): 7493–519.

2. M. Sienkiewicz, M. Wasiela, and A. Glowacka. "The Antibacterial Activity of Oregano Essential Oil (Origanum heracleoticum L.) Against Clinical Strains of Escherichia Coli and Pseudomonas Aeruginosa." *Medycyna Doswiadczalna I Mikrobiologia (Warszawa)* 64, no. 4 (2012): 297–307.

3. R. Mukkavilli et al. Agarwal R, ed. "Modulation of Cytochrome P450 Metabolism and Transport Across Intestinal Epithelial Barrier by Ginger Biophenolics." *Ketogenic Foods PLoS ONE* 9, no. 9 (2014): e108386.

4. M. Alzweiri, I. M. Alrawashdeh, and S. K. Bardaweel. "The Development and Application of Novel IR and NMR-Based Model for the Evaluation of Carminative Effect of Artemisia Judaica L. Essential Oil." *International Journal of Analytical Chemistry* (2014): 627038.

5. G. Bhaktha, B. S. Nayak, S. Mayya, and M. Shantaram. "Relationship of Caffeine with Adiponectin and Blood Sugar Levels in Subjects with and Without Diabetes." *Journal of Clinical and Diagnostic Research* 9, no. 1 (2015): BC01–3.

6. Z. Huang, B. Wang, D. H. Eaves, J. M. Shikany, and R. D. Pace. "Total Phenolics and Antioxidant Capacity of Indigenous Vegetables in the Southeast United States: Alabama Collaboration for Cardiovascular Equality Project." *International Journal of Food Sciences and Nutrition* 60, no. 2 (2009): 100–8

7. X. Zhang et al. "Cruciferous Vegetable Consumption Is Associated with a Reduced Risk of Total and Cardiovascular Disease Mortality." *The American Journal of Clinical Nutrition* 94, no. 1 (2011): 240–6.

8. G. Grosso and R. Estruch. "Nut Consumption and Age-Related Disease." *Maturitas* 84 (2016): 11–6.

9. L. R. Ledesma et al. "Monunsaturated Fatty Acid (Avocado) Rich Diet for Mild Hypercholesterolemia." *Archives of Medical Research* 27, no. 4 (1996): 519–23.

10. S. D. Phinney. "Ketogenic Diets and Physical Performance." *Nutrition & Metabolism* 1, no. 1 (2004): 2.

11. M. L. Dreher and A. J. Davenport. "Hass Avocado Composition and Potential Health Effects." *Critical Reviews in Food Science and Nutrition* 53, no. 7 (2013): 738–50.

12. S. Skrovankova, D. Sumczynski, J. Mlcek, T. Jurikova, and J. Sochor. M. Battino, ed. "Bioactive Compounds and Antioxidant Activity in Different Types of Berries." *International Journal of Molecular Sciences* 16, no. 10 (2015): 24673–706.

13. D. S. Ibrahim and M. A. E. Abd El-Maksoud. "Effect of Strawberry (Fragaria × ananassa) Leaf Extract on Diabetic Nephropathy in Rats." *International Journal of Experimental Pathology* 96, no. 2 (2015): 87–93.

14. C. N. Blesso, C. J. Andersen, J. Barona, J. S. Volek, and M. L. Fernandez. "Whole Egg Consumption Improves Lipoprotein Profiles and Insulin Sensitivity to a Greater Extent Than Yolk-Free Egg Substitute in Individuals with Metabolic Syndrome." *Metabolism* 62, no. 3 (2012): 400–10.

15. J. Ratliff et al. "Consuming Eggs for Breakfast Influences Plasma Glucose and Ghrelin, While Reducing Energy Intake During the Next 24 Hours in Adult Men." *Nutrition Research* 30, no. 2 (2010): 96–103.

16. A. De La Torre et al. "Beef Conjugated Linoleic Acid Isomers Reduce Human Cancer Cell Growth Even When Associated with Other Beef Fatty Acids." *British Journal of Nutrition* 95, no. 2 (2006): 346–52.

17. L. D. Whigham, A. C. Watras, and D. A. Schoeller. "Efficacy of Conjugated Linoleic Acid for Reducing Fat Mass: A Meta-Analysis in Humans." *The American Journal of Clinical Nutrition* 85, no. 5 (2007): 1203–11.

18. U. Tinggi. "Selenium: Its Role as Antioxidant in Human Health." *Environmental Health and Preventive Medicine* 13, no. 2 (2008): 102–8.

19. A. Ramel et al. "Beneficial Effects of Long-Chain n-3 Fatty Acids Included in an Energy-Restricted Diet on Insulin Resistance in Overweight and Obese European Young Adults." *Diabetologia* 51, no. 7 (2008): 1261–8.

20. M. C. Morris et al. "Fish Consumption and Cognitive Decline with Age in a Large Community Study." *Archives of Neurology* 62, no. 12 (2006): 1849–53.

21. J. K. Virtanen, D. Mozaffarian, S. E. Chiuve, and E. B. Rimm. "Fish Consumption and Risk of Major Chronic Disease in Men." *The American Journal of Clinical Nutrition* 88, no. 6 (2008): 1618–25.

22. G. Koren. "Polyunsaturated Fatty Acids and Fetal Brain Development: Promesses Brisées." *Canadian Family Physician* 61, no. 1 (2015): 41–2.

23. Y. Peng et al. "Nutritional and Chemical Composition and Antiviral Activity of Cultivated Seaweed *Sargassum naozhouense* Tseng et Lu." *Marine Drugs* 11, no. 1 (2013): 20–32.

24. H. Ye, K. Wang, C. Zhou, J. Liu, and X. Zeng. "Purification, Antitumor and Antioxidant Activities in vitro of Polysaccharides from the Brown *Seaweed Sargassum pallidum.*" *Food Chemistry* 111, no. 2 (2008): 428–32.

25. S. Rautiainen et al. "Dairy Consumption in Association with Weight Change and Risk of Becoming Overweight or Obese in Middle-Aged and Older Women: A Prospective Cohort Study." *The American Journal of Clinical Nutrition* 103, no. 4 (2016): 979–88.

26. H. Sharma, X. Zhang, and C. Dwivedi. "The Effect of *Ghee* (Clarified Butter) on Serum Lipid Levels and Microsomal Lipid Peroxidation." *Ayu* 31, no. 2 (2010): 134–40.

27. D. F. Hebeisen et al. "Increased Concentrations of Omega-3 Fatty Acids in Milk and Platelet Rich Plasma of Grass-Fed Cows." *International Journal for Vitamin and Nutrition Research* 63, no. 3 (1993): 229–33.

28. K. A. Page et al. "Medium-Chain Fatty Acids Improve Cognitive Function in Intensively Treated Type 1 Diabetic Patients and Support In Vitro Synaptic Transmission During Acute Hypoglycemia." *Diabetes* 58, no. 5 (2009):1237–44.

29. R. A. I. Ekanayaka, N. K. Ekanayaka, B. Perera, and P. G. S. M. De Silva. "Impact of a Traditional Dietary Supplement with Coconut Milk and Soya Milk on the Lipid Profile in Normal Free Living Subjects." *Journal of Nutrition and Metabolism* 6 (2013): 481068.

30. N. K. Hollenberg and N. D. L. Fisher. "Is It the Dark in Dark Chocolate?" *Circulation* 116 (2007): 2360–62.

31. T. K. Thorning et al. "Diets with High-Fat Cheese, High-Fat Meat, or Carbohydrate on Cardiovascular Risk Markers in Overweight Postmenopausal Women: A Randomized Crossover Trial." *The American Journal of Clinical Nutrition* 102, no. 3 (2015): 573–81.

32. A. Tremblay, C. Doyon, and M. Sanchez. "Impact of Yogurt on Appetite Control, Energy Balance, and Body Composition." *Nutrition Reviews* 73, no. Suppl 1 (2015): 23–7.

33. A. Marsset-Baglieri et al. "The Satiating Effects of Eggs or Cottage Cheese Are Similar in Healthy Subjects Despite Differences in Postprandial Kinetics." *Appetite* 90 (2015): 136–43.

34. T. P. Stein et al. "Comparison of Glucose, LCT, and LCT Plus MCT as Calorie Sources for Parenterally Nourished Septic Rats." *American Journal of Physiology* 246, no. 3 Pt 1 (1984): E277–87.

35. B. M. Kochikuzhyil, K. Devi, and S. R. Fattepur. "Effect of Saturated Fatty Acid-Rich Dietary Vegetable Oils on Lipid Profile, Antioxidant Enzymes and Glucose Tolerance in Diabetic Rats." *Indian Journal of Pharmacology* 42, no. 3 (2010): 142–5.

36. R. Barbera et al. "Sensations Induced by Medium and Long Chain Triglycerides: Role of Gastric Tone and Hormones." *Gut* 46, no. 1 (2000): 32–6.

37. M. L. Assunção et al. "Effects of Dietary Coconut Oil on the Biochemical and Anthropometric Profiles of Women Presenting Abdominal Obesity." *Lipids* 44, no. 7 (2009): 593–601.

38. L. Schwingshackl and G. Hoffmann. "Monounsaturated Fatty Acids, Olive Oil and Health Status: A Systematic Review and Meta-Analysis of Cohort Studies." *Lipids in Health and Disease* 13, no. 1 (2014): 154.

39. J. Ruano et al. "Phenolic Content of Virgin Olive Oil Improves Ischemic Reactive Hyperemia in Hypercholesterolemic Patients." *The Journal of the American College of Cardiology* 46, no. 10 (2005): 1864–8.

40. V. Goulas et al. "Phytochemicals in Olive-Leaf Extract and Their Antiproliferative Activity Against Cancer and Endothelial Cells." *Molecular Nutrition & Food Research* 53, no. 5 (2009): 600–8.

41. C. Manna et al. "Oleuropein Prevents Oxidative Myocardial Injury Induced by Ischemia and Reperfusion." *The Journal of Nutritional Biochemistry* 15, no. 8 (2004): 461–6.

42. S. H. Omar. "Oleuropein in Olive and Its Pharmacological Effects." *Scientia Pharmaceutica* 78, no. 2 (2010): 133–54.

43. M. Arumugam, M. Raman, B. Johnson, and K. Eagappan. "Dietary Fiber Isolate from Coconut Flakes—A Functional Ketogenic Food." *International Journal of Pharmaceutical Sciences Review and Research* 25, no. 2 (2014): 262–7.

44. T. P. Trinidad et al. "The Cholesterol-Lowering Effect of Coconut Flakes and Ketogenic Foods in Humans with Moderately Raised Serum Cholesterol." *Journal of Medicinal Food* 7, no. 2 (2004): 136–40.

45. J. Keithley and B. Swanson. "Glucomannan and Obesity: A Critical Review." *Alternative Therapies in Health and Medicine* 11, no. 6 (2005): 30–4.

46. V. Vuksan et al. "Konjac-Mannan (Glucomannan) Improves Glycemia and Other Associated Risk Factors for Coronary Heart Disease in Type 2 Diabetes. A Randomized Controlled Metabolic Trial." *Diabetes Care* 22, no. 6 (1999): 913–9.

47. K. Yu et al. "The Impact of Soluble Dietary Fibre on Gastric Emptying, Postprandial Blood Glucose and Insulin in Patients with Type 2 Diabetes." *Asia Pacific Journal of Clinical Nutrition* 23, no. 2 (2014): 210–8.

48. H. Liljeberg and I. Björck. (1998). "Delayed Gastric Emptying Rate May Explain Improved Glycaemia in Healthy Subjects to a Starchy Meal with Added Vinegar." *European Journal of Clinical Nutrition* 52, no. 5 (1998): 368–71.

49. K. L. Clark et al. "24-Week Study on the Use of Collagen Hydrolysate as a Dietary Supplement in Athletes with Activity-Related Joint Pain." *Current Medical Research Opinion* 24, no. 5 (2008): 1485–96.

50. C. L. Deal and R. W. Moskowitz. "Nutraceuticals as Therapeutic Agents in Osteoarthritis: The Role of Glucosamine, Chondroitin Sulfate, and Collagen Hydrolysate." *Rheumatic Disease Clinics of North America* 25, no. 2 (1999): 379–95.

51. S. Y. Choi et al. "Effect of High Advanced-Collagen Tripeptide on Wound Healing and Skin Recovery After Fractional Photothermolysis Treatment." *Clinical and Experimental Dermatology* 39, no. 8 (2014): 874–80.

52. S. Y. Choi et al. "Effects of Collagen Tripeptide Supplement on Skin Properties: A Prospective, Randomized, Controlled Study." *Journal of Cosmetic and Laser Therapy* 16, no. 3 (2013): 132–7.

Chapter 10

1. C. J. Morris, D. Aeschbach, and F. A. Scheer. "Circadian System, Sleep and Endocrinology." *Molecular and Cellular Endocrinology* 349, no. 1 (2012): 91–104.

2. S. Khani and J. A. Tayek. "Cortisol Increases Gluconeogenesis in Humans: Its Role in the Metabolic Syndrome." *Clinical Science* 101, no. 6 (2002): 739–47.

3. G. Brenta. "Why Can Insulin Resistance Be a Natural Consequence of Thyroid Dysfunction?" *Journal of Thyroid Research* 3 (2011): 152850.

4. N. L. Keim, M. D. Van Loan, W. F. Horn, T. F. Barbieri, and P. L. Mayclin. "Weight Loss Is Greater with Consumption of Large Morning Meals and Fat-Free Mass Is Preserved with Large Evening Meals in Women on a Controlled Weight Reduction Regimen." *The Journal of Nutrition* 127, no. 1 (1997): 75–82.

5. S. Sofer et al. "Greater Weight Loss and Hormonal Changes After 6 Months Diet with Carbohydrates Eaten Mostly at Dinner." *Obesity* (Silver Spring) 19, no. 10 (2011): 2006–14.

6. S. Sofer et al. "Changes in Daily Leptin, Ghrelin and Adiponectin Profiles Following a Diet with Carbohydrates Eaten at Dinner in Obese Subjects." *Nutrition, Metabolism & Cardiovascular Diseases* 23, no. 8 (2013): 744–50.

7. J. Kiefer. *Carb Back-Loading.* Accessed from LinkedIn SlideShare on July 25, 2019, https://www.slideshare.net/warehousegymexpert/carb-back-loading-54496235.

Chapter 13

1. A. Fasano. "Leaky Gut and Autoimmune Diseases." *Clinical Reviews in Allergy & Immunology* 42, no. 1 (2012): 71–8.

2. M. G. Myers et al. "Challenges and Opportunities of Defining Clinical Leptin Resistance." *Cell Metabolism* 15, no. 2 (2012): 150–6.

3. M. F. Prummel, T. Strieder, and W. M. Wiersinga. "The Environment and Autoimmune Thyroid Diseases and Hypothyroidism." *European Journal of Endocrinology* 150, no. 5 (2004): 605–18.

4. F. Economidou, E. Douka, M. Tzanela, S. Nanas, and A. Kotanidou. "Thyroid Function During Critical Illness." *Hormones* (Athens, Greece) 10, no. 2 (2011): 117–24.

5. E. M. Kaptein, J. S. Fisler, M. J. Duda, J. T. Nicoloff, and E. J. Drenick. "Relationship Between the Changes in Serum Thyroid Hormone Levels and Protein Status During Prolonged Protein Supplemented Caloric Deprivation." *Clinical Endocrinology* 22, no. 1 (1985), 1–15.

6. M. U. Yang and T. B. van Itallie. "Variability in Body Protein Loss During Protracted, Severe Caloric Restriction: Role of Triiodothyronine and Other Possible Determinants." *The American Journal of Clinical Nutrition* 40, no. 3 (1984): 611–22.

7. M. P. Rozing et al. "Low Serum Free Triiodothyronine Levels Mark Familial Longevity: The Leiden Longevity Study." *Journals of Gerontology – Series A* 65A, no. 4 (2010): 365–8.

8. L. V. Allen, Jr. "Adrenal Fatigue." *International Journal of Pharmaceutical Compounding* 17, no. 1 (2013): 39–44.

9. G. Tanaka. "The Relationships Between Sympathetic and Parasympathetic Tones and Cardiovascular Responses During Active Coping." *Shinrigaku Kenkyu* 63, no. 2 (1992): 92–9.

10. K. Hardy and H. Pollard. "The Organisation of the Stress Response, and Its Relevance to Chiropractors: A Commentary." *Chiropractic & Osteopathy* 14 (2006): 25.

11. A. Welch and R. Boone. "Sympathetic and Parasympathetic Responses to Specific Diversified Adjustments to Chiropractic Vertebral Subluxations of the Cervical and Thoracic Spine." *Journal of Chiropractic Medicine* 7, no. 3 (2008): 86–93.

12. K. K. Kesari, M. H. Siddiqui, R. Meena, H. N. Verma, and S. Kumar. "Cell Phone Radiation Exposure on Brain and Associated Biological Systems." *Indian Journal of Experimental Biology* 51, no. 3 (2013): 187–200.

13. M. N. Mead. "Benefits of Sunlight: A Bright Spot for Human Health." *Environmental Health Perspectives* 116, no. 4 (2008): A160–7.

14. H. G. Koenig. "Religion, Spirituality, and Health: The Research and Clinical Implications." *International Scholarly Research Notices: Psychiatry* 2012 (2012): 278730.

15. M. Roy et al. "HIIT in the Real World: Outcomes from a 12-Month Intervention in Overweight Adults." *Medicine & Science in Sports & Exercise* 50, no. 9 (2018).

16. J. T. Lemmer et al. "Effect of Strength Training on Resting Metabolic Rate and Physical Activity: Age and Gender Comparisons." *Medicine & Science in Sports & Exercise* 33, no. 4 (2001): 532–41.

17. C. Melby, C. Scholl, G. Edwards, and R. Bullough. "Effect of Acute Resistance Exercise on Postexercise Energy Expenditure and Resting Metabolic Rate." *Journal of Applied Physiology* 75, no. 4 (1993): 1847–53.

18. W. Crinnion. "Components of Practical Clinical Detox Programs–Sauna as a Therapeutic Tool." *Alternative Therapies in Health and Medicine* 13, no. 2 (2007): S154–6.

19. F. Raygan et al. "Comparative Effects of Carbohydrate Versus Fat Restriction on Metabolic Profiles, Biomarkers of Inflammation and Oxidative Stress in Overweight Patients with Type 2 Diabetic and Coronary Heart Disease: A Randomized Clinical Trial." *ARYA Atherosclerosis* 12, no. 6 (2006): 266–73.

20. N. Steckhan et al. "Effects of Different Dietary Approaches on Inflammatory Markers in Patients with Metabolic Syndrome: A Systematic Review and Meta-Analysis. *Nutrition* 32, no. 3 (2016): 338–48.

Chapter 14

1. E. T. Champagne. "Low Gastric Hydrochloric Acid Secretion and Mineral Bioavailability." *Advances in Experimental Medicine and Biology* 249 (1989): 173–84.

2. R. E. Cater. "Helicobacter (aka Campylobacter) pylori as the Major Causal Factor in Chronic Hypochlorhydria." *Medical Hypotheses* 39, no. 4 (1992): 367–74.

3. A. Fasano. "Leaky Gut and Autoimmune Diseases." *Clinical Reviews in Allergy & Immunology* 42, no. 1 (2012): 71–8.

4. A. R. Mansourian. "A Review of Literatures on the Adverse Effects of Thyroid Abnormalities and Liver Disorders: An Overview on Liver Dysfunction and Hypothyroidism." *Pakistan Journal of Biological Sciences* 16, no. 23 (2013): 1641–52.

5. C. Staley, A. R. Weingarden, A. Khoruts, and M. J. Sadowsky. "Interaction of Gut Microbiota with Bile Acid Metabolism and Its Influence on Disease States." *Applied Microbiology and Biotechnology* 101, no. 1 (2017): 47–64.

6. Y. M. Liu and H. S. Wang. "Medium-Chain Triglyceride Ketogenic Diet, an Effective Treatment for Drug-Resistant Epilepsy and a Comparison with Other Ketogenic Diets." *Biomedical Journal* 36, no. 1 (2013): 9–15.

7. E. A. Shaffer. "Gallbladder Sludge: What Is Its Clinical Significance?" *Current Gastroenterology Reports* 3, no. 2 (2001): 166–73.

Chapter 15

1. A. C. Bach and V. K. Babayan. "Medium-Chain Triglycerides: An Update." *The American Journal of Clinical Nutrition* 36, no. 5 (1982): 950–62.

2. Ibid.

3. T. P. Stein et al. "Comparison of Glucose, LCT, and LCT Plus MCT as Calorie Sources for Parenterally Nourished Rats." *American Journal of Physiology* 246, no. 3 Pt 1 (1984): E277–87.

4. L. K. Brahe, A. Astrup, and L. H. Larsen. "Butyrate and Obesity-Related Diseases." *Obesity Reviews* 14 (2013): 950–9.

5. M. W. Bourassa, I. Alim, S. J. Bultman, Rajiv R. Ratan. "Butyrate, Neuroepigenetics and the Gut Microbiome: Can a High Fiber Diet Improve Brain Health?" *Neuroscience Letters* 625 (2016): 56–63.

6. A. Panossian and G. Wikman, "Evidence-Based Efficacy of Adaptogens in Fatigue, and Molecular Mechanisms Related to Their Stress-Protective Activity." *Current Clinical Pharmacology* 4, no. 3 (2009): 198.

7. A. G. Panossian. "Adaptogens in Mental and Behavioral Disorders." *Psychiatric Clinics of North America* 36, no. 1 (2013): 49–64.

Chapter 16

1. M. Grembecka. "Natural Sweeteners in a Human Diet." *Roczniki Państwowego Zakładu Higieny* 66, no. 3 (2015): 195–202.

2. R. Assaei et al. "Hypoglycemic Effect of Aquatic Extract of Stevia in Pancreas of Diabetic Rats: PPARγ-Dependent Regulation or Antioxidant Potential." *Avicenna Journal of Medical Biotechnology* 8, no. 2 (2016): 65–74.

3. Y. Zhou, Y. Zheng, J. Ebersole, and C. F. Huang. (2009). "Insulin Secretion Stimulating Effects of Mogroside V and Fruit Extract of Luo Han Kuo (Siraitia Grosvenori Swingle) Fruit Extract." *Yao Xue Bao* 44, no. 11 (2009): 1252–7.

4. Q. Xu et al. "Antioxidant Effect of Mogrosides Against Oxidative Stress Induced by Palmitic Acid in Mouse Insulinoma NIT-1 Cells." *Brazilian Journal of Medical and Biological Research* 46, no. 11 (2013): 949–55.

5. M. Koubaa et al. "Current and New Insights in the Sustainable and Green Recovery of Nutritionally Valuable Compounds from *Stevia rebaudiana* Bertoni." *Journal of Agricultural and Food Chemistry* 63, no. 31 (2015): 6835–46.

6. C. Li et al. "Chemistry and Pharmacology of Siraitia grosvenorii: A Review." *Chinese Journal of Natural Medicines* 12, no. 2 (2014): 89–102.

7. S. Ghanta, A. Banerjee, A. Poddar, and S. Chattopadhyay. "Oxidative DNA Damage Preventive Activity and Antioxidant Potential of *Stevia rebaudiana* (Bertoni) Bertoni, a Natural Sweetener." *Journal of Agricultural and Food Chemistry* 55, no. 26 (2007): 10962–7.

8. A. Kozłowska and D. Szostak-Wegierek. "Flavonoids–Food Sources and Health Benefits." *Roczniki Państwowego Zakładu Higieny* 65, no. 2 (2014): 79–85.

9. V. López, S. Pérez, A. Vinuesa, C. Zorzetto, and O. Abian. "Stevia rebaudiana Ethanolic Extract Exerts Better Antioxidant Properties and Antiproliferative Effects in Tumour Cells Than Its Diterpene Glycoside Stevioside." *Food & Function* 7, no. 4 (2016): 2107–13.

10. C. Liu, L. H. Dai, D. Q. Dou, L. Q. Ma, and Y. X. Sun. "A Natural Food Sweetener with Anti-Pancreatic Cancer Properties." *Oncogenesis* 5, no. 4 (2016): e217.

11. I. Sehar, A. Kaul, S. Bani, H. C. Pal, and A. K. Saxena. "Immune Up Regulatory Response of a Non-Caloric Natural Sweetener, Stevioside." *Chemico-Biological Interactions* 173, no. 2 (2008): 115–21.

12. G. F. Ferrazzano et al. "Is *Stevia rebaudiana* Bertoni a Non Cariogenic Sweetener? A Review." *Molecules* 21, no. 1 (2015): E38.

13. P. A. Theophilus et al. (2015). "Effectiveness of *Stevia rebaudiana* Whole Leaf Extract Against the Various Morphological Forms of *Borrelia burgdorferi* in vitro." *European Journal of Microbiology and Immunology* 5, no. 4 (2015): 268–80.

14. See note 6 above.

INDEX